Vascular Disease and Affective Disorders

Edited by

Edmond Chiu AM MBBS DPM FRANZCP
Associate Professor of Psychiatry of Old Age
Academic Unit for Psychiatry of Old Age
University of Melbourne
St George's Hospital
Kew, Victoria
Australia

David Ames BA MD FRCPsych FRANZCP
Associate Professor of Psychiatry of Old Age
University of Melbourne
Department of Psychiatry
Royal Melbourne Hospital
Parkville, Victoria
Australia

Cornelius Katona MD FRCPsych
Professor of Psychiatry of the Elderly
University College London
London
UK

MARTIN DUNITZ

© Martin Dunitz Ltd 2002
First published in the United Kingdom in 2002 by
Martin Dunitz Ltd
The Livery House
7-9 Pratt Street
London NW1 0AE
UK

Tel: +44-(0)20-7482 2202
Fax: +44-(0)20-7267 0159
E-mail: info@dunitz.co.uk
Website: http://www.dunitz.co.uk

A CIP catalogue record for this book is available from the British Library

ISBN 1-84184-152-8

Distributed in the USA by
Fulfilment Center
Taylor & Francis
7625 Empire Drive
Florence, KY 41042, USA
Toll Free Tel: 1-800-634-7064
Email: cserve@routledge_ny.com

Distributed in Canada by
Taylor & Francis
74 Rolark Drive
Scarborough
Ontario M1R 4G2, Canada
Toll Free Tel: 1-877-226-2237
Email: tal_fran@istar.ca

Distributed in the rest of the world by
ITPS Limited
Cheriton House
North Way, Andover
Hampshire SP10 5BE, UK
Tel: +44- (0)1264 332424
Email: reception@itps.co.uk

Composition by 🖅 Tek-Art
Printed and bound in Great Britain by Biddles Ltd, Guildford and King's Lynn.

Contents

Concluding chapter

Contributors

David Ames BA MD FRCPsych FRANZCP
Associate Professor of Psychiatry of Old Age
University of Melbourne
Department of Psychiatry
Parkville, Victoria
Australia

Robert C Baldwin DM FRCP FRCPsych
Consultant Psychiatrist and Honorary Professor of Old Age Psychiatry
University of Manchester
Manchester Mental Health Partnership
Manchester Royal Infirmary
Manchester
UK

Eric D Caine MD
John Romano Professor and Chair
Department of Psychiatry
University of Rochester Medical Center
Rochester, NY
USA

Edmond Chiu AM MBBS DPM FRANZCP
Associate Professor of Psychiatry of Old Age
Academic Unit for Psychiatry of Old Age
University of Melbourne
St George's Hospital
Kew, Victoria
Australia

Chris Dickens MBBS MRCP MRCPsych MSc PhD
Senior Lecturer and Honorary Consultant
Department of Psychiatry
Manchester Royal Infirmary
Manchester
UK

Timo Erkinjuntti MD PhD
Professor and Head, Memory Research Unit
Department of Clinical Neurosciences
Helsinki University Central Hospital
Helsinki
Finland

David F Horrobin MA DPhil BM BCh
Medical and Research Director
Laxdale Ltd
King's Park House
Stirling
UK

Cornelius Katona MD FRCPsych
Professor of Psychiatry of the Elderly
Department Psychiatry & Behavioural Sciences
University College London
London
UK

Sirkka-Liisa Kivelä MD PhD
Professor in General Practice
University of Turku
Department of General Practice
Turku and
The Härkätie Health Centre
Lieto
Finland

K Ranga Rama Krishnan MD
Professor and Chair
Department of Psychiatry and Behavioral Sciences
Duke University Medical Center
Durham, NC
USA

Anand Kumar MD
Professor of Psychiatry
Department of Psychiatry and Biobehavioral Sciences
UCLA School of Medicine—Neuropsychiatric Institute
Los Angeles, CA
USA

Nicola T Lautenschlager MD
Senior Lecturer in Psychiatry of Old Age
Department of Psychiatry and Behavioural Science
University of Western Australia
Australia

Helen Lavretsky MD
Assistant Professor of Psychiatry
Department of Psychiatry and Biobehavioral Sciences
UCLA School of Medicine—Neuropsychiatric Institute
Los Angeles, CA
USA

Brian A Lawlor MD FRCP FRCPsych
Conolly Norman Professor of Old Age Psychiatry
St James's Hospital & Trinity College Dublin
Dublin
Republic of Ireland

Antero Leppävuori MD PhD
Head, Psychiatric Outpatient Department
Helsinki University Central Hospital
Helsinki
Finland

Jeffrey M Lyness MD
Associate Professor
Director of the Program in Geriatrics and Neuropsychiatry
Department of Psychiatry
University of Rochester Medical Center
Rochester, NY
USA

Paul Masterman BSc
Psychologist
School of Applied Psychology
Griffith University Gold Coast Campus
Queensland
Australia

Philip LP Morris MB BS BSc(**med**) PhD FRANZCP
Director of Psychiatry
Gold Coast District Integrated Mental Health Service and
Professor, Department of Psychiatry
University of Queensland
Australia

Tarja Pohjasvaara MD PhD
Head, Department of Neurology
Lohja Hospital
Lohja
Finland

Paul J Rushton BPsych MAPS
Senior Clinical Psychologist
Gold Coast District Integrated Mental Health Service
Adjunct Assistant Clinical Professor for Health Sciences
Bond University
Australia

Carol J Schramke PhD
Director of Behavioral Neurology
Department of Neurology and
Child Psychologist
Allegheny General Hospital
Pittsburgh, PA
USA

Alejandro Serbanescu MD
Buenos Aires Neuropsychiatric Center
Buenos Aires
Argentina

Kenneth I Shulman MD SM FRCPsych FRCP(C)
Professor, Department of Psychiatry
Faculty of Medicine
University of Toronto
Sunnybrook & Women's College Health Sciences Centre
Toronto, ONT
Canada

Sergio E Starkstein MD PhD
Buenos Aires Neuropsychiatric Center
Buenos Aires
Argentina

David C Steffens MD MHS
Associate Professor
Department of Psychiatry and Behavioural Sciences
Duke University Medical Center
Durham. NC
USA

Robert Stewart MD
Wellcome Trust Research Training Fellow
Section of Epidemiology
Institute of Psychiatry
London
UK

Joe Stratford MBBS BSC MRCPsych
Specialist Registrar in Old Age Psychiatry
Southmead Hospital
Bristol
UK

Greg Swanwick MD MRCPI MRCPsych
Consultant Psychiatrist in Psychiatry of Old Age
Department of Psychiatry of Later Life
The Adelaide & Meath Hospital
    Incorporating the National Children's Hospital
Dublin
Republic of Ireland

Warren D Taylor MD
Clinical Associate
Department of Psychiatry and Behavioural Sciences
Duke University Medical Center
Durham, NC
USA

Risto Vataja MD
Head, Psychogeriatric Department
Kellokoski Hospital
Kellokoski
Finland

Preface

The Cartesian dichotomy of 'mind' and 'body' has for too long divided the human person in two artificially distinct and unrelated domains, with psychiatrists and physicians falling under the influence of this mythology. In old age psychiatry, clinicians have a holistic approach in which the patient is seen as an integrated whole with all aspects of mind and body closely interacting in all anatomical, physiological, psychological and social domains.

From such a clinical background, the editors have long observed the close link between vascular diseases and affective disorders. With the advance of diagnostic technology in association with committed clinical and fundamental research, it is now clearer than ever that vascular diseases and affective disorders are linked in pathological, physiological, biochemical and social terms.

This text attempts to place before physicians of all specialties, and all health care professionals with an interest in either or both vascular disease and affective disorders the evidence of this close linkage, thereby highlighting the clinical relationship of the two and pointing to a better understanding that will lead all practitioners to provide better recognition and management of affective disorders and vascular diseases.

Rapid advances are occurring and considerable clarification of the mechanisms underlying these two sets of conditions and their rational treatment are to be expected in the next few years. This text serves as a marker of the field as it stands in 2002. We offer this compilation and integration of data to stimulate readers to further, methodologically sound research and to improve clinical practice, thus leading to better quality of life of the patients to whose care we, like our readers, remain committed.

Acknowledgement

The editors wish to thank their secretaries, Roz Seath and Marilyn Cain, for their tireless efforts.

Edmond Chiu, David Ames and Cornelius Katona

Cardiovascular Disease and Affective Disorders

1

How common are depressions and cardiovascular diseases in populations?

Sirkka-Liisa Kivelä

The occurrences of depression and coronary heart disease have interested researchers, and several studies about their point and lifetime prevalence rates as well as the incidence and mortality rates of ischaemic heart disease (coronary heart disease and myocardial infarction) have been performed. National teams of researchers have carried out most of these studies. During the past decade, some multi-centre international studies have been published about the prevalence and mortality rates of coronary heart disease and the prevalence of depression. There is marked variation in the definitions of depression and coronary heart disease and the instruments used in the studies, which renders comparisons and conclusions difficult. Other methodological differences include sampling, response rates and age range of the population. In this review, an overview of the topic is given by presenting a collection of the results of studies made among unselected populations using standardized methods.

Prevalence of depression

The occurrence of depression is usually shown by point prevalence. Lifetime prevalence rates or incidence rates have been calculated in a few studies. Suicide mortality does not represent mortality due to depression, although depression is a risk factor for suicides.

Definitions and measures

The definitions and measures of depression vary between the epidemiological studies. Some researchers have relied on measuring depressive symptoms and determined the prevalence of depression by the occurrence of an abundance of depressive symptoms. Others have tried to measure the occurrence of clinically relevant cases of depression.

Self-assessment rating scales and interview rating scales have been developed to measure depressive symptoms. Some of these have been validated in normal populations, and their sensitivity and specificity in detecting and defining diagnostic cases of depression with a certain cut-off point are known. Issues concerning sensitivities and specificities confound the comparison of data about the prevalence of depression as determined by an abundance of depressive symptoms.

Structured interviews carried out by psychiatrists, trained physicians or trained lay interviewers have been used to define diagnostic caseness. The interview schedules are computer-scored and capable of generating psychiatric diagnoses according to certain criteria. The classifications of mental disorders used in clinical medicine and epidemiological studies have been reformulated during the past 30 years, and the criteria according to which diagnoses are made vary between these instruments. Methodological differences lead to difficulties in comparing the results.

Due to the methodological differences, it is difficult to make conclusions about the variations of the prevalence of depression in different cultures, societies and geographical areas and even according to sex and age. Age groups, other socio-demographic variables of populations and participation rates vary between the studies, giving rise to new problems. Only community-based studies are included in the following review. The second criterion for inclusion is that standardized diagnostic criteria and instruments have been used in identifying depressed persons, and trials have been made to identify persons with clinically relevant depression.

Childhood and adolescence

Babies, children and adolescents may suffer from adult-like affective disorders, although the symptoms vary with the developmental stage. Preadolescents are especially likely to suffer from somatic complaints (Kazdin, 1990).

Among healthy preadolescent children, the rates of clinically significant depression vary from 0.6 to 2.5% (Kashani and Simmonds, 1979; Kashani et al, 1983; Anderson et al, 1987; Fleming et al, 1989; Velez et al, 1989).

The prevalence rates are higher among adolescents. The point prevalence rates of major depression in the western countries vary from 1.8 to 5% (Kashani et al, 1987; Fleming et al, 1989; Garrison et al, 1989, 1992; McGee et al, 1990; Bailly et al, 1992; Lewinsohn et al, 1993; Polaino-Lorente and Domenech, 1993; Blazer et al, 1994; Canals et al, 1995), and the 1-year prevalence varies from 4 to 5.8% (Ferguson et al, 1993; Olsson and von Knorring, 1999). At the age of 18 years, the lifetime prevalence of major depression is 11.5–3.7% for girls and 2.8–5.1% for boys (Reinherz et al, 1993; Olsson and von Knorring, 1999). The prevalence rate of dysthymic disorder is 2–6.4% (Polain-Lorente and Domenech, 1993; Olsson and von Knorring, 1999). A consistent finding is that depressions are more common among girls than boys.

There is some evidence to suggest that depression was more common in the young age cohorts in the late 1980s and 1990s than in the previous decades (Olsson & von Knorring, 1999).

Working-aged population

Only the results of studies using the DSM-III criteria in defining the occurrence of major depression and dysthymic disorder are presented in Table 1.1. Although the prevalence rates show some variation, there exist no great cross-cultural or geographical differences in the prevalence rates for major depression between the western countries when similar criteria have been applied. In different cultures, the rate of major depression varies from 1.3 to 3.8% among men and from 2.6 to 8.8% among women. The results consistently show the prevalence to be higher for women than for men.

There may be differences between the age groups, as shown by Blazer et al. (1994). In men aged 45–54 years the rate was lower (2.3%) than in men aged 15–44 years (4.0–4.3%). In women, the prevalence was highest among those aged 15–24 years (8.2%) and next highest among those aged 35–44 years (6.4%). Somewhat lower rates were found for women aged

Table 1.1   Prevalence of major depression and dysthymic disorder in working-aged populations according to community-based studies using DSM-III (*Diagnostic and Statistical Manual of Mental Disorders*, 3rd edn) criteria.

Author(s) and year	Country	N	Age	Prevalence %	
Major depression					
Hällström, 1984	Sweden	800 women	38–54	Women only	6.9
Myers et al, 1984	USA	9543	18+	Men	1.3–2.2
				Women	3.0–4.6
Regier et al, 1988	USA		18+	Men	1.6
				Women	2.9
Bland et al, 1988	Canada	3258	18+	Men	2.5
				Women	3.9
Faravelli et al, 1990	Italy	1000	15+	Men	3.5
				Women	8.8
Narrow et al, 1990	USA	1481	20–74	Men	1.5
				Women	2.6
Wittchen et al, 1992	West Germany	657	25–64	All	3.0
Blazer et al, 1994	USA	8098	15–54	Men	3.8
				Women	5.9
Dysthymic disorder					
Bland et al, 1988	Canada	3258	18+	Men	2.2
				Women	5.2
Weissman et al, 1988	USA	18572	18+	All	3.1
Faravelli et al, 1990	Italy	1000	15+	Men	2.2
				Women	3.7
Wittchen et al, 1992	West Germany	657	25–64	Men	2.5
				Women	5.4

45–54 years (5.0%) or 25–34 years (4.3%) (Blazer et al, 1994). The differences in the age distributions of the study series shown in Table 1.1 may partly explain the differences in the prevalence rates of major depression.

The lifetime prevalence of major depression (DSM-III criteria) is about 12% for men and nearly 22% for women at the age of 45–54 years (Blazer et al, 1994).

The total annual incidence of DSM-III major depression per 100 persons at risk as calculated from the figures in the USA is 1.10 for working-aged men, and 1.98 for women. This study shows the maximum debut for men to be in the age group 18–29 years, while for women there was a rise up to the peak years in the mid-forties (Eaton et al, 1989).

Nor are there any significant differences in the prevalence rates of dysthymic disorder between certain European or North American countries when the DSM-III criteria are applied. Lower rates are consistently found for men (2.2–2.5%) than for women (3.7–5.4%).

Older population

The methodologies of the studies determining the prevalence of major depression among older people have not been uniform. Considering the results of all studies shown in Table 1.2, the variation of the prevalence rate is from 0.4% (Japan) to 10.2% (Australia). Even when similar criteria have been used, viz. the DSM-III classification, the studies have given a notable range of variation. A constant finding is that men have lower rates than women.

Quite high rates of minor depressions have been found in the United Kingdom, Finland, the Netherlands and, in the early 1980s, in the USA. The findings from Japan and from the US in the late 1990s show lower rates.

Ischaemic heart disease patients

Clinical studies have shown the prevalence of major depression to be high (from 9 to 17%) among patients hospitalized due to acute myocardial infarction and among patients with severe coronary heart disease before coronary surgery (Kavanagh et al, 1975; Crowe et al, 1996; Carney et al, 1997).

Depression and sociodemographic variables

The prevalence of depression is higher in women than in men, beginning at mid-puberty and persisting throughout adult life (Piccinelli and Wilkinson, 2000). Sex differences are smallest among children and in the oldest age groups (Jorm, 1987). Psychosocial, social or genetic and biological factors may explain the differences. Women may be more apt than men to report symptoms of depression. Adverse experiences in childhood, socio-cultural

Table 1.2   Prevalence of major depression and minor depressions in older populations according to community-based studies using standardized diagnostic criteria and instruments.

Author(s) and year	Country	N	Age	Criteria/ Instrument	Prevalence	%
Major depression						
Essen-Möller and Hagnell, 1961	Sweden	443	60+	Psychiatric interview		2.0
Parsons, 1965	UK	228		Psychiatric interview		0.9
Weissman and Myers, 1978	USA	111	66+	SADS-RDC		5.4
Blazer and Williams, 1980	USA	997		DSM-III		1.8
Kay et al, 1985	Australia	274	70+	DSM-III	Total	10.2
					70–79 years	6.3
					80 years	15.5
O'Hara et al, 1985	USA	3159		RDC		1.2
Copeland et al, 1987	UK	1070	65+	GMS-AGECAT		2.9
Ben-Arie et al, 1987	South Africa	139	65+	CATEGO		9.4
Bland et al, 1988	Canada	358	65+	DIS		1.2
Kivelä et al, 1988	Finland	1529	60+	DSM-III	Total	3.7
Lindesay et al, 1989	UK	890	65+	SHORT-CARE		4.3
Madianos et al, 1992	Greece	251	65+	DSM-III		1.5
Henderson et al, 1993	Australia	945		CIE		1.0
Komahashi et al, 1994	Japan	1914		DSM-III		0.4
Beekman et al, 1995	Netherlands	3056	55+	DIS		2.0
Pahkala et al, 1995	Finland	1086	65+	DSM-III	Total	2.2
Steffens et al, 2000	USA	4559	65+	DSM-IV	Total	3.7
Minor depressions						
Copeland et al, 1987	UK	1070	65+	GMS-AGECAT		8.3
Kivelä et al, 1988	Finland	1529	60+	DSM-III	Total	23.2
Lindesay et al, 1989	UK	890	65+	SHORT-CARE		13.5
Komahashi et al, 1994	Japan	1914		DSM-III		2.4
Beekman et al, 1995	Netherlands	3056	55+	CES-D/DIS		12.9
Pahkala et al, 1995	Finland	1086	65+	DSM-III	Total	14.3
Steffens et al, 2000	USA	4559	65+	DSM-IV	Total	0.9

Abbreviations:
CES-D   Center for Epidemiologic Studies Depression Scale
DIS   Diagnostic Interview Schedule
DSM-III   *Diagnostic and Statistical Manual of Mental Disorders*, 3rd edn.
DSM-IIIR   *Diagnostic and Statistical Manual of Mental Disorders*, 3rd edn, revised.
DSM-IV   *Diagnostic and Statistical Manual of Mental Disorders*, 4th edn.
ICD   International Classification of Diseases

roles with related adverse experiences, psychological attributes related to vulnerability to life events and coping skills may be involved (Piccinelli and Wilkinson, 2000).

Although the association between age and depression has attracted considerable interest, there exists no consensus regarding the age differences in prevalence rates. Some studies have shown an increase in depressive symptoms with higher age among the older populations. However, after adjustment for the confounding effects of physical illnesses, bereavement and sex, an inverse association between age and depression has been detected (Beekman et al, 1999). Some results among older populations have shown the prevalence to decrease with increasing age. Major depression is a rare disorder among the oldest-old (Kivelä et al, 1988; Pahkala et al, 1995). The confounding factor here may be the exclusion of mildly, moderately or severely demented persons from the series. The prevalence of dementia increases with increasing age, and depression is common in mildly or moderately demented persons. Thus, the exclusion of demented persons leads to an underestimation of the occurrence of depression among the oldest-old.

Mortality, incidence and prevalence of cardiovascular diseases

Definitions and measures

Coronary heart disease, myocardial infarction, hypertension, cardiac failure and peripheral atherosclerosis are the most common cardiovascular diseases in the industrialized western countries. Their occurrence is associated with age, and with the exception of some very rare cases of hypertension and cardiac failure due to congenital anomalies or other congenital causes, they do not occur in babies, children or adolescents. They are also rare in early adulthood, but their incidence increases along with increasing age from middle adulthood onwards. Due to the rareness of cardiovascular diseases in preadolescence and adolescence, only adult and older populations are included in the following description of the mortality, incidence and prevalence of cardiovascular diseases.

Mortality statistics and age-specific death rates are commonly used to answer the question of how common cardiovascular diseases, coronary heart disease or myocardial infarctions are in populations. Routine mortality statistics provide a reasonably reliable source of information for investigating death rates and trends in these rates in countries with adequate death-reporting systems. Although between-country comparisons are more prone to errors than trends over time in one country, cross-cultural comparisons are commonly made. About one-third of the population in the world is covered by an adequate system for reporting deaths and causes of deaths, and no descriptive mortality data are available from many countries (WHO, 1995).

A majority of myocardial infarctions are treated in hospitals in the developed countries, and hospital discharge registers are usually used in calculating their incidences. Routine hospital discharge registers are only collected in a few countries, and specific monitoring systems have been developed in order to register myocardial infarctions in international multi-centre studies (Tunstall-Pedoe et al, 1994).

Standardized interviews about symptoms, diagnosed diseases, medications and previous operations; clinical diagnoses collected from medical records; and findings in electrocardiograms recorded during examinations are usually used in defining the prevalence of coronary heart disease or myocardial infarctions in epidemiological studies. The definitions of coronary heart disease or myocardial infarction and the methods used in collecting data vary between these studies, and cross-cultural or other comparisons of results are problematic.

The occurrence of hypertension has been determined either exclusively based on interviews about diagnosed hypertension and medications used or by combining standardized measurements of blood pressure with interviews. Even here, the methodologies vary between studies.

Mortality – a world-wide perspective

In mortality statistics, cardio- and cerebrovascular diseases are usually presented as one group, and mortality from all cardiovascular diseases has not been presented separately. Mortality due to ischaemic heart disease (coronary heart disease, myocardial infarction) is usually separated from overall cardio- and cerebrovascular diseases.

Cardio- and cerebrovascular diseases constitute the leading group of causes of deaths in the developed countries. In 1990, a total of 10.9 million deaths occurred in the developed countries, and 5.3 million of these were attributed to cardio- and cerebrovascular diseases, primarily ischaemic heart disease (2.7 million) and cerebrovascular disorders (1.4 million). The time trends during the past three decades show significant declines in total mortality associated with cardio- and cerebrovascular diseases among middle-aged populations, especially in Japan, Australia, Canada, France and the USA. The declines in Scandinavia, Ireland, Portugal and Spain have been quite impressive, too. In the Eastern European countries, especially in Hungary, former Czechoslovakia, Poland and Bulgaria, and the former Soviet Union, the development has been opposite in direction and the death rates have risen. Cardio- and cerebrovascular diseases still account for about 50% of all deaths in the developed countries (Lopez, 1993; Tunstall-Pedoe et al, 1994).

The cause of death statistics are unreliable in the developing countries. It is estimated that 8–9 million deaths can be attributed annually to cardio- and cerebrovascular diseases in these countries, and they constitute a smaller proportion of all deaths than in the developed countries. In 1993, their share out of all deaths was estimated to be 30% in China, 10% in India, 20–45% in the Eastern Mediterranean, 25% in Latin America and 15–20% in SubSaharan Africa. General mortality is decreasing in these countries, but cardio- and cerebrovascular mortality is increasing, and relative increases in the prevalence rates of coronary heart disease and hypertension have also been reported (Bertrand, 1997).

Working-aged population

The occurrence of coronary heart disease varies greatly between working-aged populations, and the trends in morbidity and mortality from coronary heart disease also differ between countries. The researchers of the Monica Project have collected data about non-fatal and fatal myocardial infarctions and fatal coronary events among populations aged 35–64 years in several European countries, the US, Canada, China and Russia and calculated the annual incidences of these events. In all these countries, the incidence rates are higher among men than women (Table 1.3). According to European data from 1985 to 1987, coronary heart disease was most common in the United Kingdom and Finland and least common in Spain, Italy, France, Germany and Switzerland. Quite high rates were found in the Eastern European countries. A low rate of events was found in China, while the rates in Canada, the

Table 1.3   Age-standardized annual rates of nonfatal and fatal myocardial infarctions and coronary deaths per 100 000 population among men and women aged 35–64 years in selected countries according to Monica Project (Tunstall-Pedoe et al, 1994).

Country	Men Rate/100 000	Women Rate/100 000
Australia	561	188
Belgium	514	118
Canada	605	138
China	76	37
Czech Republic	495	89
Denmark	529	141
Finland	824	129
France	336	77
Germany	353	70
Iceland	540	94
Italy	305	48
Lithuania	492	84
Poland	583	110
Russia	500	109
Spain	187	30
Sweden	406	91
Switzerland	321	Not presented
United Kingdom	823	256
USA	508	139
Yugoslavia	423	81

Based on coronary event registration in 1985 through 1987.

USA and Russia were nearly similar to those in Eastern Europe. There was a 12-fold difference in the rates of events among men and an 8.5-fold difference among women (Tunstall-Pedoe et al, 1994).

According to the Framingham Heart Study, the lifetime risk for developing coronary heart disease at the age of 40 years is 48.6% for men and 31.7% for women (Lloyd-Jones et al, 1999).

The prevalence of hypertension varies between countries, but no great variation between sexes has been found. The following prevalence rates from the 1970s and 1980s have been presented by the Interhealth Steering Committee (1991): Finland, males 39%, females 35%; the USA, males 11–23%, females 9–22%; Malta, males 36%, females 33%; Chile, males 9%, females 9%; China, males 25%, females 22%; Tanzania, males 8–9%, females 9–11%.

Older population

Age-specific death rates from cardio- and cerebrovascular diseases are higher in older populations than in middle-aged ones. Among older populations, the rates increase dramatically with increasing age (Table 1.4). The highest mortality rates for the 65–74-year-old European populations in 1990 were recorded in the Eastern European countries (2924 per 100 000 population in men in former Czechoslovakia and 1836 per 100 000 women in Romania), while the lowest rate was recorded in France (men: 818 per 100 000 population, and women: 350 per 100 000 population). Outside Europe, a very low rate for both men and women was found in Japan. According to a cross-cultural comparison, the highest rate was about four times higher than the lowest for both men and women. Within each country, age-specific death rates for all cardio- and cerebrovascular diseases show at least a twofold increase between the age groups of 65–74 years and 75–84 years, and the differences between countries show a similar pattern in both age groups (WHO, 1995).

In most countries, coronary heart disease was the leading cause of cardio- and cerebrovascular deaths in both older men and women in 1990. Exceptions in Europe were Bulgaria, Greece, Portugal and former Yugoslavia, and outside Europe Argentina, China and Japan, where the death rates of stroke were higher than those of coronary heart disease. The highest death rates of coronary heart disease for men aged 65 years and over were seen in the former Soviet Union, Finland, Ireland, the United Kingdom and Denmark and those for women in the former Soviet Union, former Czechoslovakia, Bulgaria and Romania.

In the majority of countries for which time-trend data are available, the overall cardio- and cerebrovascular mortality rates have declined both in middle-aged and in older populations during the past three decades. The declines in the death rates of coronary heart disease among older populations have been remarkable in many of these countries, being the principal reason for the overall increases in life expectancy at older ages (WHO, 1995).

Table 1.4   Age-specific death rates of all cardio- and cerebrovascular diseases (CVD) and of coronary heart disease (CHD) per 100 000 population among older men and women in 1990 in selected countries according to mortality statistics (WHO, 1995).

Country	CVD				CHD			
	Men		Women		Men		Women	
	65–74	75–84	65–74	75–84	65–74	75–84	65–74	75–84
Argentina	1915	5080	981	3824	506	1106	198	702
USA	1512	3763	790	2505	898	2130	415	1288
Chile	1316	3686	781	2829	543	1453	286	1007
Canada	1298	3399	603	2219	879	2059	365	1217
Czechoslovakia	2924	7582	1551	5735	1658	3725	744	2526
Soviet Union	2820	7274	1758	5802	1597	3950	878	2874
Bulgaria	2742	7936	963	2667	1760	6759	529	2160
Hungary	2612	7075	1570	5642	1171	2523	581	1732
Poland	2609	7156	1407	5250	750	1022	292	535
Romania	2444	7753	794	2094	1836	7056	529	1824
Ireland	2126	5160	1026	3486	1446	2958	578	1714
Finland	2085	5270	1006	3655	1458	3255	589	1908
United Kingdom	1920	4568	987	3114	1352	2743	594	1586
Norway	1794	4605	754	2995	1220	2507	404	1373
Germany	1699	5351	848	3853	893	2237	343	1303
Portugal	1642	5010	970	4015	485	987	221	677
Sweden	1620	4868	1120	2698	678	2977	386	1397
Netherlands	1497	3880	849	1809	628	2505	302	978
Greece	1356	4055	932	3723	566	1037	247	653
Switzerland	1270	3805	518	2502	687	1570	211	850
Italy	1144	3875	590	2842	520	1235	196	739
Spain	1056	3422	595	2825	427	912	159	555
France	818	2762	350	1878	344	879	114	508
Australia	1621	4265	818	3043	1115	2540	507	1605
China	1592	4704	1135	3478	274	834	189	589
Japan	780	2837	456	2075	175	517	83	345

Although mortality from coronary heart disease has declined among older persons, ischaemic heart diseases are still common in these age groups. The prevalence of coronary heart disease varies between 17 and 38% in older men and between 14 and 42% in older women according to the results of the studies performed (Table 1.5). The prevalence rate is high in Finland among both men and women. A low rate has been reported from Hong Kong. Methodological differences between studies partly explain the variation, but there are also true differences between countries as shown by the mortality statistics.

When the occurrence of ischaemic heart disease has been determined by the occurrence of symptoms of angina pectoris, the rates have varied between 3 and 20% among older men and between 2 and 17% among older women. The lowest rates have been reported from Hawaii and Denmark, and the highest from Finland.

Table 1.5   Prevalence of ischaemic heart diseases (angina, AP; coronary heart disease, CHD; or myocardial infarction, MI) among populations according to community studies using standardized diagnostic criteria and instruments.

Author(s) and year	Country	N	Age	Prevalence %		
Caird et al, 1974	UK	2254	65+	AP		14
				MI		9
Kennedy et al, 1977	UK	401	65+	CHD	Men	25
					Women	21
				AP	Men	16
					Women	8
Jensen, 1984	Denmark	3255	60–69	AP	Men	4
					Women	2
Lernfelt et al, 1989	Sweden	973	70–79	CHD	70 years	
					Men	17
					Women	22
				CHD	79 years	
					Men	35
					Women	29
Aromaa et al, 1989	Finland	8000	30–99	AP	65–99 years	
					Men	20
					Women	17
				MI	65–99 years	
					Men	6
					Women	3
Nadelmann et al, 1990	USA	390	75–85	MI		19
Curb et al, 1990	Hawaii (Japanese)	1379	60–81	AP		3
				MI		6
Smith et al, 1990	UK (Scotland)	10359	40–59	AP	Men	5.5
					Women	3.9
				MI	Men	4.3
					Women	1.4
Simons et al, 1991	Australia	2805	60+	CHD	60–69 years	
					Men	21
					Women	12
					70–79 years	
					Men	30
					Women	24
					80 years	
					Men	23
					Women	25
					60 years	
					Men	24
					Women	18
Dewhurst et al, 1991	UK	295	65–95	AP	Men	16
					Women	11
				MI	Men	9
					Women	5
Bild et al, 1993	USA	5201	60+	CHD	65–74 years	
					Men	28
					Women	19
					75–84 years	
					Men	35
					Women	26

▶

Table 1.5   (Continued)

Author(s) and year	Country	N	Age	Prevalence %		
					85 years	
					Men	32
					Women	37
					65 years	
					Men	29
					Women	19
				MI	65–74 years	
					Men	11
					Women	4
					75–84 years	
					Men	16
					Women	6
					85 years	
					Men	7
					Women	9
Sigurdsson et al, 1993	Iceland	9141 (men)	30–79	Years 1967–1968 CHD		
					30–34 years	3.6
					50–54 years	7.9
					55–59 years	9.7
					60–64 years	25.3
					Years 1983–1987 CHD	
					50–54 years	9.0
					55–59 years	9.1
					60–64 years	11.4
Woo et al, 1993	Hong Kong	197	70+	CHD	Men	17
					Women	14
Howard et al, 1995	USA	4549 (Indians)	45–74	Non-diabetics		
				CHD	Men	2.8
					Women	0.4
				Diabetics		
				CHD	Men	5.3
					Women	1.4
de Bruyne et al, 1997	Netherlands	3272	55+	MI	Men	16
					Women	7
Ahto et al, 1998	Finland	1196	65+	CHD	Men	38
					Women	42
				MI	Men	14
					Women	7
Glader and Stegmayr, 1999	Sweden	2459	35–64	Year 1986		
				AP	Men	3.4
					Women	5.9
				Year 1994		
				AP	Men	3.1
					Women	2.8
Ford et al, 2000	USA	17 705	17+	CHD		
					40–64 years	8.2
					65 years	18.7

The prevalence of previous myocardial infarction in older populations varies between 2 and 20% among men and between 3 and 13% among women. As for the prevalence of angina pectoris, the rates are lowest in Hawaii and Denmark. A higher rate has been recorded in the USA.

As in the younger age groups, coronary heart disease is more common among men than women in older age. An exception here is the oldest old age group. Some studies have shown that the rate is higher for women in those aged 85 years or over.

Calculated on the basis of the data collected in the Framingham Heart Study, the lifetime risk of coronary heart disease at the age of 70 years is 34.9% for men and 24.2% for women (Lloyd-Jones et al, 1999).

If hypertension is defined as either taking hypertensive medications or having a systolic blood pressure of 160 mmHg or over and/or a diastolic blood pressure of 95 mmHg or over, a notable proportion of the older population are hypertensive. There is marked variation in the prevalence of hypertension between countries, but up to nearly one-half of all persons 65 years of age or over have elevated blood pressure by the above criteria (WHO, 1995).

The hospitalization registers from 1976 to 1980 in the USA have shown that, each year, about 1% of the population aged 65 years or over experience cardiac failure requiring hospital treatment. More women than men are hospitalized for cardiac failure, and the rates of hospitalization have increased during the recording period (Ghali et al, 1990).

Conclusions

Both depression and coronary heart disease are common among the population. Depression is no rare disorder even among adolescents, and its prevalence rate is higher among women than among men in all age groups. No critical conclusions about the differences in the prevalence rates for depression in the different age groups can be made. Cross-cultural comparisons about its prevalence are problematic due to the differences of the methods applied. However, it seems that there are cross-cultural differences, especially among the aged. These findings merit further studies.

The occurrence of coronary heart disease is closely connected with increasing age. With the exception of the oldest-old population, coronary heart disease is more common among men than women. The heavy burden of coronary heart disease on populations and societies is shown by both morbidity and mortality data. Changes in the occurrence of coronary heart disease have been monitored in terms of mortality data, and some comprehensive international comparisons about the incidence of ischaemic heart disease have been performed. In developed societies, the incidence, prevalence and mortality rates of ischaemic heart disease have decreased among the middle-aged and even the older populations. The rates have increased in the former socialist countries of Eastern Europe, the former Soviet Union and the developing countries.

In order to improve the comparability of epidemiological researches, there is a need to conduct large international multi-centre studies by using similar methods in all centres. Researchers focusing on cardiovascular epidemiology have been more active than researchers of psychiatric epidemiology to develop international research teams and to apply similar methodologies in many countries. One reason for this may be the obvious burden caused by cardiovascular diseases on healthcare systems. Politicians have been apt to allocate resources to monitor the burden and to fund trials to find the causes of coronary heart disease. Depressed patients are less visible than patients with coronary heart disease. Considering the relatively high occurrence of depression in all age groups and the importance of depression for public health, there is a need to improve the comparability of epidemiological data and to perform studies with similar methodologies in many countries.

Acknowledgement

The Lions Organization has, through the Foundation of Nordic Red Feather, supported studies about coronary heart disease and associations between coronary heart disease and depression carried out by Professor Sirkka-Liisa Kivelä and her research team in Finland.

References

Ahto M, Isoaho R, Puolijoki H et al, Prevalence of coronary heart disease, associated manifestations and electrocardiographic findings in elderly Finns, *Age Ageing* (1998) **27**: 729–37.

Anderson JC, Williams S, McGee R, Silva PA DSM-III disorders in preadolescent children: Prevalence in a large sample from the general population, *Arch Gen Psychiatry* (1987) **44**: 69–76.

Aromaa A, Heliövaara M, Impivaara O et al, (1989) *Terveys, toimintakyky ja hoidontarve Suomessa. Mini-Suomi-terveystutkimuksen perustulokset. English summary: Health, functional limitations and need for care in Finland. Basic results from the Mini-Finland Health Survey.* (The Social Insurance Institution, Publication No. 32. Kuntoutustutkimuskeskus ja Sosiaaliturvan tutkimuslaitos: Helsinki, Turku).

Bailly D, Beuscart R, Collinet C, Alexandre JY, Parquet PJ Sex differences in the manifestations of depression in young people. A study of French high school students. Part I. Prevalence and clinical data, *Eur Child Adolesc Psychiatry* (1992) **1**: 135–45.

Beekman ATF, Deeg DJH, van Tilburg T et al, Major and minor depression in later life: a study of prevalence and associated factors, *J Affect Disord* (1995) **36**: 65–75.

Beekman ATF, Copeland JRM, Prince MJ, Review of community prevalence of depression in later life, *Br J Psychiatry* (1999) **174**: 307–11.

Ben-Arie O, Swarte L, Dickman BJ, Depression in the elderly living in the community: its presentation and features, *Br J Psychiatry* (1987) **150**: 169–74.

Bertrand E, Cardiovascular disease stoppable in developing countries? *Wld Hlth Forum* (1997) **18**: 163–5.

Bild D, Fitzpatrick A, Fried L et al, Age-related trends in cardiovascular morbidity and physical functioning in the elderly: the Cardiovascular Health Study, *J Am Geriatr Soc* (1993) **41**: 1047–56.

Bland RC, Newman SC, Orn H, Period prevalence of psychiatric disorders in Edmonton, *Acta Psychiatr Scand* (1988) **77**: 57–63.

Blazer DG, Williams CD, Epidemiology of dysphoria and depression in an elderly population, *Am J Psychiatry* (1980) **137**: 439–44.

Blazer DG, Kessler RC, McGonagle KA, Swartz MS, The prevalence and distribution of major depression in a national community sample: the national comorbidity survey, *Am J Psychiatry* (1994) **151**: 979–86.

Caird FI, Campbell A, Jackson TFM, Significance of abnormalities of electrocardiogram in old people, *Br Heart J* (1974) **36**: 1012–8.

Canals J, Marti-Henneberg C, Fernandez-Ballart J, Domenech E, A longitudinal study of depression in an urban Spanish pubertal population, *Eur Child Adolesc Psychiatry* (1995) **4**: 102–11.

Carney RM, Freedland KE, Sheline YI, Weiss ES, Depression and coronary heart disease: a review for cardiologist, *Clin Cardiol* (1997) **20**: 196–200.

Copeland JRM, Dewey ME, Wood N et al, Range of mental illness among the elderly in the community. Prevalence in Liverpool using the GMS-AGECAT package, *Br J Psychiatry* (1987) **150**: 815–23.

Crowe JM, Runions J, Ebbesen LS, Oldridge NB, Streiner DL, Anxiety and depression after acute myocardial infarction, *Heart Lung* (1996) **25**: 98–107.

Curb JD, Reed DM, Miller FD, Yano K, Health status and life style in elderly Japanese men with a long life expectancy, *J Gerontol* (1990) **45**: S206–11.

de Bruyne MC, Mosterd A, Hoes AW et al, Prevalence, determinants and misclassification of myocardial infarction in the elderly, *Epidemiology* (1997) **8**: 495–500.

Dewhurst G, Wood DA, Walker F et al, A population survey of cardiovascular disease in elderly people: design, methods and prevalence results, *Age Ageing* (1991) **20**: 353–60.

Eaton WW, Kramer M, Anthony JC et al, The incidence of specific DIS/DSM-III mental disorders: data from the NIMH Epidemiologic Catchment Area Program, *Acta Psychiatr Scand* (1989) **79**: 163–78.

Essen-Möller E, Hagnell O, The frequency and risk of depression within a rural population group in Scania, *Acta Psychiatr Scand* (1961) (Suppl) **162**: 28–32.

Faravelli C, Guerrini Degl'Innocenti B et al, Epidemiology of mood disorders: a community survey in Florence, *J Affect Disord* (1990) **20**: 135–41.

Ferguson DM, Horwood LJ, Lynskey MT, Prevalence and comorbidity of DSM-III-R diagnoses in a birth cohort of 15-year-olds, *J Am Acad Child Adolesc Psychiatry* (1993) **32**: 1127–34.

Fleming JE, Offord DR, Boyle MH, Prevalence of childhood and adolescent depression in the Community Ontario Child Health Study, *Br J Psychiatry* (1989) **55**: 647–54.

Ford ES, Giles WH, Croft JB, Prevalence of nonfatal coronary heart disease among American adults, *Am Heart J* (2000) **139**: 371–7.

Garrison CZ, Schluchter MD, Shoenbach VJ, Kaplan BK, Epidemiology of depressive symptoms in young adolescents, *J Am Acad Child Adolesc Psychiatry* (1989) **28**: 343–51.

Garrison CZ, Addy CL, Jackson KL, McKeown RE, Waller JL, Major depressive disorder and dysthymia in young adolescents, *Am J Epidemiol* (1992) **135**: 792–802.

Ghali JK, Cooper R, Ford E, Trends in hospitalization rates for heart failure in the United States, 1975–1986; evidence for increasing population prevalence, *Arch Int Med* (1990) **150**: 769–73.

Glader EL, Stegmayr B, Declining prevalence of angina pectoris in middle-aged men and women. A population- based study within the Northern Sweden

MONICA Project, *J Int Med* (1999) **246**: 285–91.

Henderson AS, Jorm AF, McKinnon A et al, The prevalence of depressive disorders and the distribution of depressive symptoms in later life: a survey using the draft ICD-10 and DSM-III-R, *Psychol Med* (1993) **23**: 719–29.

Howard BV, Lee ET, Cowan LD et al, Coronary heart disease prevalence and its relation to risk factors in American Indians. The Strong Heart Study, *Am J Epidemiol* (1995) **142**(3): 254–68.

Hällström T, Point prevalence of major depressive disorder in a Swedish urban female population, *Acta Psychiatr Scand* (1984) **69**: 52–9.

Interhealth Steering Committee (members: McAlister A, Nissinen A, Berrios X, Alberti KGMM, Khaltaev N), Demonstration projects for the integrated prevention and control of noncommunicable diseases (Interhealth Programme): epidemiological background and rationale, *Wld Hlth Statist Quart* (1991) **44**: 48–54.

Jensen G, Epidemiology of chest pain and angina pectoris – with special reference to treatment needs, *Acta Med Scand* (1984) (Suppl) **680**: 1–120.

Jorm AF, Sex and age differences in depression: a quantitative synthesis of published research, *Aust NZ J Psychiatry* (1987) **21**: 46–53.

Kashani JH, Simmonds JF, Incidence of depression in children, *Am J Psychiatry* (1979) **136**: 1203–5.

Kashani JH, McGee R, Clarkson R et al, Depression in a sample of 9–year-old children: Prevalence and associated characteristics, *Arch Gen Psychiatry* (1983) **40**: 1217–23.

Kashani JH, Beck NC, Hoeper EW et al, Psychiatric disorders in a community sample of adolescents, *Am J Psychiatry* (1987) **144**: 584–9.

Kavanagh T, Shephard RJ, Tuck JA, Depression after myocardial infarction, *Can Med J* (1975) **113**: 25–7.

Kay DWK, Henderson AS, Scott R et al, Dementia and depression among the elderly living in the Hobart community: the effect of the diagnostic criteria on the prevalence rates, *Psychol Med* (1985) **15**: 771–88.

Kazdin AE, Childhood depression, *J Child Psychol Psychiatry* (1990) **31**: 121–60.

Kennedy RD, Andrews GR, Caird FI, Ischaemic heart disease in the elderly, *Br Heart J* (1977) **39**: 1121–7.

Kivelä S-L, Pahkala K, Laippala P, Prevalence of depression in an elderly Finnish population, *Acta Psychiatr Scand* (1988) **78**: 401–13.

Komahashi M, Ohmori K, Nakano T, Epidemiological survey of dementia and depression among the aged living in the community in Japan, *Jpn J Psychiat Neurol* (1994) **48**: 517–26.

Lernfelt B, Landahl S, Svanborg A, Koronarhjärtsjukdom, *Läkartidningen* (1989) **86**: 2768–71.

Lewinsohn PM, Hops H, Roberts RE, Seeley JR, Andrews JA, Adolescent psychopathology. I. Prevalence and incidence of depression and other DSM-III-R disorders in high school students, *J Abnorm Psychol* (1993) **102**: 133–44.

Lindesay J, Briggs K, Murphy E, The Guy's/Age Concern Survey. Prevalence rates of cognitive impairment, depression and anxiety in an urban elderly community. *Br J Psychiatry* (1989) **155**: 317–29.

Lloyd-Jones D, Larson MG, Beiser A, Levy D, Lifetime risk of developing coronary heart disease, *Lancet* (1999) **353**: 89–92.

Lopez AD, Assessing the burden of mortality from cardiovascular diseases, *Wld Hlth Statist Quart* (1993) **46**: 91–6.

Madianos MG, Gournas G, Stefanis CN, Depressive symptoms and depression among elderly people in Athens, *Acta Psychiat Scand* (1992) **86**: 320–6.

McGee R, Feehan M, Williams S et al, DSM-III disorders in a large sample of adolescents, *J Am Acad Child Adolesc Psychiatry* (1990) **29**: 611–9.

Myers JK, Weissman MM, Tischler GL et al, Six-month prevalence of psychiatric disorders in three communities, *Arch Gen Psychiatry* (1984) **41**: 959–67.

Nadelmann J, Frishman WH, Ooi WL et al, Prevalence, incidence and prognosis of recognized and unrecognized myocardial infarction in persons aged 75 years or older: the Bronx Aging Study, *Am J Cardiol* (1990) **66**: 533–7.

Narrow WE, Rae DS, Moscicki EK, Locke BZ, Regier DA, Depression among Cuban Americans. The Hispanic health and nutrition examination survey, *Soc Psychiatry Psychiatr Epidemiol* (1990) **25**: 260–8.

O'Hara MW, Kohout FJ, Wallace RB, Depression among the rural elderly, *J Nerv Ment Dis* (1985) **173**: 582–9.

Olsson GI, von Knorring A-L, Adolescent depression: prevalence in Swedish high-school students, *Acta Psychiatr Scand* (1999) **99**: 324–31.

Pahkala K, Kesti E, Kongas-Saviaro P, Laippala P, Kivelä S-L, Prevalence of depresssion in an aged population in Finland, *Soc Psychiat Psychiatric Epidemiol* (1995) **30**: 99–106.

Parsons PL, Mental health of Swansea's old folk, *Br J Prevent Med* (1965) **19**: 43–7.

Piccinelli M, Wilkinson G, Gender differences in depression, *Br J Psychiatry* (2000) **177**: 486–92.

Polaino-Lorente A, Domenech E, Prevalence of childhood depression: results of the first study in Spain, *J Child Psychol Psychiatry* (1993) **34**: 1007–17.

Regier DA, Boyd JH, Burke JD Jr et al, One month prevalence of mental disorders in the United States: based on five Epidemiologic Catchment Area sites, *Arch Gen Psychiatry* (1988) **45**: 977–86.

Reinherz HZ, Giaconia RM, Pakiz B et al, Psychosocial risks for major depression in late adolescence: a longitudinal community study, *J Am Acad Child Adolesc Psychiatry* (1993) **32**: 1155–63.

Sigurdsson E, Thorgeirsson G, Sigvaldason H, Sigfusson N, Prevalence of coronary heart disease in Icelandic men 1968–1986. The Reykjavik Study, *Eur Heart J* (1993) **14**: 584–91.

Simons LA, Friedlander Y, McCallum J et al, The Dubbo Study of the health of the elderly: correlates of coronary heart disease at study entry, *J Am Geriatr Soc* (1991) **39**: 584–90.

Smith WCS, Kenicer MD, Tunstall-Pedoe H, Clark EC, Crombie IK, Prevalence of coronary heart disease in Scotland: Scottish Heart Health Study, *Br Heart J* (1990) **64**: 295–8.

Steffens DC, Skoog I, Norton MC et al, Prevalence of depression and its treatment in an elderly population. The Cache County Study, *Arch Gen Psychiatry* (2000) **57**: 601–7.

Tunstall-Pedoe H, Kuulasmaa K, Amonyel P et al, Myocardial infarction and coronary deaths in the World Health Organization MONICA Project, *Circulation* (1994) **90**: 583–612.

Velez CN, Johnson J, Cohen P, A longitudinal analysis of selected risk factors for childhood psychopathology, *J Am Acad Child Adolesc Psychiatry* (1989) **28**: 861–4.

Weissman MM, Myers JK, Affective disorders in a US urban community, *Arch Gen Psychiatry* (1978) **35**: 1304–11.

Weissman MM, Leaf PJ, Livingston Bruce M, Florio L, The epidemiology of dysthymia in five communities: rates, risks, comorbidity and treatment, *Am J Psychiatry* (1988) **145**: 815–9.

WHO Study Group, *Epidemiology and prevention of cardiovascular diseases in elderly people*, Report of a WHO Study Group. WHO Technical Report Series 853x (WHO: Geneva, (1995).

Wittchen H-U, Essau CA, Zerssen D von, Krieg J-C, Zaudig M, Lifetime and six-month prevalence of mental disorders in the Munich follow-up study, *Eur Arch Psychiatry Clin Neurosci* (1992) **241**: 247–58.

Woo J, Ho S, Lau J, Yuen Y, Chan S, Masarei J, Cardiovascular symptoms, electrocardiographic abnormalities and associated risk factors in an elderly Chinese population, *Int J Cardiol* (1993) **42**: 249–55.

2
Affective disorders and cardiovascular disease

Chris Dickens

Introduction

In this chapter the impact of affective disorders on the development and course of cardiovascular disease (CaVD) will be reviewed. Since anxiety is dealt with in a separate chapter (Chapter 4), the scope of this section will be limited mainly to depression. It should be recognized, however, that few studies manage to separate the effects of depression from those of anxiety effectively, so discriminating between these two related dimensions/constructs is somewhat artificial. Where data are available, evidence for the association of mania and CaVD will be mentioned also, though such data are extremely limited in the published literature. The impact of affective disorders on the aetiology and course of CaVD will be considered, along with effects of CaVD on the natural history of affective disorders.

The impact of affective disorders on the aetiology of CaVD

Depression is a common disorder affecting 3–5% of the general population at any given time (Regier et al, 1988). For some time it has been recognized that depression is associated with increased mortality, a proportion of which is attributable to CaVDs.

Cardiovascular mortality in psychiatric patients

Malzberg et al compared psychiatric patients with healthy subjects from the general population and found increased rates of mortality attributable to CaVDs in the psychiatric group (Malzberg, 1937). This study, though unique at the time, failed to control for the effects of chronic institutionalization on the development of CaVD and, as a result, its findings were inconclusive. With changes in the treatments for psychiatric conditions, later studies were largely free from the confounding effects of long-term institutionalization.

Weeke used the Danish National Registries to identify a cohort of patients with either major depression or manic depressive disorder and followed them over a period of 5 years (Weeke, 1979). The vast majority of her subjects had not been institutionalized for any prolonged period. Compared to the general population, subjects with major depression or manic depression were found to have a 50% higher death rate from CaVD. This greater number of deaths from CaVD among depressed and manic-depressed patients has been confirmed in other studies (Tsuang et al, 1980; Norton and Whalley, 1984; Rabins et al, 1985; Vestergaard and Aargaard, 1991; Sharma and Marker, 1994).

Though these studies were free from the effects of chronic institutionalization, the use of antidepressant drugs constituted another potential confounding factor on cardiovascular mortality. None of these early studies controlled for the differences in the use of antidepressant drugs between the depressed and non-depressed populations. Consequently they could not determine whether the increase in cardiovascular mortality in the depressed patient groups was attributable to depression, per se, or due to the use of antidepressant drugs.

Weeke et al recognized this failure to control for drug usage as a methodological shortcoming and published a later study comparing the cardiovascular mortality rates of depressed subjects before and after the introduction of antidepressant drugs (Weeke et al, 1987). This study showed an increased risk of cardiovascular mortality in depressed patients both before and after the introduction of antidepressant medication, though the risk of death was lower in the latter group. This evidence suggested that the raised cardiovascular mortality in subjects with affective disorders could not be attributed solely to the use of antidepressant drugs.

Cardiovascular mortality associated with depression in population samples

The recruitment of depressed subjects from the general population, as opposed to psychiatric patient populations, represented a substantial methodological advance in this area of research. Identification of depressed subjects by screening large numbers of the general population has the advantage that the majority of such depressed subjects have not received any psychiatric treatment. Thus, the potential confounding/moderating effects of chronic institutionalization and antidepressant drugs on cardiovascular mortality are minimized. Furthermore, the study of a community sample of depressed subjects offers the opportunity to look at the effects of depression of lesser severity than that seen in psychiatric patients, who represent the severe end of the spectrum of affective disorders.

Hallstrom et al recruited a cohort of 795 Swedish women aged 38–54 years, subjected them to detailed physical and psychiatric assessment at baseline, and reviewed them 6 and 12 years later (Hallstrom et al, 1986). After controlling for age, marital status and social class, severity of depressive symptoms at baseline (Hamilton Rating Scale for Depression) predicted the development of angina, though not the rate of myocardial infarction (MI) or mortality during the follow-up period. A number of conventional coronary risk factors were related to the development of CaVD also (physical activity, waist-to-hip circumference ratio and triglyceride levels), and controlling for these did not diminish the association of severity of depression with angina. Interestingly, subjects meeting standardized diagnostic criteria for major depressive disorder (DSM-III) at baseline were not more likely to experience angina, which demonstrates how the choice of depression assessment can affect study outcome. Furthermore, exclusion of men and subjects over 54 years old at baseline may have greatly affected the apparent effects of depression on outcome.

Murphy et al studied 1003 subjects from the general population and followed them for 16 years (Murphy et al, 1987). Using a computerized algorithm they had devised themselves, affective disorders (anxiety and depression) were identified in 12% of the study population. Compared with subjects without a psychiatric disorder at baseline, subjects with an affective disorder at baseline were 1.5 times as likely to die from CaVD during follow-up. Regrettably, details of the independent effects of depression on cardiovascular mortality were not presented and there was no control for other cardiovascular risk factors which could potentially confound this association.

No reliable conclusions regarding the impact of depression on the development of CaVD can be drawn from either of these studies. The inclusion of subjects with demographic characteristics that are not representative of most populations at risk from CaVD and the use of idiosyncratic assessments means that it is not advisable to generalize the findings of these studies. A further problem with these early community-based studies was their failure to control adequately for other cardiovascular risk factors such as the existence of CaVD at baseline. In addition, a history of depression, past or present, is associated with an increased likelihood of smoking and increased likelihood of failing to give up smoking (Glassman and Sharma, 1998). Since smoking is also a major predictor of CaVD, differences in smoking behaviour between depressed and non-depressed subjects might account for the apparent effects of depression on the development of CaVD.

Anda et al were the first to study the effects of depression on outcome in a large community sample (2832 subjects) and to control for the effects of smoking and other major cardiovascular risk factors (Anda et al, 1993). Their study population was selected to exclude subjects with CaVD at baseline based on history and physical assessment. Furthermore, subjects developing CaVD with 2.5 years of entering the study were excluded to reduce further the chance of them having suffered from occult CaVD at baseline. Over a 12-year follow-up period subjects with raised depression scores (depression subscale of the General Well-Being Schedule) at baseline had an increased risk of fatal and non-fatal ischaemic heart disease (IHD). This association remained even after controlling for differences in demographic characteristics and other cardiovascular risk factors including smoking [relative risk for fatal IHD 1.5, 95% Confidence Intervals (CI) 1.0–2.3].

Since the study by Anda et al at least seven other large, community-based studies have examined the association between depression and the development of CaVD (Aromaa et al, 1994; Vogt et al, 1994; Barefoot and Schroll, 1996; Everson et al, 1996; Pratt et al, 1996; Ford et al, 1998; Pennix et al, 2001). All except one of these studies (Vogt et al, 1994) has shown an association between depression and the development of CaVDs after controlling for pre-existing CaVD, antidepressant medication, and other coronary risk factors such as smoking. Overall, these studies show that depression predicts:

i) deaths from CaVD (any cause): relative risk of 1.5–3.9 (Aromaa et al, 1994; Pennix et al, 2001),
ii) deaths from coronary (ischaemic) heart disease specifically: relative risk of 1.3–5.2 (Anda et al, 1993; Aromaa et al, 1994; Pennix et al, 2001),
iii) myocardial infarction: relative risk of 1.7–4.5 (Aromaa et al, 1994; Barefoot et al, 1996; Pratt et al, 1996; Ford et al, 1998), and
iv) the development of symptomatic ischaemic heart disease/angina: relative risk of 2.12–4.59 (Aromaa et al, 1994; Ford et al, 1998).

In general, these studies have shown significant effects of both major depression and minor depression on the development of CaVD. Individual studies that have identified both major and minor depression in their subjects show a greater effect with major depression than minor depression (Pratt et al, 1996; Pennix et al, 2001). There is some evidence that this association between depression and CaVD may be less marked in women, the elderly and higher socio-economic classes.

Antidepressant medication and myocardial infarction

The above studies provide convincing evidence that the development of CaVD in depressed subjects cannot be attributed to the effects of antidepressant medications alone. There is considerable concern, however, that antidepressant medication may make an important contribution to the development of CaVD in this group of patients.

Tricyclic antidepressants have been shown to change cardiac conductivity and contractility, and to cause orthostatic hypotension (Giardina et al, 1981; Glassman and Bigger, 1981; Glassman et al, 1987; Pary et al, 1989; Warrington et al, 1989). Specific serotonin re-uptake inhibitors (SSRIs) to a much lesser extent have been associated with cardiac arrhythmias (Sheline et al, 1997). A number of studies have indicated that antidepressants, particularly the tricyclic group, are associated with the development of ischaemic heart disease and increased risk of cardiovascular mortality (Cohen et al, 2000; Hippisley-Cox et al, 2001). Since none of these studies have adequately controlled for the effects of depression on the development of CaVD, no firm conclusions can be drawn regarding the direct effects of antidepressants on the development of ischaemic heart disease.

Pratt et al performed a large, prospective study of subjects free from CaVD at baseline (Pratt et al, 1996). A standardized psychiatric assessment was used to identify a lifetime history of major depression (DSM-III criteria) and details of previous antidepressant use were recorded. At follow-up 13 years later, though depression predicted MI, there was no association between use of tricyclic antidepressants and later MI (crude Odds Ratio 1.62; 95% CI 0.68–3.85).

Thus the balance of evidence to date indicates that tricyclic antidepressants, and to a much lesser extent SSRIs, are associated with cardiac toxicity in the short term. There is no convincing evidence, however, that antidepressants have any long-term effects on the development of ischaemic heart disease.

The impact of affective disorders on the course of established CaVD

The prevalence of depression is higher among subjects with CaVD. The inclusion in studies of subjects with different types of CaVD, different severities of disease, recruited from varying settings has resulted in discrepant prevalence figures, however. Differing gender and age mixes in the populations studied and the use of a wide range of depression assessments have contributed to this variability in prevalences.

Depression has been found in 37% of outpatients with angiographically confirmed coronary artery disease using a self-rating questionnaire: 11% had moderate to severe depression and 26% had mild depression (Barefoot et al, 1996). In a similar study using a standardized clinical interview, the gold standard of research tools, Valkamo et al identified major depression (DSM-III-R criteria) in 7.2% of outpatients with angiographically confirmed coronary heart disease in Finland (Valkamo et al, 2001). This latter figure, obtained by more careful assessment, is likely to represent the prevalence of depression that a psychiatrist would consider as being clinically significant. Similar rates for depression were obtained using the higher cut-off on a self-rating questionnaire (Barefoot et al, 1996). Thus in ambulant patients with ischaemic heart disease the prevalence of major depression exceeds that in the general population by a factor of approximately 1.5.

Depressive disorder, as defined by standardized research criteria, has been recorded in 13–19% of patients at the time of myocardial infarction (MI) (Schleifer et al, 1989; Ladwig et al, 1991, 1994; Silverstone, 1991; Forrester et al, 1992; Frasure-Smith et al, 1993, 1995). So in this group the prevalence of depression is 3–4-fold that seen in the general population.

In subjects admitted to hospital with congestive cardiac failure the prevalence of depression may be greater still. From a consecutive series of cardiac patients admitted to a hospital, Koenig et al found that major depression, diagnosed using a psychiatric research interview, was present in 26% of those in cardiac failure (Koenig, 1998). In the same study 17% of inpatients with cardiological disorders other than cardiac failure met criteria for major depression. This latter prevalence compares well with results in inpatients following myocardial infarction.

Thus, despite the methodological variability in the studies performed, a pattern emerges that strongly suggests that prevalence rates of depression are higher in patients with CaVD. Conservative estimates, from studies using standardized interview assessments, indicate that these rates may be lowest in outpatients, in whom the prevalence may be little more than in the general population. Prevalence rates are higher in inpatient populations, e.g. following MI, and may be particularly high in inpatients with cardiac failure.

This graded increment in the prevalence of depression with increasing severity of heart disease may reflect a true graduation in the severity of depression with increasing severity of CaVD. Another possible explanation for this, however, is that subjects with severe cardiac disease may be more likely to report physical symptoms that might be regarded as being the result of depression. In other words cardiac symptoms might contribute towards a subject meeting diagnostic criteria for depression in the more severe cases. Diagnosing depression in the medically ill is fraught with problems for exactly this reason. This problem is greatest when self-rated questionnaires are used. Fortunately, most interview assessments enable researchers to determine whether symptoms arise as the result of a physical or psychological condition, which minimizes this confusion. Thus prevalences of depression established using standardized interviews are reasonably reliable.

Depression is important in these groups of CaVD patients because it is associated with several adverse outcomes: increased mortality; increased morbidity, including angina, arrhythmic events, re-hospitalization, and delayed return to work; and reduced health-related quality of life.

Depression and mortality

In the most widely quoted paper on depression and mortality following myocardial infarction, major depression (diagnosed using standardized interview) was associated with a significantly increased risk of mortality at 6 months (hazard ratio 4.3) (Frasure-Smith et al, 1993). This association remained even after controlling for severity of physical factors related to infarct (severity of MI and occurrence of previous MI). Similar results have been found in other studies, with the magnitude of the relative risk varying from 1.4 to 2.5 after adjustment for physical risk factors (Ahern et al, 1990; Irvine et al, 1999; Welin et al, 2000).

Despite the magnitude of the effect of post-infarct depression on mortality in the above studies, a number of studies have failed to show that depression is associated with increased risk of post-infarct mortality once the severity of physical risk factors are controlled for, even when sample size has been adequate (Schleifer et al, 1989; Ladwig et al, 1991; Denollet and Brutsaert, 1998; Kaufmann et al, 1999; Lane et al, 2001; Mayou et al, 2000).

Methodological differences between studies are likely to account for the variability in findings, notably the measure of depression used and the duration of follow-up. In the original Frasure-Smith study it was found that major depressive disorder strongly predicted mortality 6 months after infarct (Frasure-Smith et al, 1993). At 18 months follow-up this measure of depression was not associated with mortality in the same population but the number of depressive symptoms at baseline [Beck Depression Inventory (BDI) score $\geq$ 10], predicted mortality once physical factors were controlled for (OR = 6.64, P < 0.01) (Frasure-Smith et al, 1995). It is not clear why different measures are related to different outcomes in this way.

One possible explanation for this difference in outcome with differing measures of depression is that the increased risk associated with an episode of major depression is finite in duration. Subjects identified as depressed by less stringent criteria may have included those with increased depressive symptoms but who did not meet criteria for major depression. Such subjects would be at high risk of developing a serious depressive illness over subsequent months (Judd et al, 2000). In other words, in a proportion of such subjects with raised depressive symptoms their risk of cardiac mortality may not have been immediate but may be deferred until an episode of major depression developed months or years later.

A further complicating issue is that different measures assess depression over differing time periods. It is not always clear whether previous studies have measured chronic depression, which was present before the infarct, or post-MI depression. This is important because the former, not the latter, is associated with social difficulties, previous psychiatric history and continued smoking after MI (Lloyd and Cawley, 1982, 1983).

Some studies have selected especially high-risk populations exhibiting multiple physical risk factors such as cardiac failure and multiple premature ventricular contractions. Ahern et al included only subjects with $\geq$ 10 ventricular premature complexes per hour or $\geq$ 5 episodes of non-sustained ventricular tachycardia recorded between 6 and 60 days post MI. Denollet and Brutsaert included only subjects with a left ventricular ejection fraction of $\leq$ 50% following infarction. Irvine et al included only subjects with frequent ($\geq$ 10/hour) or repetitive ventricular depolarizations on ambulatory electrocardiogram. In fact, of the four independent studies* that showed that depression predicted mortality after controlling for physical variables two have included subjects with an increased tendency for ventricular arrhythmias (Ahern et al, 1990; Irvine et al, 1999). This suggests that depression, or something associated with depression, may be particularly related to mortality in subjects at high risk of ventricular arrhythmias.

---

* the two published reports of Frasure-Smith et al represent repeated follow-ups on the same population and are considered to be one study.

Other important methodological differences in these studies are the proportions of women included (0–46%), the variety of physical factors entered into the multivariate analyses, and whether subjects with previous MI are included. All of these factors may be associated with depression and the likelihood of death, thus affecting the outcome of the studies.

Research evidence also suggests that depression may be associated with mortality in subjects with cardiovascular problems other than myocardial infarction. Recruiting outpatients with angiographically confirmed CaVD and following them for up to 19 years, Barefoot et al confirmed that depression, assessed using the Zung Depression Scale, was associated with an increase in mortality (Barefoot et al, 1996). This increase was present for mild depression (38% increase in mortality during follow-up compared with non-depressed subjects), and moderate to severe depression (69% increase in mortality during follow-up compared with non-depressed subjects). Furthermore, the impact of depression on the risk of mortality was maintained throughout the prolonged follow-up. Lesperance et al studied patients admitted to hospital with unstable angina. Depression (Beck Depression Inventory scores $\geq$ 10) at baseline was associated with increase risk of cardiac mortality over the 12-month follow-up period (OR 3.30; 95% CI 1.0–10.9) Lesperance et al, 2000). This increased risk remained even after controlling for other cardiac risk factors.

Fewer studies have examined subjects with cardiac failure. As has been suggested already, this patient group may have higher levels of depression compared to patients with other CaVDs. Denollet and Brutsaert identified 87 subjects who had experienced a myocardial infarction within the previous 2 months and who had global ejection fraction $\leq$ 50% (Denollet et al, 1998). Subjects underwent a detailed physical and psychological assessment at baseline and were followed up for between 6 and 10 years. Subjects experiencing a fatal cardiac event during follow-up were more depressed at baseline than survivors, though this relationship failed to reach statistical significance when other physical and psychological risk factors were controlled for. Koenig et al studied 107 subjects admitted to hospital with cardiac failure as a primary or secondary diagnosis (Koenig, 1998). Once again subjects underwent a detailed physical and psychological assessment at baseline and were followed up for 12 months. Twenty-nine per cent of subjects who were depressed at baseline died during follow-up compared to 20% of the non-depressed subjects. This difference failed to reach statistical significance.

Both of these studies were relatively small by comparison with the other studies reviewed. The group of Denollet and Brutsaert had only 13 fatal cardiac events, while Koenig et al had 27 deaths among their cardiac failure subjects. Thus the lack of statistical significance may simply reflect the fact that there were too few subjects to assess the association. Alternatively, in view of the seriousness of the physical condition in subjects with cardiac failure, physical factors may be even more important in determining mortality, thus reducing the apparent impact of depression in this group.

Depression and morbidity

With regard to the impact of depression on health outcomes other than death, Ladwig et al showed that severe depression predicted more frequent angina in the 6 months following MI but that moderate depression had no significant effect (Ladwig et al, 1994). Schleifer et al found no significant differences in frequency of chest pain post-MI in subjects with major depression (Schleifer et al, 1989). They also studied frequency of re-infarction, though the number of subjects with re-infarction over the 3 months following MI was too small to give meaningful results. Denollet and Brutsaert found that depression at the time of infarction predicts all later cardiac events (fatal and non-fatal), though depression failed to contribute to cardiac events once severity of cardiac failure, negative emotionality and social withdrawal were controlled for (Denollet and Brutsaert 1998).

Of subjects admitted to hospital with unstable angina, Lesperance et al found that those who were depressed were more likely to suffer a further non-fatal MI during the 12-month follow-up period (6.7%) compared with those who were not depressed (1.2%) (OR 6.0; 95% CI 1.67–21.58, $P<0.0005$) (Lesperance et al, 2000). There was also a non-significant trend for depressed subjects to be re-admitted with unstable angina (32.6% vs 25%) (OR 1.45; 95% CI 0.95–2.22, $P=0.09$). These results represent univariate analyses, and it is not clear whether depression still predicted outcome for these non-fatal events once other risk factors were controlled for.

Three studies have indicated that emotional distress following MI might predict subsequent re-hospitalization (Schleifer et al, 1989; Havik et al, 1990; Stern et al, 1977). Stern et al found that subjects with Zung depression ratings over 40 following MI were significantly more likely to be re-admitted over the 12 months after MI compared to non-depressed subjects. Havik et al found that subjects with a high level of emotional upset (anxiety, depression, irritability measured using a multiple adjective checklist) showed a non-significant trend for more frequent re-hospitalizations over the 6 months after infarction compared to those with lower levels of distress. Schleifer et al found that subjects meeting Research Diagnostic Criteria for major depressive disorder had a non-significant trend to be re-admitted to hospital more frequently than the non-depressed (13% vs 7%, respectively) in the 3 months following MI. These studies suggest that depression may be important in predicting re-hospitalization over the months following a myocardial infarction, though the effect seen over short periods of follow-up appears to be small.

In subjects admitted to hospital with cardiac failure, depression predicted degree of functional impairment in the weeks following discharge (Friedman et al, 2001). Furthermore, depression on admission with cardiac failure predicts number of medications prescribed on discharge from hospital, and later re-admission to hospital, though not use of outpatient services (Koenig, 1998). These differences in medication use and re-admission rates became non-significant on controlling for the severity of failure during index admission.

There may also be economic implications of depression in subjects suffering from CaVD. Allinson et al found that depression was associated with higher levels of hospitalization and interventions, even when severity of ischaemic heart disease was controlled for; this led to greatly increased healthcare costs (Allinson et al, 1995). Frasure-Smith et al examined the healthcare costs of 848 subjects for the 12-month period following their admission to hospital with an acute MI and confirmed these findings (Frasure-Smith et al, 2000a). Total costs for subjects who were depressed at baseline were 41% higher than for the non-depressed. The majority of this excess cost arose from a greater likelihood of being re-admitted, longer stays in hospital when re-admitted, and more emergency room visits. After controlling for other sociodemographic factors and cardiac risk factors (smoking, hypertension and severity of MI), the costs of depressed subjects still exceeded those of the non-depressed by 11%, though this difference failed to reach statistical significance.

Depression and quality of life

The majority of studies of the impact of depression on outcome in subjects with CaVD have focused on *hard* outcomes such as mortality and morbidity. Increasingly quality of life is being considered as an important outcome in this group. The development of quantitative assessments of quality of life has greatly facilitated this research.

Lane et al considered the quality of life of subjects surviving for 12 months following a myocardial infarction using a multidimensional measure, though excluding the section measuring emotional factors (it was anticipated that these would bear a direct relation with depression) (Lane et al, 2001). Subjects with depression (Beck Depression Scores $\geqslant$ 10) had worse global quality of life 12 months following index myocardial infarction. Since a number of physical factors also predicted worse quality of life at follow-up (gender, social support, employment status, severity of index MI and length of initial hospital stay), multivariate analyses were performed entering these potential confounding variables onto the model. Depression was the strongest predictor of quality of life ($R^2 = 0.11$, $P = 0.001$). Severity of infarction ($R^2 = 0.07$, $P = 0.001$), living alone ($R^2 = 0.07$, $P = 0.001$) and anxiety ($R^2 = 0.03$, $P = 0.008$) also entered the model, whereas the other sociodemographic and physical risk factors failed to make a significant contribution.

A number of studies have recorded outcome variables, such as mood state, life stresses, social adjustment, return to work, and sexual functioning, which are likely to be highly related to quality of life. Five studies confirm that depression following MI is associated with significant continued depression in the months after the event (Stern et al, 1976; Lloyd and Cawley 1982; Schleifer et al, 1989; Garcia et al, 1994; Lesperance et al, 1996). Such depression is associated with impaired health-related quality of life, more pain and reduced activity. This impact of depression on outcome may, in part, be mediated by more negative health beliefs. Depressed subjects have more negative views regarding their levels of functional ability and the degree of control they have over their life (Cassem and Hackett, 1971; Stern et al, 1976).

Depression is associated with delayed return to work in subjects with CaVD. Cay et al found that 'emotional upset' was a highly significant predictor of return to work at 4 months and 12 months following index MI (Cay et al, 1972). Stern studied 68 subjects following MI and reassessed them 6 and 12 months later, finding that depressed subjects at baseline were less likely to be at work at 12 months ($P < 0.05$) (Stern et al, 1977). Three other studies support the finding that depressed subjects are slower to return to work in the 3–6 months following MI (Maeland and Havik, 1987; Trelawny-Ross and Russell, 1987; Schleifer et al, 1989). Furthermore, depressed subjects are slower to return to normal sexual functioning and are more likely to experience life stresses 6 months later, particularly in the domains of health, work, and finance (Stern et al, 1977; Rosal et al, 1994).

Overall, the evidence for depression being a secondary risk factor in subjects with CaVD is somewhat mixed. With regard to *hard* outcomes such as cardiac mortality and re-infarction there are approximately equal numbers of studies identifying an association between depression and adverse outcome as those that do not. As already mentioned, there are many methodological differences between studies which might account for this variability.

Where other, more subjective, outcomes such as functional impairment, quality of life, return to work and sexual functioning are concerned, there appears to be a clearer link between depression and adverse outcome. It remains possible that depression is having an adverse effect on these functional outcomes by influencing the progression of the CaVD process itself. In the absence of clear evidence that depression has a clinically significant effect on these processes, however, it seems more likely that ongoing functional impairment is mediated by maladaptive health behaviours and health cognitions which have been shown to be associated with depression in subjects with CaVD.

Despite the wealth of research in this area, certain questions remain unanswered. Though this review has focused on depression as a risk factor for CaVDs, a number of studies have indicated that it may not be depression per se but something associated with depression that results in adverse outcome. Social support, or rather its absence, has been proposed as one candidate for confounding the association between depression and mortality. A number of studies have shown that social stress and social isolation are linked to an increased risk of MI and/or subsequent increased mortality (Ruberman et al, 1984; Case et al, 1992; Jenkinson et al, 1993).

Some studies indicate that the effects of social support and depression interact, however. Two studies have emphasized that the greatest effect of depression on mortality is among women, especially those recently divorced

(Stern et al, 1977; Powell et al, 1993). Lesperance et al reported that low social support was only associated with increased mortality in those who were also depressed (Lesperance et al, 1995) and conversely that depression had its greatest effect in subjects with least social support (Frasure-Smith et al, 2000b). Denollet's construct of 'Type D personality', which appears to be particularly closely related to increased mortality or recurrent myocardial infarction, consists of depression combined with social inhibition (Denollet and Brutsaert 1998). These studies indicate that social support may act to buffer the adverse effects of depression.

A further candidate for predicting adverse outcome is 'vital exhaustion'. Vital exhaustion is characterized by lack of energy in addition to demoralization and irritability, and has been shown to predict myocardial infarction and a negative outcome following angioplasty (Appels et al, 1987, 1995; Appels and Mulder, 1988). This construct of vital exhaustion is clearly related to depression and may also reflect premonitory symptoms of cardiac disease. Further research is required to disentangle the relative importance of physical, emotional and psychosocial risk factors in CaVD.

Even if depression is the key predictive factor, the role of so-called minor depression, i.e. depressive symptoms that fail to reach diagnostic criteria for major depression, has not been established. Minor depression is one of the strongest predictors of the development of major depression (Judd et al, 2000). None of the above studies can truly differentiate whether minor depression has importance in the development of CaVD or whether it is only those subjects who develop major depression during follow-up who experience cardiovascular problems.

Also, depression is a highly heterogeneous condition and it is not clear whether particular aspects of this disease have greater likelihood of predicting the development of CaVD than others. Finally, the mechanisms by which depression leads to CaVD remain obscure. Numerous physiological and behavioural mechanisms have been proposed (Blumenthal et al, 1982; Musselman et al, 1998). However, it is not beyond the realms of possibility for both depression and CaVD to be caused by some hitherto unsuspected confounding factor, e.g. childhood deprivation or a viral infection.

The nature and course of depression in CaVD patients

So far this chapter has focused on the impact of depression on the evolution of CaVD. No mention has yet been made of factors that influence the development of depression or its natural history in subjects with CaVD. As with other areas considered in this chapter, most relevant research has been performed in subjects with myocardial infarction. Data from these studies will be reviewed here.

The psychological well-being of individuals following myocardial infarction appears to be of two main types transient or persistent / recurrent.

Transient emotional disturbances following myocardial infarction

Lloyd et al investigated 100 men who were admitted to hospital consecutively following myocardial infarction (Lloyd and Cawley, 1982; Lloyd et al, 1983). Using a standardized psychiatric interview they found that 35% of their study population had a diagnosable psychiatric disorder 1 week following their MI; of this group 19% appeared to develop the disturbance following the MI and the other 16% reported symptoms starting prior to the MI. Those subjects developing a psychiatric disorder following their MI had similar demographic and personality characteristics to those who did not develop a psychiatric disorder. Furthermore, in subjects developing a post-MI psychiatric disorder, the disorder tended to be transient in the majority: 75% of cases had remitted by 4 months after the MI.

Subjects reporting that the psychiatric disorder pre-dated their MI were substantially different to those who became disturbed subsequently. Compared with the other subjects, those in whom the psychiatric disorder began before the MI were more likely to be unmarried and to report social, relationship, and occupational stress. These stresses tended to persist well beyond their MI. They suffered from a greater range of psychiatric disorders and were more likely to have received previous psychiatric treatment. When compared with subjects who developed a psychiatric disorder following their MI, those with a pre-morbid psychiatric problem tended to have a more persistent psychiatric disorder: only 8% had remitted by 4 months compared to 75% of those developing psychiatric problems post-MI.

Major depression following myocardial infarction

Lesperance et al studied 222 male and female patients admitted with myocardial infarction to Montreal Heart Institute and limited their psychiatric assessments to identifying major depression according to the criteria of DSM-III-R (Lesperance et al, 1996). They found that 15.8% of subjects met criteria for major depression during their hospital admission. Taken in conjunction with the findings of Lloyd et al this would indicate that approximately half of all subjects suffering from a psychiatric disorder following myocardial infarction meet diagnostic criteria for major depression.

Subjects with major depression in the Lesperance et al study were more likely to be female, to lack close friends and to have a history of depression. There were no other demographic factors or markers of severity of MI which were found to be associated with depression. Ladwig et al confirmed the lack of any association between depression and markers of the size / severity of MI, though they did find that subjects experiencing major cardiac complications or dyspnoea during admission were more likely to be depressed (Ladwig et al, 1992). Other factors predicting depression in hospital in their study were more significant life events in the 2 years preceding MI, work stresses, prolonged pre-MI angina, exhaustion and fatigue.

Of their subjects, Lesperance et al found that 61 (27.5%) had a lifetime history of major depression, 17 (22.1%) of whom had suffered from the depression within the 12 months preceding the MI and 12 (5.4%) of whom had an episode less than 6 months preceding their MI (Lesperance et al, 1996). Subjects with a lifetime history of depression were more likely to be female and less likely to take regular exercise. Lesperance et al also found that subjects with a lifetime history of major depression were more likely to have a severe MI (high Killip Class) on admission and were more likely to develop depression in hospital (24.6% vs 12.4%) or in the year following infarct.

Lesperance et al did not find that subjects with a lifetime history of depression were more likely to die during the 18-month follow-up period compared to subjects without a lifetime history of depression, however (Lesperance et al, 1996). Interestingly, though the numbers studied were small, subjects whose in-hospital episode of major depression represented a relapse or recurrence of a previous episode of depression were four times more likely to die in the 12 months of follow-up: 40% mortality in those with a previous episode of depression vs 10% mortality in subjects whose depression in hospital represented a first episode.

Just under half of the subjects with major depression following MI (15 out of the 35 depressed subjects) went on to suffer from persistent or recurrent depression post-infarct. Subjects developing persistent or recurrent depression tended to be younger, to have a history of depression, and higher BDI scores during admission. Similarly, Stern et al found that depression was not transient and was associated with lower social class (Stern et al, 1976).

In summary, psychiatric disorders following MI are common, being detectable in approximately one third of sufferers whilst in hospital. Half of these subjects will have major depression that is likely to persist and that may be associated with adverse outcomes such as increased mortality, morbidity and delayed return of functioning in the months/years following MI. Major depression following MI is particularly common in subjects with a prolonged history of cardiac disease prior to MI, multiple psychosocial stresses and a past history of depression. This depression may be particularly likely to be associated with adverse outcomes when it is not the first episode of depression but represents a relapse or recurrence of a previous depressive illness.

Conclusions

There can be little doubt that depression is associated with CaVD. Depression is a predictor of later CaVD in otherwise healthy individuals even after controlling for other cardiovascular risk factors. Many questions remain unanswered about this association, however. More studies are required to determine the roles of potential confounding factors and to investigate mechanisms by which depression might influence outcome.

The role of depression as a predictor of outcome in subjects with established CaVD is less clear, probably due to the influence of a multitude of other physical and behavioural factors on outcome. However, there is clear evidence that approximately one in six myocardial infarction patients have depression, that this depression is independent of severity of heart disease and may persist for many months or years. Depression is associated with poor outcomes, including poor quality of life, impaired function, continued cardiac symptoms, and possibly increased heart disease and mortality. For these reasons cardiologists, like other physicians, need to incorporate assessments of mood and treat concurrent depression in order to improve quality of life and potentially to improve survival in patients with CaVD.

References

Ahern DK, Gorkin L, Anderson JL et al, Biobehavioral variables and mortality of cardiac arrest in the Cardiac Arrhythmia Pilot Study (CAPS), *Am J Cardiol* (1990) **66**:59–62.

Allinson, TG, Williams DE, Miller TD et al, Medical and economic costs of psychological distress in patients with coronary artery disease, *Mayo Clin Proc* (1995) **70**:734–42.

Anda R, Williamson D, Jones D et al, Depressed affect, hopelessness and the risk of ischaemic heart disease in a cohort of US adults, *Epidemiology* (1993) **4**:285–94.

Appels A, Mulder P, Excess fatigue as a precursor of myocardial infarction, *Eur Heart J* (1988) **9**:758–64.

Appels A, Hoppener P, Mulder P, A questionnaire to assess premonitory symptoms of myocardial infarction, *Int J Cardiol* (1987) **17**:15–24.

Appels A, Kop W, Bar F, de Swart H, Mendes de Leon C, Vital exhaustion, extent of atherosclerosis, and the clinical course after successful percutaneous transluminal coronary angioplasty, *Eur Heart J* (1995) **16**:1880–5.

Aromaa A, Raitasalo R, Reunanen A et al, Depression and cardiovascular diseases, *Acta Psychiatr Scand* (1994) (Suppl) **377**:77–82.

Barefoot JC, Schroll M, Symptoms of depression, acute myocardial infarction and total mortality in a community sample, *Circulation* (1996) **93**:1976–80.

Barefoot JC, Helms MJ, Mark DB, Blumenthal JA, Califf RM et al Depression and long-term mortality risk in patients with coronary artery disease, *Am J Cardiol* (1996) **78**:613–7.

Blumenthal JA, Williams RS, Wallace AG, Williams RB, Needles TL, Physiological and psychological variables predict compliance to prescribed exercise therapy in patients recovering from myocardial infarction, *Psychosom Med* (1982) **44**:519–27.

Case RB, Moss AJ, Case N, McDermott M, Eberly S, Living alone after myocardial infarction: impact on progress, *JAMA* (1992) **267**:515–9.

Cassem NH, Hackett TP, Psychiatric consultations in a coronary care unit, *Ann Intern Med* (1971) **75**:9–14.

Cay EL, Vetter N, Philip A, Dugard P Return to work after a heart attack, *J Psychosom Res* (1972) **17**:231–43.

Cohen HW, Gibson G, Alderman MH, Excess risk of myocardial infarction in patients treated with antidepressant medications: Association with use of tricyclic, *Am J Med* (2000) **108**:2–8.

Denollet J, Brutsaert DL, Personality, disease severity, and risk of long-term cardiac events in patients with a decreased ejection fraction after myocardial infarction, *Circulation* (1998) **97**:167–73.

Everson SA, Goldberg DE, Kaplan GA et al, Hopelessness and the risk of mortality and incidence of myocardial infarction and cancer, *Psychosom Med* (1996) **58**:113–21.

Ford D, Mead L, Chang P et al, Depression is a risk factor for coronary artery disease in men: the precursor study, *Arch Intern Med* (1998) **158**:1422–6.

Forrester AW, Lipsey JR, Teitelbaum ML, DePaulo JR, Andrzejewski PL, Depression following myocardial infarction, *Int J Psychiatry Med* (1992) **22**:33–46.

Frasure-Smith N, Lesperance F, Talajic M, Depression following myocardial infarction. Impact on 6-month survival, *JAMA* (1993) **270**:1819–25.

Frasure-Smith N, Lesperance F, Talajic M, Depression and 18-month prognosis after myocardial infarction, *Circulation* (1995) **91**:999–1005.

Frasure-Smith N, Lesperance F, Gravel G et al, Depression and health-care costs during the first year following myocardial infarction, *J Psychosom Res* (2000a) **48**:471–8.

Frasure-Smith N, Lesperance F et al, Social support, depression, and mortality during the first year after myocardial infarction, *Circulation* (2000b) **101**:1919–24.

Friedman MM, Griffin JA, Relationship of physical symptoms and physical functioning to depression in patients with heart failure, *Heart Lung* (2001) **30**:98–104.

Garcia L, Valdes M, Jodar I, Riesco N, de Flores T, Psychological factors and vulnerability to psychiatric morbidity after myocardial infarction, *Psychother Psychosom* (1994) **61**:187–94.

Giardina EG, Bigger JT, Johnson LL, The effects of imipramine and nortriptyline on ventricular premature depolarizations and left ventricular function, *Circulation* (1981) **64**:316.

Glassman AH, Bigger JT, Cardiovascular effects of therapeutic doses of tricyclic antidepressants: a review, *Arch Gen Psychiatry* (1981) **38**:815–20.

Glassman AH, Roose S, Giardina EG, Cardiovascular effects of tricyclic antidepressants. In: Meltzer HY, ed, *Psychopharmacology: The Third Generation of progress* (Raven Press: New York 1987) 1437–42.

Glassman AH, Sharma R, Depression and the course of cardiovascular disease, *Am J Psychiatry* (1998) **155**:4–11.

Hallstrom T, Lapidus L, Bengtsson C, Edstrom K, Psychosocial factors and risk of ischaemic heart disease and death in women: a 12 year follow up of participants in the population study of women in Gothenburg, Sweden, *J Psychosom Res* (1986) **30**:451–9.

Havik OE, Maeland JG, Patterns of emotional reactions after a myocardial infarction, *J Psychosom Res* (1990) **34**:271–85.

Hippisley-Cox J, Pringle M, Crown N et al, Antidepressants as risk factor for ischaemic heart disease: case-control study in primary care, *BMJ* (2001) **323**:666–9.

Irvine J, Basinski A, Baker B et al, Depression and risk of sudden cardiac death after acute myocardial infarction: testing for the confounding effects of fatigue, *Psychosom Med* (1999) **61**:729–37.

Jenkinson CM, Madeley RJ, Mitchell JRA, Turner ID, The influence of psychosocial factors on survival after myocardial infarction, *Public Health* (1993) **107**:305–17.

Judd LL, Akiskal HS, Delineating the longitudinal structure of depressive illness: beyond clinical subtypes and duration thresholds, *Pharmacopsychiatry* (2000) **33**:3–7.

Kaufmann MW, Fitzgibbons JP, Sussman EJ, et al, Relation between myocardial infarction, depression, hostility, and death, *Am Heart J* (1999) **138**:549–54.

Koenig HG, Depression in hospitalized older patients with congestive heart failure, *Gen Hosp Psychiatry* (1998) **20**:29–43.

Ladwig K, Lehmacher W, Roth R et al, Factors which provoke post-infarction depression: results from the post-infarction late potential study (PILP), *J Psychosom Res* (1992) **36**:723–9.

Ladwig KH, Kieser M, Konig J, Breithardt G, Borggrefe M, Affective disorders and survival after acute myocardial infarction. Results from the post-infarction late potential study, *Eur Heart J* (1991) **12**:959–64.

Ladwig KH, Roll G, Breithardt G, Budde T, Borggrefe M, Post-infarction depression and incomplete recovery 6 months after acute myocardial infarction [see comments], *Lancet* (1994) **343**:20–3.

Lane D, Carroll D, Ring C, Beevers DG, Lip GY, Mortality and quality of life 12 months after myocardial infarction: effects of depression and anxiety, *Psychosom Med* (2001) **63**:221–30.

Lesperance F, Frasure-Smith N, Talajic M, Depression and beyond: affect, arteriosclerosis and death, *Eur Neuropsychopharmacol* (1995) **3**:219–20.

Lesperance F, Frasure-Smith N, Talajic M, Major depression before and after myocardial infarction: its nature and consequences, *Psychosom Med* (1996) **58**:99–110.

Lesperance F, Frasure-Smith N, Juneau M, Theroux P, Depression and 1-year prognosis in unstable angina, *Arch Intern Med* (2000) **160**:1354–60.

Lloyd GG, Cawley RH, Psychiatric morbidity after myocardial infarction, *Q J Med* (1982) **201**:33–42.

Lloyd GG, Cawley RH Distress or illness? A study of the psychological symptoms after myocardial infarction, *Br J Psychiatry* (1983) **142**:120–5.

Maeland JG, Havik OE, Psychological predictors of return to work after myocardial infarction, *J Psychosom Res* (1987) **4**:471–81.

Malzberg B, Mortality among patients with melancholia, *Am J Psychiatry* (1937) **93**:1231–8.

Mayou RA, Gill D, Thompson DR et al, Depression and anxiety as predictors of outcome after myocardial infarction, *Psychosom Med* (2000) **62**:212–9.

Murphy JM, Monson RR, Olivier DC, Sobol AM, Leighton AH, Affective disorders and mortality: a general population study, *Arch Gen Psychiatry* (1987) **44**:473–80.

Musselman DL, Evans DL, Nemeroff CB, The relationship of depression to cardiovascular disease, *Arch Gen Psychiatry* (1998) **55**:580–92.

Norton B, Whalley EJ, Mortality of a lithium-treated population, *Br J Psychiatry* (1984) **145**:277–82.

Pary RP, Tobias CR, Lippman S, Antidepressants and the cardiac patient: selecting an appropriate medication, *Postgrad Med* (1989) **85**:267–9.

Pennix BWJH, Beekman ATF, Honig A et al, Depression and cardiac mortality, *Arch Gen Psychiatry* (2001) **58**:221–7.

Powell LH, Shaker LA, Jones BA et al, Psychosocial predictors of mortality in 83 women with premature acute myocardial infarction, *Psychosom Med* (1993) **55**:426–33.

Pratt LA, Ford D, Crum RM et al, Coronary heart disease / myocardial infarction: depression, psychotropic medication and risk of myocardial infarction: prospective data from the Baltimore ECA follow-up, *Circulation* (1996) **94**:3123–9.

Rabins PV, Harvis K, Koven S, High fatality rates of late-life depression associated with cardiovascular disease, *J Affect Disord* (1985) **9**:165–7.

Regier DA, Boyd JH, Rae DS et al, One month prevalence of mental disorders in the United States, *Arch Gen Psychiatry* (1988) **45**:977–86.

Rosal MC, Downing J, Littman AB, Ahern D, Social functioning post-myocardial infarction: effects of beta-blockers, psychological status and safety information, *J Psychosom Res* (1994) **38**:655–67.

Ruberman W, Weinblatt E, Goldberg JD, Chaudhary BS, Psychosocial influences on mortality after myocardial infarction, *N Eng J Med* (1984) **311**:552–9.

Schleifer SJ, Macari-Hinson MM, Coyle et al, The nature and course of depression following myocardial infarction, *Arch Intern Med* (1989) **149**:1785–9.

Sharma R, Markar HR, Mortality rates and affective disorders, *J Affect Disord* (1994) **31**:91–6.

Sheline YI, Freedland KE, Carney RM, How safe are serotonin re-uptake inhibitors for depression in patients with coronary heart disease?, *Am J Med* (1997) **102**:54–9.

Silverstone PH, Depression increases mortality and morbidity in acute life-threatening medical illness, *J Psychosom Res* (1991) **34**:651–7.

Stern MJ, Pascale L, McLoone JB, Psychosocial adaptation following an acute myocardial infarction, *J Chron Dis* (1976) **29**:513–26.

Stern MJ, Pascale L, Ackerman A, Life adjustment postmyocardial infarction. Determining predictive variables, *Arch Intern Med* (1977) **137**:1680–5.

Trelawny-Ross C, Russell O, Social and psychological responses to myocardial infarction: multiple determinants of outcome at six months, *J Psychosom Res* (1987) **31**:125–30.

Tsuang MT, Woolson RF, Fleming JA, Premature deaths in schizophrenia and affective disorders: an analysis of survival curves and variables affecting the shortened survival, *Arch Gen Psychiatry* (1980) **37**:979–83.

Valkamo M, Hintikka J, Honkalampi K et al, Alexithymia in patients with coronary heart disease, *J Psychosom Res* (2001) **50**:125–30.

Vestergaard P, Aargaard J, Five-year mortality in lithium treated manic depressive patients, *J Affect Disord* (1991) **21**:33–8.

Vogt T, Pope C, Mullooly J, Hollis J, Mental health status as a predictor of morbidity and mortality: a 15 year follow-up of members of a health maintenance organization, *Am J Public Health* (1994) **84**:227–31.

Warrington SJ, Padgham C, Lader M, The cardiovascular effects of antidepressants, *Psychol Med* (1989) (Suppl) **16**:1–40.

Weeke A, Causes of death in manic-depressives. In: Schou M, Stromgren E, eds, *Origin, Prevention and Treatment of Affective Disorders* (Academic Press: London 1979) 289–99.

Weeke A, Juel K, Vaeth M, Cardiovascular deaths and manic-depressive psychosis, *J Affect Disord* (1987) **13**:287–92.

Welin C, Lappas G, Wilhelmsen L, Independent importance of psychosocial factors for prognosis after myocardial infarction, *J Intern Med* (2000) **247**:629–39.

3
Panic disorder and cardiovascular disease

Paul J Rushton, Philip LP Morris and Paul Masterman

Introduction

Panic disorder and cardiovascular disease have symptoms in common. These similarities pose difficulties in detection and treatment for medical and mental health practitioners. Beyond the diagnostic issues, there is a possible interaction between panic disorder and coronary artery disease that has implications for the pathophysiology of both conditions, and panic disorder has a role as a risk factor for cardiovascular disease. To address these issues, panic disorder will first be briefly described and the overlap in the clinical features of this disorder and cardiovascular disease will be discussed. Second, the association between panic disorder and more specific conditions, such as coronary artery disease, will be explored. Third, the pathophysiology of panic disorder and its role as a risk factor for cardiovascular disease will be discussed. Fourth, implications for assessment and treatment will be outlined. Lastly, future research initiatives will be suggested.

Panic disorder

Panic disorder is a common, highly symptomatic and disabling anxiety disorder characterized by recurrent, unpredictable episodes of sudden, intense fear or discomfort known as panic attacks. Panic attacks may also occur in psychiatric disorders other than panic disorder (e.g. other anxiety disorders, mood disorders, adjustment disorders, and substance use and withdrawal). Panic attacks may be observed in non-psychiatric medical conditions such as cardiovascular disease.

Panic attacks are experienced as intense physiological reactions with accompanying cardiovascular symptoms. Indeed, symptoms such as chest pain, palpitations, sweating, shortness of breath (dyspnoea), sensation of choking, numbness or tingling sensations (paraesthesia), and hot flushes are not only present in panic disorder but are also cardinal features of cardiovascular disease. In addition to panic attacks, panic disorder also requires a number of other features to be present. The full *Diagnostic and Statistical Manual of Mental Disorders,* 4th edn (DSM-IV) criteria

(American Psychiatric Association, 1994) for panic disorder can be found in Table 3.1.

Panic disorder is associated with the high rates of use of general, emergency and psychiatric services compared with other psychiatric disorders or non-psychiatric conditions (Katon et al, 1992). Because of the similarities in symptoms between panic disorder and cardiovascular disease, patients are often referred incorrectly, and when these conditions co-exist one condition is often missed. Two studies estimate that around 50% of panic disorder patients remain undiagnosed (Sartorius et al, 1996; Lecrubier and Uston, 1998). Canadian researchers found that of patients who presented with chest pains in the emergency department of a major hospital and who met criteria for panic disorder, up to 98% were not recognized by cardiologists as suffering from this condition (Fleet et al, 1996). Unfortunately, many people with panic disorder undergo elaborate, expensive, but inconclusive medical workups or receive ineffective treatment for non-specific anxiety (Kaplan and Sadock, 1995). Consequently, many patients remain undiagnosed and untreated, resulting in a significant individual distress and cost to health-care systems.

Table 3.1   DSM-IV diagnostic criteria for panic disorder.

Panic disorder
a.   Recurrent unexpected panic attacks as described below
b.   At least one of the attacks has been followed by 1 month (or more) of one (or more) of the following:
  • Persistent concern about having additional attacks
  • Worry about the implications of the attack or its consequences, e.g. losing control
  • A significant change in behaviour related to the attacks

Panic attack
A discrete period of intense fear or discomfort, in which four (or more) of the following symptoms developed abruptly and reached a peak within 10 minutes
  1. Palpitations, pounding heart or accelerated heart rate
  2. Sweating
  3. Trembling or shaking
  4. Sensations of shortness of breath or smothering (dysponea)
  5. Feelings of choking
  6. Chest pain or discomfort
  7. Nausea or abdominal discomfort
  8. Dizziness, light-headiness, or faintness
  9. Derealization (feelings of unreality) or depersonalization (feeling detached from oneself)
  10. Fear of losing control or going crazy
  11. Fear of dying
  12. Numbness or tingling sensations (paresthesias)
  13. Chills or hot flushes

The attacks are not better accounted for by another mental disorder such as social phobia, and are not due to the direct physiological effects of a substance, e.g. a medication, or a general medical condition, e.g. hyperthyroidism.

Many patients with panic disorder become preoccupied with the possibility of experiencing further attacks in particular situations in the future. This anticipation of future panic attacks may cause patients to avoid these feared situations, leading to the development of agoraphobia. Consequently, the presentation of panic disorder in the presence of agoraphobia is more common than panic disorder alone. In a US community prevalence study, in which over 11 000 people were interviewed, the 6-month prevalence of panic disorder was found to be 0.8% without agoraphobia, but 3.8% with agoraphobia (Myers et al, 1984). More recently, panic disorder, with or without agoraphobia, has been estimated to affect approximately 1–5% of the general population of the USA (Kessler et al, 1994).

Specific diagnostic dilemmas

Non-cardiac chest pain

Chest pain is a common complaint among patients seen in primary care practice, yet no specific medical aetiology is found in 80–90% of patients reporting chest pain in this context (Katon, 1990). While some patients with chest pain who have normal angiograms have been found to have a number of other problems (e.g. oesophageal motility disorders and mitral valve prolapse) many of these people have psychiatric disorders. In a review of the literature, Fleet et al (1994) concluded that at least a third of patients in cardiology practice who present with atypical chest pain and normal coronary arteries meet criteria for panic disorder. Several studies have also examined the prevalence of panic disorder among patients with chest pain who have been seen in a hospital emergency room. Between 16 and 25% of emergency room patients with a chief complaint of chest pain suffer from panic disorder (Yingling et al, 1993; Fleet et al, 1996; Zaubler and Katon, 1996).

These findings indicate that cardiologists are frequently confronted with panic disorder in their daily practice. As previously mentioned, a large number of panic disorder sufferers will remain undiagnosed in primary care settings and will continue to seek explanation and reassurance for their symptoms through costly repeat consultations with physicians (Jeejeebhoy et al, 2000). Given that panic disorder is treatable with specific pharmacological agents and cognitive behaviour therapy, cardiologists should be trained to detect panic disorder and make referrals for psychiatric or psychological treatment.

Heart palpitations/arrhythmias

Palpitations are reported by up to 16% of outpatients in a general medical setting (Kroenke et al, 1990). The prevalence of panic disorder in patients reporting palpitations has been found to be around 30% (Barsky et al, 1995; Weber and Kapoor, 1996). Jeejeebhoy et al (2000) point out that for patients who report palpitations and have panic disorder there is little correlation between palpitations and cardiac rhythm irregularities. A study by Barsky et al (1994) showed that patients with a documented arrhythmia were less likely to somatise and to have hypochondriacal concerns and psychiatric disorders than those without measurable arrhythmia. These results point to cognitive theories of panic that propose that panic sufferers have an enduring tendency to be hyper-aware of internal bodily sensations and possess a predisposition to interpret minor somatic symptoms and physiological activity in a catastrophic way.

Coronary artery disease

Panic disorder may also occur in patients with existing coronary artery disease. A study by Fleet et al (1998) showed that 34% (25 of 74) of emergency department chest pain patients with a documented history of coronary artery disease who were discharged with a non-cardiac chest pain diagnosis suffered from panic disorder.

A recent review of studies concluded that the frequency of panic disorder ranges from 10 to 50% in both general cardiology outpatients and patients with documented coronary artery disease (Fleet et al, 2000). Patients who have symptoms that cannot be explained by their coronary status or who have atypical chest pain are more likely to be found to have panic disorder.

Panic disorder and sudden cardiac death

Given that panic disorder may be comorbid with coronary artery disease, there is some concern that panic disorder may be a risk factor for increased cardiac morbidity and mortality. One retrospective study examined mortality rates over a 35-year period for 113 former inpatients diagnosed with panic disorder and unipolar depression. This group was then compared to expected mortality rates based on relevant vital statistics from the state of Iowa, USA. It was found that 12 males from the inpatient group died from circulatory disease while only six deaths were expected from the Iowa statistics. However, mortality due to cardiovascular disease among women diagnosed with panic disorder was no different than expected from the population statistics (Coryell et al, 1982).

Prospective studies have shown an association between anxiety (not panic specifically) and sudden cardiac death. One study, in which the participants were all male, found that participants with high levels of phobic anxiety had a three-fold increase in their relative risk of sudden cardiac death compared to participants with the lowest levels of anxiety (Kawachi et al, 1994a).

In the Normative Aging Study, Kawachi et al (1994b) also observed an association between anxiety and subsequent coronary heart disease. The population for this study consisted of 2,280 male community respondents from the Boston area in the USA. Results showed that after adjusting for possible confounding factors such as age, smoking, alcohol use, family history of coronary heart disease, body mass and blood pressure, men reporting two or more symptoms of anxiety had a greater risk of sudden cardiac death compared with men reporting no symptoms of anxiety.

While the above studies appear to show an association between anxiety and cardiovascular death, they should be interpreted with caution as they suffer from several methodological limitations. First, by their very nature, retrospective studies do not allow for the exclusion of confounding factors such as the development of other psychiatric or somatic disorders, or the engagement by participants in behaviours such as cigarette smoking that are separate risk factors for cardiovascular disease. Second, the diagnosis of panic disorder was taken from medical chart reviews and not validated self reports or structured psychiatric interviews. The prospective studies of Kawachi et al (1994a) managed to overcome many of the problems just mentioned, however their studies did not specifically focus on panic disorder. Third, the association between panic disorder and mortality in women has had little study.

Myocardial infarction

It is well known that anxiety levels increase after the experience of myocardial infarction. The reader is directed to Jacob and Waldstein (1991) for a comprehensive review. However, as these authors point out, all of the studies are retrospective and are also biased by the inclusion of patients who have survived a myocardial infarction. Only one study has examined the association between a diagnosis of coronary artery disease and subsequent development of panic disorder. Goldberg et al (1990) interviewed 52 cardiology outpatients to assess the prevalence of panic disorder using criteria from the *Diagnostic and Statistical Manual of Mental Disorders*, 3rd edn, revised (DSM III-R) (American Psychiatric Association, 1987). Twenty-three of these patients were found to have documented history of coronary heart disease in the form of previous myocardial infarction, positive angiogram, or bypass surgery, and 16 of these patients had panic disorder. Among the patients who had panic disorder, two identifiable groups existed based on duration of panic symptoms. For patients who had panic disorder for an average of only 4 years (the short duration group, $N = 9$), panic developed after they received a diagnosis of coronary artery disease. For patients who had panic disorder for an average of 33 years (the long duration group, $N = 7$), the diagnosis of coronary artery disease occurred subsequent to the development of having panic disorder.

Fleet et al (2000) suggest that once patients receive a diagnosis of coronary artery disease or have suffered a myocardial infarction they may become hypervigilant to further cardiac symptoms that could be interpreted as signalling an impending heart attack or death. Such catastrophic thinking may lead to an intensification of physiological symptoms, creating a vicious cycle that could culminate in the development of panic disorder. However, while this sequence of events might be plausible, the study mentioned above suffered from the use of retrospective data and a small sample size.

Evidence suggesting a causal relationship between the diagnosis of coronary artery disease and the development of panic disorder is not yet conclusive.

Pathophysiology of panic disorder and risk for cardiovascular disease

Reduced heart rate variability

While no conclusive pathophysiological pathway producing panic disorder has been found to date (Jeejeebhoy et al, 2000), recent research has elaborated on the notion that overstimulation of the sympathetic nervous system might be responsible for a number of the symptoms of panic attacks. This work also suggests that decreased parasympathetic autonomic regulation or vagal activity may play a role in the pathophysiology of panic disorder. During normal breathing, the heart speeds up on inspiration and slows down during expiration. This pattern of variability in heart rate is known as respiratory sinus arrhythmia and is achieved through variation in vagal excitation of the sinus node. Measuring the respiratory sinus arrhythmia can therefore provide an indication of the degree of vagal activity in the heart. Variability in heart rate will decrease if vagal activity is decreased (Zaubler and Katon, 1996).

Recent studies have found that reduced heart rate variability is associated with sudden cardiac death among patients with documented coronary artery disease (Wulsin et al, 1999). Kawachi et al (1995) reported a similar relationship in the Normative Ageing Study, and also an inverse relationship between heart rate variability and phobic anxiety: as phobic anxiety increased, heart rate variability decreased. Kawachi et al (1995) suggest that reduced heart rate variability is a marker for ventricular arrhythmia and confers a risk for sudden cardiac death, although there is no definitive mechanism to explain this association.

In order to explore the idea that panic disorder patients may have decreased vagal tone and thereby be at risk of sudden cardiac death, Yeragini et al (1993) investigated vagal tone in 21 patients with panic disorder and 21 normal controls. Patients were tested in sitting and standing postures. In both positions patients with panic disorder had lower heart rate variability than controls. In a smaller study of only 10 patients with panic disorder, Klein et al (1995) reported similar findings. However, both these studies were cross-sectional. There have been no longitudinal studies of the possible relationship between panic disorder, lowered heart rate variability and cardiac events. Consequently, it remains to be seen whether reduced heart rate variability is a consequence of panic disorder or vice versa. It would also be of interest to determine whether heart rate variability returned to normal levels after patients were successfully treated for panic disorder.

Mitral valve prolapse

The symptoms of mitral valve prolapse and of panic disorder share similar characteristics and as a result the association between these two conditions has been of interest. A review of the literature by Zaubler and Katon (1996) found that mitral valve prolapse and panic disorder often co-occur. However, it has also been shown that patients with mitral valve prolapse do not have increased rates of panic disorder compared to patients with other cardiac symptoms (Margraf et al, 1988; Alpert et al, 1991). Furthermore, Yang et al (1997) concluded that, while both mitral valve prolapse and panic disorder appear to present with similar symptoms and occur in similar populations, there is no causal relationship between the two. Despite this, due to the similarity in symptoms, patients with mitral valve prolapse should be assessed for panic disorder for two reasons. First, if panic disorder remains undiagnosed and untreated the risk of further complicating psychiatric comorbidity (e.g. depression) is increased. Second, patients with panic disorder and mitral valve prolapse respond equally as well to treatment for panic disorder as do patients with panic disorder alone (Zaubler and Katon, 1996).

Myocardial ischaemia

Fleet et al (2000) argue that panic disorder may be associated with myocardial ischaemia. This proposal is based on laboratory studies that show that mental stress induces myocardial ischaemia in patients with coronary artery disease. Because panic disorder and coronary artery disease can occur together, and panic attacks could be conceptualized as potent stressors, there might be a link between panic attacks and transient ischaemia, at least in patients with concomitant coronary artery disease. At present the proposed mechanisms linking mental stress and myocardial ischaemia in panic disorder are not well understood, although Esler (1998) suggests that pronounced sympathetic outflow to the heart can produce coronary artery spasm and infarction during panic attacks. Future research should be directed at investigation of possible panic-induced myocardial ischaemia in patients with and without coronary artery disease.

Catecholamines and idiopathic cardiomyopathy

While a number of studies show conflicting results regarding increased catecholamine levels in patients with panic disorder, an interesting link has been found between noradrenaline, panic disorder and idiopathic cardiomyopathy (Jacob and Waldstein, 1991). A study by Kahn et al (1987) found that among patients waiting for cardiac transplants, those whose heart disease was due to idiopathic cardiomyopathy (a form of left ventricular hypertrophy) had a much higher prevalence of panic disorder (51%) than those needing transplants for post-infarction cardiac failure (5.5%), or rheumatic or congenital heart disease (0%). Kahn et al (1990) followed this study by comparing 35 patients who had panic disorder with 35 controls on subclinical cardio-myopathic changes in the heart. Twenty-three percent of patients with panic disorder had significant increases in left ventricular mass and chamber size which were consistent with more advanced idiopathic cardiomyopathy. Only 3% of the controls showed similar increases. Studies have shown that left ventricular hypertrophy can be induced by infusion with noradrenaline in dogs (Laks et al, 1973) and that elevations in baseline levels of noradrena-line are related to left ventricular hypertrophy in groups of people with hypertension (Wollam et al, 1983).

Therefore, if panic disorder is characterized by high levels of circulating catecholamines and consequent subclinical cardiomyopathy, then this may provide one explanation for the link to cardiovascular disease. However, much more research is required to validate this association and provide explanations of causal mechanisms.

Hypertension and hyperventilation

In a review of the literature, Jacob and Waldstein (1991) concluded that despite several methodological problems (including small sample sizes, inad-equate assessments of anxiety, confounding effects of medications and no direct investigations of panic disorder) there appears to be modest support for a relationship between panic disorder and hypertension. One study by Noyes et al (1980) that was not included in Jacob and Waldstein's review showed that patients with normal blood pressure who were diagnosed with panic disorder had significantly more hypertension at 6-year follow-up than did a control group. However, further studies are needed to examine the strength and extent of this relationship.

Panic disorder is associated with labile hypertension and tachycardia. Several studies using ambulatory monitoring of heart rate and blood pres-sure have shown heart rate elevations and increased blood pressure during panic attacks (Shear, 1986; White and Baker, 1987; Woods et al, 1987). It has also been shown that hyperventilation can be observed during panic attacks (Jacob and Waldstein, 1991). When healthy individuals are forced to hyperventilate under experimental conditions, increases in heart rate, reduc-tion in coronary blood flow, and rises in blood pressure have resulted (Todd et al, 1995). Hyperventilation can also be used to induce panic attacks in patients with panic disorder (Jeejeebhoy et al, 2000). Hyperventilation, then, might be the aetiological pathway linking panic disorder to hypertension and coronary ischaemia. A combination of repeated episodes of labile hyperten-sion, exaggerated adrenal activity, and increased cardiac and peripheral catecholamine levels might lead to enduring peripheral vasoconstriction and hypertension (Zaubler and Katon, 1998).

Implications for assessment and treatment

As noted above, panic disorder remains largely undiagnosed in patients who present with cardiovascular symptoms in primary care and general hospital settings. It is imperative for making an accurate diagnosis that the physician be aware of the possibility of a psychiatric aetiology for cardiovascular presentations and make time for careful, specific questioning (Kaplan and Sadock, 1995). Jeejeebhoy et al (2000) suggest that panic disorder should be considered in patients with:

- Chest pain and no evidence of organic disease.
- Atypical chest pain when there is coronary artery disease but the symptoms are not consistent with the organic disease.
- Palpitations and no evidence of a significant arrhythmia found on monitoring.
- Palpitations and no symptom–rhythym correlation found on monitoring.
- Mitral valve prolapse and significant cardiovascular symptoms.

It is important to note that panic disorder and cardiovascular disease are not mutually exclusive, and determining which symptoms relate to panic disorder and which are due to an organic disease is often challenging (Jeejeebhoy et al, 2000).

If panic disorder is not diagnosed and treated, sufferers can develop agoraphobia. When this avoidance pattern becomes severe the patient is often housebound, which restricts their social and work interactions and affects quality of life. Chronic panic disorder is also a risk factor for alcoholism, depression and suicide (Fleet et al, 1996). These complications might be avoided if panic disorder is diagnosed early and effective treatments are given for this condition.

There have been a number of randomized, controlled trials reported in the literature showing the effectiveness of both specific pharmacotherapy and cognitive behaviour therapy (CBT) for the treatment of panic disorder. Initial pharmacological treatment of panic disorder included tricyclic antidepressants such as imipramine, and benzodiazepines such as alprazolam and clonazepam. Unfortunately, imipramine is poorly tolerated and potentially dangerous for patients with both panic disorder and cardiac illness as it may induce arrhythmia, as well as raising blood pressure and heart rate in some patients (Jeejeebhoy et al, 2000). While benzodiazepines have a faster onset of action and fewer side-effects than tricyclics and were widely used to treat panic disorder, there is concern over their abuse potential and the consequences of sudden withdrawal (Rizley et al, 1986). More recently antidepressants such as the monoamine oxidase inhibitors (MAOIs) and selective serotonin reuptake inhibitors (SSRIs) have been found useful. As SSRIs have fewer side-effects and drug interactions than either tricyclics, benzodiazepines or MAOIs, and are incompatible with many cardiac medications, SSRIs such as paroxetine, fluvoxamine and sertraline are now considered to be the treatment of choice for chronic panic disorder in the general population and for patients with cardiovascular disease (Clum and Surls, 1993; American Psychiatric Association, 1998).

CBT is highly effective in the treatment of panic disorder. Recent reviews of methodologically sound treatment studies of CBT show that around 80% of patients will be treated successfully. Moreover, these treatment gains (including panic-free status and significant reductions in agoraphobic avoidance, lower general anxiety levels, and less depression) continue to persist at 2-year follow-up (Margraf et al, 1993; Barlow, 1997). Overall, treatment with either CBT or SSRIs, or treatment with both, produces notable symptom improvements within 6–8 weeks and successfully treats the majority of patients diagnosed with panic disorder (American Psychiatric Association, 1998).

Conclusions and directions for future research

Panic disorder is present in many patients who undergo cardiac assessment and interventions, especially patients with non-cardiac chest pain and coronary artery disease. Due to the similarities in symptoms between panic disorder and cardiovascular disease, panic disorder is often undetected and therefore untreated in patients who present with cardiovascular symptoms. Professionals working in the cardiovascular area should be trained to detect panic disorder and make referrals for psychological and psychiatric treatment. Whilst evidence suggests a relationship between panic disorder and cardiovascular disease, prospective studies examining the nature and extent of this association, as well as research into the pathophysiological pathways linking these conditions, are required before causal connections can be established.

References

Alpert MA, Mukerjee V, Sabeti M, Russell JL, Beitman BD, Mitral valve prolapse, panic disorder and chest pain. *Med Clin N Am* (1991) **75**: 1119–33.

American Psychiatric Association, *Diagnostic and Statistical Manual of Mental Disorders, 3rd edn, Revised* (American Psychiatric Association: Washington, DC, (1987).

American Psychiatric Association, *Diagnostic and Statistical Manual of Mental Disorders*, 4th edn (American Psychiatric Association: Washington, DC, (1994).

American Psychiatric Association, Practice guidelines for the treatment of patients with panic disorder. Work group on panic disorder, *Am J Psychiatry* (1998) (Suppl. 5) **155**: 1–34.

Barlow DH, Cognitive behavioural therapy for panic disorder: current status, *J Clin Psychiatry* (1997) (Suppl 2) **58**: 32–6.

Barsky AJ, Cleary PD, Barnett MC, Christiansen CL, Ruskin JN, The accuracy of symptom reporting by patients complaining of palpitations, *Am J Med* (1994) **97**: 214–21.

Barsky AJ, Cleary PD, Coeytaux RR, Ruskin JN, The clinical course of palpitations in medical outpatients, *Arch Intern Med* (1995) **155**: 1782–8.

Clum GA, Surls R, A meta-analysis of treatments for panic disorder, *J Cons Clin Psychol* (1993) **61**: 317–26.

Coryell W, Noyes R, Clancy J, Excess mortality in panic disorder: a comparison with primary unipolar depression, *Arch Gen Psychiatry* (1982) **39**: 701–3.

Esler M, Stress, stressors and cardiovascular disease. In Morris P, Raphael B, Bordujenko, A, eds, *Stress and Challenge. Health and Disease. Proceedings of the RMA Consensus Conference 1998*, Canberra (Repatriation Medical Authority, (1998).

Fleet RP, Dupuis G, Marchand A et al, Panic disorder, chest pain and coronary artery disease: Literature review, *Can J Cardiol* (1994) **10**: 827–34.

Fleet RP, Dupuis G, Marchand A et al, Panic disorder in emergency department chest pain patients: prevalence, comorbidity, suicidal ideation and physical recognition, *Am J Med* (1996) **101**: 371–80.

Fleet RP, Dupuis G, Marchand A et al, Panic disorder in coronary artery disease patients with non-cardiac chest pain, *J Psychosom Res* (1998) **44**: 81–90.

Fleet RP, Lavoie K, Beitman BD, Is panic disorder associated with coronary artery disease? A critical review of the literature, *J Psychosom Res* (2000) **48**: 347–56.

Goldberg R, Morris P, Christian F et al, Panic disorder in cardiac outpatients, *Psychosomatics* (1990) **31**: 168–73.

Jacob RG, Waldstein SR, Panic disorder, anxiety, and the cardiovascular system. In Shapiro AP, Baum A, eds, *Behavioral Aspects of Cardiovascular Disease. Perspectives in Behavioral Medicine*, (Lawrence Erlbaum Associates Inc.: Hillsdale, NJ, 1991).

Jeejeebhoy FM, Dorian P, Newman DM, Panic disorder and the heart: a cardiology perspective, *J Psychosom Res* (2000) **48**: 393–403.

Kahn JP, Drusin RE, Klein DF, Idiopathic cardiomyopathy and panic disorder: Clinical association in cardiac transplant candidates, *Am J Psychiatry* (1987) **144**: 1327–30.

Kahn JP, Gorman JM, King DL et al, Cardiac left ventricular hypertrophy and chamber dilatation in panic disorder patients: implications for idiopathic cardiomyopathy, *Psychiatry Res* (1990) **32**: 55–61.

Kaplan H I, Sadock B, *Comprehensive Textbook of Psychiatry*, 6th edn (Williams & Wilkins: New York 1995).

Katon W, Chest pain, cardiac disease, and panic disorder, *J Clin Psychiatry* (1990) **51**: 27–30.

Katon WJ, Von Korff M, Lin E, Panic disorder, relationship to high medical utilisation, *Am J Med* (1992) **92**: 1A–11S.

Kawachi I, Colditz GA, Ascherio A et al, Prospective study of phobic anxiety and risk of coronary heart disease in men, *Circulation* (1994a) **89**: 1992–7.

Kawachi I, Sparrow D, Vakonas PS, Weiss ST, Symptoms of anxiety and risk of coronary heart disease: the Normative Ageing Study, *Circulation* (1994b) **90**: 2225–9.

Kawachi I, Sparrow D, Vakonas PS, Weiss ST, Decreased heart rate variability in men with phobic anxiety (data from the Normative Ageing Study), *Am J Cardiol* (1995) **75**: 882–5.

Kessler RC, McGonagle KA, Zhao S, Lifetime and 12 months prevalence of DSM-III-R psychiatric disorders in the United States: results from the National Comorbidity Survey, *Arch Gen Psychiatry* (1994) **51**: 8–19.

Klein E, Cnaami E, Harel T, Braun S, Ben Haim SA, Altered heart rate variability in panic disorder patients, *Biol Psychiatry* (1995) **37**: 18–24.

Kroenke K, Arrington ME, Mangelsdorff AD, The prevalence of symptoms in medical outpatients and the adequacy of therapy, *Arch Intern Med* (1990) **150**: 1685–9.

Laks MM, Morady F, Swan HJC, Myocardial hypertrophy produced by chronic infusion of subhypertensive doses of norepinephrine in the dog, *Chest* (1973) **64**: 75–8.

Lecrubier Y, Uston TB, Panic and depression: a worldwide primary care perspective, *Int Clin Psychopharmacol* (1998) (Suppl 4) **13**: 7–11.

Margraf J, Ehlers A, Roth WT, Mitral valve prolapse and panic disorder: A review of their relationship, *Psychosom Med* (1988) **50**: 93–113.

Margraf J, Barlow DH, Clark DM, Telch MJ, Psychological treatment of panic: work in progress on outcome, active ingredients, and follow-up, *Behav Res Ther* (1993) **31**: 1–8.

Myers JK, Weissman MM, Tischler GL, Holzer CE, Leaf PJ, Six months prevalence of psychiatric disorders in three communities, *Arch Gen Psychiatry* (1984) **49**: 949–67.

Noyes R, Clancy J, Hoenk PR, Slymen DJ, The prognosis of anxiety neurosis, *Arch Gen Psychiatry* (1980) **37**: 173–8.

Rizley R, Kahn R, McNair D, Frankenthaler LM, A comparison of alprazolam and imipramine in the treatment of agoraphobia and panic disorder, *Psychopharmacol Bull* (1986) **22**: 167–72.

Sartorius N, Uston TB, Lecrubier Y, Wittchen HU, Depression comorbid with anxiety: results from the WHO study on psychological disorders in primary health care, *Br J Psychiatry* (1996) (Suppl 30) **168**: 38–43.

Shear MK, Pathophysiology of panic: a review of pharmacologic provocative tests and naturalistic monitoring data, *J Clin Psychiatry* **47**: 18–26.

Todd GP, Chadwick IG, Yeo WW, Jackson PR, Ramsay LE, Pressor effect of hyperventilation in healthy subjects, *J Hum Hypertens* (1995) **9**: 119–22.

Weber BE, Kapoor WN, Evaluation and outcomes of patients with palpitations, *Am J Med* (1996) **100**: 138–48.

White WB, Baker LH, Ambulatory blood pressure monitoring in patients with panic disorder, *Arch Intern Med* (1987) **147**: 1973–5.

Wollam GL, Hall WD, Porter VD, Douglas MB, Unger DJ, Time course of regression of left ventricular hypertrophy in treated hypertensive patients, *Am J Med* (1983) **75**: 100–10.

Woods SW, Charney DS, Goodman WK, Heninger GR, Carbon-dioxide-induced anxiety, *Arch Gen Psychiatry* (1987) **45**: 43–52.

Wulsin LR, Vaillant GE, Wells VE, A systematic review of the mortality of depression, *Psychosom Med* (1999) **61**: 6–17.

Yang S, Tsai CH, Hou ZY, Chen CY, Sim CB, The effect of panic attack on mitral valve prolapse, *Acta Psychiatr Scand* (1997) **96**: 408–11.

Yeragani VK, Pohl R, Berger R et al, Decreased heart rate variability in panic disorder patients: a study of power-spectral analysis of heart rate, *Psychiatry Res* (1993) **46**: 89–103.

Yingling KW, Wulsin LR, Arnold LM, Rouan GW, Estimated prevalence of panic disorder and depression among consecutive patients seen in an emergency department with acute chest pain, *J Gen Intern Med* (1993) **8**: 231–5.

Zaubler TS, Katon W, Panic disorder and medical commodity: a review of the medical and psychiatric literature, *Bull Menninger Clin* (1996) (Suppl A) **60**: 13–39.

Zaubler TS, Katon W, Panic disorder in the general medical setting, *J Psychosom Res* (1998) **44**: 25–42.

4
Anxiety disorders and cardiovascular disease

Nicola T Lautenschlager

'Out of the abundance of the heart the mouth speaketh'. It is a common perception that the heart and emotions are linked closely together and this is reflected in many sayings that are part of our everyday language: 'with all my heart, it wrings my heart, it will break his heart, open one's heart, take heart, at the bottom of his heart, be half-hearted about something, come from the heart, be heartfelt, be without a heart, have something at heart, take something to heart, take someone to one's heart, heart's delight, kind-hearted, heart-stirring, heartless, heart-rending'. For centuries it has been suggested that negative emotions may affect cardiac health. And one of the most prominent negative emotions is anxiety. This chapter provides a review of the relationship between anxiety disorders (for panic disorder see Chapter 3) and cardiovascular disease (CaVD). This relationship is complex and most of it is not yet unravelled. We can look at it from both ends, like a bi-directional highway. Can suffering from CaVD lead to an anxiety disorder, and can a sick heart trigger anxiety via somatic pathways? Can experiencing anxiety or an anxiety disorder increase one's risk of developing CaVD, and, if so, how could this be explained?

Anxiety disorders are amongst the most prevalent psychiatric disorders in almost all the populations studied (Kessler et al, 1994; WHO International Consortium in Psychiatric Epidemiology, 2000). They are correlated with high frequencies of mortality, functional impairment and utilization of health care (Rice et al, 1998). The positive message is that available treatment options are amongst the most successful in psychiatry (Ballenger, 1999). In the ICD-10 these disorders are listed in chapter F4 under the heading 'neurotic, stress-related and somatoform disorders (F40–F48)' (WHO, 1994). Table 4.1 lists the different subtypes of anxiety disorders as they appear in the ICD-10 and in the *Diagnostic and Statistical Manual of Mental Disorders of the American Psychiatric Association* (DSM-IV) (American Psychiatric Association, 1994).

The prevalence rates for the different subtypes of anxiety disorders vary depending on the inclusion criteria and the study design. But it has been shown that the prevalence rates can change in the aged population. Table 4.2 shows prevalence rates among individuals aged 15–54 years compared to prevalence rates in individuals above age 65 years.

Anxiety disorders frequently coexist with or accompany organic symptoms, most prominently in panic disorder, but also in other subtypes.

Table 4.1   Subtypes of anxiety disorders in the two most commonly used psychiatric classification systems.

ICD-10	DSM-IV
Phobic anxiety disorder	Panic disorder
Agoraphobia	Agoraphobia
Social phobia	Specific phobia
Specific phobias	Social phobia
Panic disorder	Obsessive–compulsive disorder
Generalized anxiety disorder	Acute stress disorder
Mixed anxiety and depressive disorder	Post-traumatic stress disorder
Obsessive–compulsive disorder	Generalized anxiety disorder
Acute stress reaction	
Post-traumatic stress disorder	

Table 4.2   Shows prevalence rates (%) for people under 65 years of age compared to prevalence rates in subjects above age 65 years.

< 65 years	> 65 years
Panic disorder: 3.5	Panic disorder: 0.1
Agoraphobia: 5.3	Agoraphobia: 1.4 – 7.9
Specific phobia: 11.3	Specific phobia: 4.0
Social phobia: 13.3	Social phobia: 1.0
Generalized anxiety disorder: 5.1	Generalized anxiety disorder: 4.0

Krasucki et al, 1998; Kessler et al, 1999.

Phobic anxiety disorders and agoraphobia include organic symptoms in their list of criteria. Table 4.3 presents somatic symptoms listed in the ICD-10.

Comorbidity between psychiatric and somatic diseases is common and expensive (high direct and indirect costs due to high utilization of health

Table 4.3   Somatic symptoms of anxiety disorder according to ICD-10.

Autonomic arousal symptoms
Palpitation, pounding heart, accelerated heart rate
Sweating, trembling or shaking
Dry mouth

Symptoms involving chest and abdomen
Difficulty in breathing
Feeling of choking
Chest pain or discomfort
Nausea or abdominal distress

General symptoms
Hot flushes or cold chills
Numbness or tingling sensations

services, increased disability, poor prognosis). It is not unexpected that patients with severe or life-threatening cardiac diseases have a higher prevalence of anxiety disorder than the general population. In a Canadian study, 69% of 785 hospitalized patients with acute myocardial infarction experienced significant anxiety symptoms (Frasure-Smith et al, 1995).

The effect of comorbid anxiety on quality of life was studied in 875 community patients who received general medical care in the USA (Sherbourne et al, 1996). Interestingly, patients with heart disease and comorbid anxiety reported better physical health on quality of life scales compared to patients with heart disease without comorbid anxiety. Within the 2-year observation period, however, patients with heart disease and comorbid anxiety experienced a decline in emotional well-being and social functioning compared to patients with heart disease without comorbid anxiety. How can the better physical health of patients with comorbid anxiety be explained? The authors present the theory that comorbid anxiety could serve as coping strategy, encouraging patients to seek help much earlier when physical symptoms occur.

Anxiety in this scenario would function as a preventive strategy through the seeking of earlier intervention in serious pathological cardiac events, such as myocardial infarction. Over time, this may lead to an improved quality of life.

A limitation of this study is that anxiety disorders were diagnosed with the help of questionnaires and not on the basis of a clinical assessment. The information on the level of functioning was based on self-report. These results apply mainly to generalised anxiety disorder, since phobia and panic disorder were rare in this sample.

The anxious and their heart

Symptoms of anxiety and of CaVD have a broad and well-known overlap. Roughly 10–20% of coronary angiograms performed in patients with chest pain reveal normal or non-relevant narrowed coronary arteries (Chambers and Bass, 1990). Underlying psychiatric disorders are suspected to be responsible for cardiac symptoms in these patients. Anxiety disorders are significantly more frequent in patients with negative angiogram results compared to those with evidence of CaVD in their angiogram. Their mortality over time is low. Potts and Bass (1995) report a 91% survival after 11 years follow-up in 41 patients with negative angiogram (mean age: 46.3 years) among whom 39% patients suffered from an anxiety disorder.

The chest pain symptoms in the angiogram negative patients with anxiety disorders may be explained as psychosomatic symptoms triggered by anxiety via pathophysiological mechanisms like hyperventilation, autonomic arousability or muscular tension (Bass, 1991; Lynch et al, 1991). In these patients there seems to be little evidence for the presence of a somatic cardiac disease. But there is also evidence that anxiety can lead to the long-term presence of CaVD.

In the Northwick Park Heart Study 1457 healthy men were followed over 10 years. High levels of phobic anxiety, assessed with the Crown–Crisp index, were associated with a relative risk of fatal coronary heart disease of 3.77 (95% CI: 1.64–8.64) compared to low levels of phobic anxiety. Those men with a history of myocardial infarction at study entry ($N = 49$) had higher scores on the subscale free-floating anxiety (Haines et al, 1987). In 2001 additional data on the same study was presented (Haines et al, 2001), and showed that the significant association between phobic anxiety and fatal ischaemic heart disease was only evident for the first 10 years of follow-up and decreased thereafter to 1.07 (95% CI: 0.99–1.15). Kawachi et al (1994a) present data on the Health Professional Follow-Up Study in which 33 999 healthy male health professionals were followed. Again, the relative risk for fatal coronary heart disease was elevated in men with high phobic anxiety (measured with the Crown–Crisp index) to 2.45 (95% CI: 1.00–5.06).

More generalized symptoms of anxiety have been shown to be associated with fatal coronary heart disease. Eaker et al (1992) showed that in female homemakers from the Framingham Heart Study the presence of anxiety symptoms increased the risk for myocardial infarction and cardiac death to 7.8 (95% CI: 1.9–32.3). Kawachi et al (1994b) demonstrated in the Normative Aging Study that men who considered themselves to be nervous had a significantly higher risk for sudden cardiac death (OR = 4.46; 95% CI: 0.92–21.60). In the same study sample Kubzansky et al (1997) reported an association between worry, a common cognitive sign of anxiety disorder, and coronary heart disease. Specifically, worries regarding health, finances and social conditions increased the risk for non-fatal myocardial infarction significantly with a dose-dependent relationship. The higher the level of worries, the higher the risk. In their conclusion of a review article asking the question 'Can negative emotions cause coronary heart disease?' Kubzansky and Kawachi (2000) stated that anxiety shows a stronger association with onset of coronary heart disease than anger and depression. The authors observed that prospective population-based studies found positive results whereas studies concentrating on psychiatric patients tended to report negative results. One suggested reason for this was that the latter tended to have weaker study designs.

Some review articles on this topic conclude that higher levels of general anxiety in initially healthy individuals cannot be viewed as a robust risk factor for CaVD (Booth-Kewley et al, 1987; Glassman et al, 1998).

There are far too few prospective studies to provide the answer to the question of whether anxiety could be a risk factor for CaVD. The limited number of studies on this topic are often difficult to compare, since different study designs and instruments were used. It also remains unclear how many of the study subjects who experienced symptoms of anxiety actually suffered from an anxiety disorder or had subclinical anxiety levels since a psychiatric assessment was not performed in some cases.

Another problem is mixed psychopathology, especially between depression and anxiety. There is very often a combination present and most of the studies on anxiety as a potential risk factor for CaVD did not adjust for this. The isolated influence of anxiety, without depression, on cardiac health is therefore unclear.

But how can the presence of an anxiety disorder increase the risk for CaVD? There are several physiological pathways from generated emotions to the heart and they are in themselves not necessarily pathological. From an evolutionary perspective, it makes for the survival of the human race that anxiety triggers an activation of the sympathetic-adrenal-medullary system. This activation helps the organism to escape in the event of a life-threatening risk.

Other physiological pathways triggered by anxiety include the autonomic regulation of the heart and the hypothalamic–pituitary–adrenocorticol (HPA) axis (Kamarck and Jennings, 1991; Friedman and Thayer, 1998).

Chronic over-activation of these systems due to anxiety would help to explain the increased frequency of cardiovascular risk factors in patients with anxiety disorders. Reduced variability of heart rate has been proposed as a risk factor for sudden cardiac death. Kawachi et al (1995) report that for men in the Normative Aging Study higher levels of phobic anxiety reduce the heart rate variability after adjusting for age, body mass index and mean heart rate ($P = 0.03$ for linear trend). The authors conclude that this finding could reflect an altered cardiac autonomic control in patients with phobic anxiety as a risk factor for sudden cardiac death. Wells et al (1989) reported in a large cross-sectional study a high association between hypertension and anxiety disorders. Yakovlevitch and Black (1991) suggested that in 8% of patients with treatment-resistant hypertension, the hypertension could be attributed to underlying psychological causes, including severe anxiety. Others could not find this strong relationship (Toner et al, 1990; Isaksson et al, 1991, 1992). Davies et al (1997) could find no difference between 136 cases with treatment-resistant hypertension compared to 136 controls with non-treatment-resistant hypertension with regard to the presence of panic disorder, anxiety and depression. Symptoms of these psychiatric conditions were assessed with the help of a self-completed questionnaire, the Hospital Anxiety and Depression Scale.

In the hypertensive state a chronic anxiety disorder may trigger increased levels of epinephrine and norepinephrine which could also increase the heart rate, the total peripheral resistance and even increase the circulating fatty acids (Schneidermann, 1987).

This interaction is consistent with the positive clinical association of elevated cholesterol levels and anxiety in three of the four existing studies (Hayward, 1995).

Another, less direct pathway from anxiety disorder to CaVD could be the tendency to behaviours like smoking, consumption of high-fat food or lack of exercise in patients with anxiety disorders. Several studies found a higher prevalence of behaviour-related cardiovascular risk factors such as smoking, low physical activity, high body mass index, and alcohol consumption, in patients with anxiety disorders (Hayward, 1995).

Another indirect behavioural risk factor for CaVD is lack of social support and social isolation (Thoits, 1995; Kawachi et al, 1996). Patients with a chronic anxiety disorder may be at higher risk of having an inadequate social network and would therefore score positive for this risk factor.

The 'weak hearted' and their anxiety

Anxiety, independent from depression, was shown to increase the risk of patients with myocardial infarction suffering further cardiac complications two- to five-fold compared to non-anxious myocardial infarction patients. This effect could be found in the acute post myocardial infarction period as well as 18 months later (Frasure-Smith et al, 1995).

Moser and Dracup (1996) confirmed that patients with high anxiety levels, as measured with the Brief Symptom Inventory, had a 4.9 times higher risk (19.6% vs 6%; $P = 0.001$) than post-myocardial infarction patients with low anxiety levels of having further cardiological complications within the first 48 hours after acute myocardial infarction.

For patients with CaVD without myocardial infarction there exist positive findings related to anxiety. It has been suggested that in patients already suffering from CaVD subjective stress with emotions like anger and anxiety can reduce the coronary artery blood flow, which can be fatal. The reduced blood flow is linked to coronary spasms and abnormal ventricular wall motion (Blumenthal et al, 1995). Emotionally induced coronary artery spasm has been reported in patients with angina pectoris (Schiffer et al, 1980). This has been suggested as a possible underlying mechanism, with cross-sectional and prospective design studies comparing patients with healthy controls showing a significant association between subjective stress and angina pectoris (Hagman et al, 1987). Hyperventilation, a common symptom associated with subjective stress and anxiety disorders, can provoke vaso-spastic angina (Mortensen et al, 1981).

A prospective study with a 5-year follow-up of 144 men with positive angiograms investigated the association of psychosocial risk factors and further pathological cardiac events like angina frequency, myocardial infarction, revascularizations and death (Ketterer et al, 1998).

Each patient was asked to complete, amongst other questionnaires, the Ketterer Stress Symptom Frequency Checklist (KSSFC), which provides scores on depression, anger and anxiety. A close relative or friend (selected by the patient) was asked to complete the same questionnaires about the patient. The only factor showing a significant relationship with angina frequency was the level of anxiety in the patients rated by the relative/friend (R = 0.267, F = 10.9, df = 142, $P = 0.001$). Interestingly, the result correlated negatively with the subjective anxiety score of the patient ($P = 0.003$). The authors concluded that this could be interpreted as 'denial' of emotional distress by the patient; such denial of emotional distress has already been observed as common in cardiac patients (Ketterer et al, 1996). This result is of importance because it highlights one of the major measurement errors in population-based prospective studies on emotional distress, which rely on self-assessment screening tools.

However, not all the studies report a significant positive association between high anxiety levels and unfavourable outcome in patients with CaVD. Some found only a very small correlation (Ahern et al, 1990) no correlation at all (Glassman, 1998) or even an inverse relationship (Blumenthal et al, 1979). Herrmann et al (2000) conducted a prospective follow-up study with 5017 patients with CaVD over 5.7 years. Depression and generalized anxiety were measured with the Hospital Anxiety and Depression Scale (HADS). Surprisingly, depression and anxiety showed independent opposite effects in the adjusted logistic regression model with mortality as outcome.

With every increase in the HADS anxiety by 1 SD, survival improved by 19% (95% CI = 8 – 28%; P = 0.0014), whereas for every 1 SD increase in HADS depression, survival decreased by 14% (95% CI = 1 – 30%; P = 0.041). The authors suggest as explanation that anxious behaviour regarding somatic symptoms could provide some protection since concerned patients tend to see their doctors more frequently and are more likely to receive coronary angiography (Schocken et al, 1987; Simon et al, 1995). Furthermore, the authors stress that generalized anxiety might have a different prognostic influence in patients with CaVD than phobic anxiety, which has different underlying psychophysiological mechanisms. These study results have to be considered carefully since less than half of the patients received a coronary angiogram. Therefore, it cannot be excluded that some of the patients might in fact not have suffered from CaVD, but rather from somatic symptoms, like chest pain, related to an anxiety disorder.

Another approach to the problem of CaVD and experienced anxiety during the course of disease is the concept of post-traumatic stress disorder. Ladwig et al (1999) investigated whether the prevalence of emotional disability in cardiac arrest survivors influences their level of functioning and quality of life. Forty-five patients were followed up for 39 months and compared to 35 patients with CaVD who did not experience cardiac arrest.

There was no overall increased frequency of anxiety or depression (measured with the Hospital Anxiety and Depression Scale) in the cardiac arrest group compared to the non-cardiac-arrest group. This is surprising since their mortality rate after 39 months was 33% compared to 8% in the non-cardiac-arrest patients. But 38% of the cardiac arrest survivors had significantly more intrusive thoughts (P < 0.001), avoidant states (P < 0.0001), increased arousal (P < 0.03) and anxiety (P < 0.003) than the comparison group and were diagnosed with post-traumatic stress disorder. Consequently, they had a lower quality of life and lower level of functioning. It is remarkable that sedation at the onset of illness significantly predicted a favourable outcome and reduced the risk of developing post-traumatic stress disorder by five-fold.

Conclusion

The body of literature on the topic of anxiety and CaVD is limited and inconclusive. This is remarkable considering the high prevalence of both diseases and the common clinical wisdom on the substantial overlap between them. The majority of prospective studies concentrate on the association between symptoms of anxiety and CaVD. These symptoms of anxiety are assessed with a wide variety of different criteria. Recent prospective studies have not concentrated on patients with a psychiatric diagnosis of an anxiety disorder. Therefore it is unclear to what extent the results for anxiety symptoms could apply to patients with a clinical anxiety disorder. The same problem arises with studies investigating anxiety symptoms in patients with CaVD. This leaves us with a number of open questions, which invite future research.

It is to be hoped that such research should emerge as a combined effort from the different disciplines of cardiology, geriatric medicine, psychiatry, old age psychiatry and psychology. With a collaborative approach, the quality of diagnosis for the somatic as well as the psychiatric disorders involved could be guaranteed. Once the body of evidence is stronger on the association between anxiety and CaVD, an era of preventive medicine might begin in which routine screening for negative emotions and undiagnosed psychiatric disorders would be included in assessments for cardiovascular risk factors. Psychiatric risk factors could then join already well-established organic risk factors like hypertension, elevated lipid levels, low exercise, increased body mass index, diabetes, alcohol consumption and smoking.

References

Ahern DK, Gorkin L, Anderson JL et al, Biobehavioural variables and mortality or cardiac arrest in the Cardiac Arrythmia Pilot Study (CAPS), *Am J Cardiol* (1990) **66**: 59–62.

American Psychiatric Association, *Diagnostic and Statistical Manual of Mental Disorders, 4th edn, DSM-IV* (American Psychiatric Association, Washington, DC, (1994).

Ballenger JC, Current treatments of the anxiety disorders in adults, *Biol Psychiatry* (1999) **46**: 1579–94.

Bass C, Unexplained chest pain and breathlessness, *Med Clin North Am* (1991) **75**: 1157–73.

Blumenthal JA, Thompson LW, Williams RB Jr, Kong Y, Anxiety-proneness and coronary heart disease, *J Psychosom Res* (1979) **23**: 17–21.

Blumenthal JA, Jiang W, Waugh RA et al, Mental stress-induced ischaemia in the laboratory and ambulatory ischaemia during daily life. Association and haemodynamic features, *Circulation* (1995) **92**: 2102–8.

Booth-Kewley S, Friedman HS, Psychological predictors of heart disease: a quantitative review, *Psychol Bull* (1987) **101**: 343–62.

Chambers JB and Bass C, Chest pain with normal coronary anatomy: a review of natural history and possible etiologic factors, *Prog Cardiovasc Dis* (1990) **33**: 161–84.

Davies SJC, Ghahramani P, Jackson PR et al, Panic disorder, anxiety and depression in resistant hypertension – a case-control study, *J Hypertens* (1997) **15**: 1077–82.

Eaker ED, Pinsky J, Castelli WP, Myocardial infarction and coronary death among women: Psychosocial predictors from a 20-year follow-up of women in the Framingham Heart Study, *Am J Epidemiol* (1992) **135**: 854–64.

Frasure-Smith N, Lesperance F, Talajic M, Depression following myocardial infarction, *Circulation* (1995) **91**: 999–1005.

Friedman BH, Thayer JF, Anxiety and autonomic flexibility: a cardiovascular approach, *Biol Psychol* (1998) **49**: 303–23.

Glassman AH, Shapiro PA, Depression and the course of coronary artery disease, *Am J Psychiatry* (1998) **155**: 4–11.

Hagman M, Wilhelmsen L, Wedel H, Pennert K, Risk factors for angina pectoris in a population study of Swedish men, *J Chron Dis* (1987) **140**: 265–75.

Haines AP, Imeson JD, Meade TW, Phobic anxiety and ischaemic heart disease, *BMJ* (1987) **295**: 297–99.

Haines AP, Cooper J, Meade TW, Psychological characteristics and fatal ischaemic heart disease, *Heart* (2001) **85**: 385–9.

Hayward C, Psychiatric illness and cardiovascular disease risk, *Epidemiol Rev* (1995) **17**: 129–38.

Herrmann C, Brand-Driesthorst S, Buss U, Rüger U, Effects of anxiety and depression on 5-year mortality in 5057 patients referred for exercise testing, *J Psychosom Res* (2000) **48**: 455–62.

Isaksson H, Danielsson M, Rosenhammer G, Konarski-Svensson JC, Ostergren J, Characteristics of patients resistant to antihypertensive drug therapy, *J Intern Med* (1991) **229**: 421–6.

Isaksson H, Konarski K, Theorell T, The psychological and social conditions of hypertension resistant to pharmacological treatment, *Soc Sci Med* (1992) **35**: 869–75.

Kamarck T, Jennings JR, Biobehavioral factors in sudden cardiac death, *Psychol Bull* (1991) **109**: 42–5.

Kawachi I, Colditz GA, Ascherio A, et al, Prospective study on phobic anxiety and the risk of coronary heart disease in men, *Circulation* (1994a) **89**: 1992–7.

Kawachi I, Sparrow D, Vokonas PS, Weiss ST, Symptoms of anxiety and risk of coronary heart disease. The Normative Aging Study, *Circulation* (1994b) **90**: 2225–9.

Kawachi I, Sparrow D, Vokonas PS, Weiss ST, Decreased heart rate variability in men with phobic anxiety, *Am J Cardiology* (1995) **75**: 825–82.

Kawachi I, Colditz GA, Ascherio A et al, A prospective study of social networks in relation to total mortality and cardiovascular disease incidence in men, *J Epidemiol Commun Hlth* (1996) **50**: 245–51.

Kessler RC, McGonagle KA, Zhao S et al, Lifetime and 12-month prevalence of DSM-III-R psychiatric disorders in the United States. Results from the National Comorbidity Survey, *Arch Gen Psychiatry* (1994) **51**: 8–19.

Ketterer MW, Kenyon L, Foley BA et al, Denial of depression as an independent correlate of coronary artery disease, *J Hlth Psychol* (1996) **1**: 93–105.

Ketterer MW, Huffman J, Lumley MA et al, Five-year follow-up for adverse outcomes in males with at least minimally positive angiograms: Importance of 'denial' in assessing psychosocial risk factors, *J Psychosom Res* (1998) **44**: 241–50.

Krasucki C, Howard R, Mann A, The relationship between anxiety disorders and age, *Int J Ger Psychiatry* (1998) **13**: 79–99.

Kubzansky LD, Kawachi I, Spiro A III et al, Is worrying bad for your heart? A prospective study on worry and coronary heart disease in the Normative Aging Study, *Circulation* (1997) **95**: 818–24.

Kubzansky LD, Kawachi I, Going to the heart of the matter: do negative emotions cause coronary heart disease? *J Psychosom Res* (2000) **48**: 323–37.

Ladwig K-H, Schoefinius A, Dammann G et al, Long-acting psychosomatic properties of a cardiac arrest experience, *Am J Psychiatry* (1999) **156**: 912–9.

Lynch P, Bakal DA, Whitelaw W, Fung T, Chest muscle activity and panic anxiety: a preliminary investigation, *Psychosom Med* (1991) **53**: 80–9.

Mortensen SA, Vilhelmsen R, Sandoe E, Prinzmetal's variant angina (PVA). Circardian variation in response to hyperventilation, *Acta Med Scand* (1981) (Suppl) **644**: 38–41.

Moser DK, Dracup K Is anxiety early after myocardial infarction associated with subsequent ischaemic and arrhythmic events? *Psychosom Med* (1996) **58**: 395–401.

Potts SG, Bass CM, Psychological morbidity in patients with chest pain and normal or near-normal coronary arteries: a long-term follow-up study, *Psychol Med* (1995) **25**: 339–47.

Rice DP, Miller LS, Health economics and cost implications of anxiety and other mental disorders in the United States, *Br J Psychiatry* (1998) (Suppl) **34**: 4–9.

Schiffer F, Hartley HL, Schulman CL, Abelmann WH, Evidence for emotionally-induced coronary arterial spasm in patients with angina pectoris, *Brit Heart J* (1980) **44**: 62–6.

Schneidermann N, Psychophysiologic factors in atherogenesis and coronary artery disease, *Circulation* (1987) **76**: I-41–7.

Schocken DD, Greene AF, Worden TJ, Harrison EE, Spielberger CD, Effects of age and gender on the relationship between anxiety and coronary artery disease, *Psychosom Med* (1987) **49**: 118–26.

Sherbourne CD, Wells KB, Meredith LS, Jackson CA, Camp P, Comorbid anxiety disorder and the functioning and well-being of chronically ill patients of general medical providers, *Arch Gen Psychiatry* (1996) **53**: 889–95.

Simon G, Ormel J, Von Korff M, Barlow W, Health care costs associated with depressive and anxiety disorders in primary care, *Am J Psychiatry* (1995) **151**: 352–7.

Thoits PA, Stress, coping, and social support processes: Where are we? What next? *J Health Soc Behav* (1995) (Special Issue)**:** 53–79.

Toner JM, Close CF, Ramsay LE, Factors related to treatment resistance in hypertension, *Q J Med* (1990) **283**: 1195–1204.

Wells KB, Golding JM, Buman MA, Chronic medical conditions in a sample of the general population with anxiety, affective, and substance use disorders, *Am J Psychiatry* (1989) **146**: 1440–6.

World Health Organization ICD-10, *Classification of mental and behavioural disorders* (World Health Organisation, Geneva, (1994).

WHO International Consortium in Psychiatric Epidemiology, Cross-national comparison of the prevalences and correlates of mental disorders, *Bull WHO* (2000) **78**: 413–26.

Yakovlevitch M, Black HR, Resistant hypertension in a tertiary care clinic, *Arch Intern Med* (1991) **151**: 176–92.

5
Cardiac surgery and affective disorders

Joe Stratford and David Ames

"By my troth, he'll yield the crow a pudding one of these days. The King has killed his heart."

The hostess, speaking of Sir John Falstaff, whose spirit has been crushed by Henry V's rejection of him at the Coronation (Henry V, II, i, William Shakespeare).

Introduction

The concept of the heart has long carried great emotional significance. It is no coincidence that in many languages the word 'heart' has meanings relating both to the cardiac organ and also to a much wider emotional context. Like concepts such as the soul or spirit, the heart is considered the very essence of what it is to be human. The notion, then, of a surgeon actually opening up one's chest and cutting into this 'heart' or even removing it is likely to have a huge emotional impact. Any discussion of heart surgery needs to acknowledge these implications.

In this chapter, we examine the relationship between affective disorders and cardiac surgery, both in general terms and, where possible, with specific reference to four of the most common cardiac surgical procedures performed in adults. Following this introduction, the history of cardiac surgery is outlined. Mention is then made of cognitive deficits that may occur after cardiac surgery, leading on to a review of the literature regarding cardiac surgery and depressive disorders. Finally, an approach to the psychological management of a patient undergoing cardiac surgery will be presented, and consideration given to future areas of research in this rapidly developing field.

Both depression and mania will be considered in this chapter under the umbrella of affective disorders, but less mention will be made of mania. Mania prior to cardiac surgery would be a significant contraindication, but also pure 'non-organic' mania appears to be exceedingly rare as a sequel of cardiac surgery and published data consist solely of case reports (Isles and Orrel, 1991). Indeed, according to the current literature, manic symptomatology following cardiac surgery seems to occur only in the context of post-operative delirium and therefore cannot be considered as true mania.

History of cardiac surgery

Cardiac surgery has evolved rapidly, with developments in technology and knowledge of physiology, to stand at the forefront of modern medicine. An overview will be presented of the history of four major cardiac surgical procedures – angioplasty, valve surgery, bypass grafting and transplantation.

Cardiac angioplasty

The history of angioplasty has its origins up to 5000 years ago when the Egyptians performed the first catheterizations using metal pipes to gain access to the bladder in cases of retention. Approximately 4700 years later, in 1733, the first cardiac catheterization was performed by the English physiologist Stephen Hales. This was done in a horse using brass pipes, a glass tube and the trachea of a goose.

A breakthrough came in 1929 when Werner Forssmann, a young surgical resident working in Eberswald, Germany, performed the first human cardiac catheterization – on himself! He anaesthetized his left ante-cubital fossa and inserted a catheter into his ante-cubital vein. Next he carefully threaded the catheter along the venous system before X-raying his chest, which identified the tip of the catheter sitting in what he assumed (correctly) to be his right atrium. This milestone was followed in 1941 by Andre Cournand and Dickinson Richards, working at the Bellevue Hospital, New York, who utilized Forssmann's basic technique to measure pressures and cardiac output as a diagnostic and research tool. The importance of this work was recognized by the joint award of a Nobel Prize to all three pioneers.

In 1958, the technique of coronary angiography was discovered, by accident, by Mason Stones, an American radiologist. Stones was experimenting on aortic angiography when 30 ml of contrast solution was accidentally injected into the left anterior descending artery of the heart (LAD). Far from killing the patient, the angiograms revealed vital information about coronary perfusion and paved the way for the first coronary angioplasties.

Another American radiologist, Charles Dotter, introduced the concept of angioplasty, performing the first recorded procedure by dilating a narrowed renal artery in 1964. Further work continued and, together with the developments in angiography, Andreas Gruentzig and his team in Zurich performed the world's first human coronary angioplasty in 1977. The technique involved the use of a 'balloon' that Gruentzig had helped develop.

Balloon angioplasty is widely practised today, as are the insertion of stents to preserve the patency of the arterial lumen. The numbers of these procedures performed have gradually increased since the late 1970s and by a factor of 248% from 1987 to 1998, during which latter year over 500 000 cardiac angioplasties took place in the USA alone (American Heart Association, 2001). As an interventional procedure, performed under local anaesthesia, angioplasty probably has less potential to affect cognition or mood than the more invasive and traumatic open heart surgical techniques discussed below.

Valve surgery

The first successful cardiac operation for mitral valve disease was performed in London by Elliott Cutler and Henry Souttar in the early 1920s. Of 10 early patients suffering from mitral stenosis treated with 'finger dilatation', only two survived. The major obstacle was difficulty gaining access to the interior of a beating heart and the associated risks, the greatest being that of air embolism.

The next development came as a result of World War II. Dwight Harken, an American army surgeon, developed techniques for opening up beating hearts in order to remove fragments of shrapnel. In 1948, within days of each other but working separately, Charles Bailey (another US surgeon) and Harken reported the earliest successful 'trans-atrial commissurotomies' to treat mitral valve stenosis.

The science of heart surgery received a huge boost from the invention of the heart–lung machine by the American John Gibbon in 1953. This machine subsumed the role of circulation and oxygenation of the blood from the heart, enabling the organ to be slowed (or stopped) and thus allowing various cardiac procedures to be undertaken more easily and with less risk. However, early machines were cumbersome and dangerous. They regularly leaked blood and caused clotting and air emboli, but as the design improved over subsequent years, so did the results of using such machines.

The first report of a successful mitral valve replacement was by Chesterman in the UK in 1955. Since then, the number of cardiac valve procedures has increased to approximately 100,000 per year in the USA (American Heart Association, 2001).

Coronary artery bypass grafting

The first reports of coronary artery bypass grafting (CABG) go back to 1910 when Alexis Carrel reported to the American Surgical Association that he had sutured a carotid artery graft to the left coronary system in a dog. Few developments occurred until 1951 when Vineberg and Miller directly implanted the internal mammary artery (IMA) into the myocardium of a human subject. In 1964 Vasilii Kolesov, working in Leningrad, was the first to anastomose the IMA to the left anterior descending coronary artery. Three years later Favoloro and Effler at the Cleveland Clinic began the technique of reversed saphenous leg vein bypass grafting, which remains one of the preferred models of this procedure today.

Building on the experience gained over the last 50 years, CABGs have become very common cardiac surgical procedures. Up to four separate grafts are anastomosed on each patient. Some patients receive 'off pump' surgery where the internal mammary artery is connected to the coronary artery while the heart is still beating. There have been continuous reductions in both mortality and stroke rate which both now run at about 1%. Hospital stay is usually no more than 7 days. Whereas surgery was once reserved for those for whom medical treatment had failed, it is now offered to some people with few or mild symptoms purely for its prognostic benefit. Surgery is now offered both to older and sicker patients than was the case 20 years ago. In 1998, over 500 000 CABG operations were carried out in the USA (American Heart Foundation, 2001). This compares to a figure of 28 000 in 1997 in the UK (British Heart Foundation, 2001) and 15 000 in Australia in 1994 (National Heart Foundation of Australia, 2001).

Cardiac transplantation

The history of heart transplantation began in 1960 when Richard Lower and Norman Shumway first described the technique while working at Stanford University. Two years later they performed the first successful heart transplant in a dog. The dog lived for a few hours, but this was enough to demonstrate that heart transplantation was possible and provide encouragement that one day it might be a viable option for human subjects.

In December of 1967, a South African surgeon, Christiaan Barnard, transplanted the heart of a 23-year-old Cape Town woman who had been killed in a motor vehicle accident into the body of a middle-aged man suffering from severe cardiac failure. The recipient lived for just 18 days before succumbing to iatrogenic pneumonia, which occurred as a result of the powerful immunosuppressive medication prescribed to prevent tissue rejection.

Barnard's next transplant patient lived for 18 months, giving hope to thousands more potential patients. However, the early days of transplantation were dogged by tissue rejection, until the discovery of cyclosporin and its ability to prevent rejection without excessive immunosuppression.

The numbers of transplant operations increased from the early 1970s to the mid-1990s, when they peaked at around 4000 per year worldwide. This figure has since fallen to approximately 3000 in 1999, a major limiting factor being the lack of suitable donor hearts (Hunt, 2000).

Cognitive impairments following cardiac surgery

No discussion of the relationship between cardiac surgery and affective disorders would be complete without mention of the cognitive sequelae of such surgery. Of course, depression itself can have a significant impact on cognition resulting in a variety of impairments in domains such as attention and memory (Cassens et al, 1990).

There is a large volume of literature examining the cognitive effect of both general and cardiac surgery. This dates back to when Bedford reported cognitive changes following anaesthesia (Bedford, 1955). Subsequent studies have looked at specific procedures and types of anaesthesia used. There is a wealth of data on cognitive changes (particularly in the elderly) following non-cardiac surgery. For the rest of this section only cardiac surgery will be considered.

Four major neurological/cognitive sequelae are associated with cardiac surgery – stroke, post-operative delirium, short- and long-term cognitive changes. In a study of 312 patients, Shaw et al (1985) found neurological changes in 61% of the sample following CABG surgery. These included primitive reflexes and ophthalmic abnormalities as well as stroke. We shall concentrate on cognitive changes only.

The proposed aetiological mechanisms for such cognitive changes (recently and somewhat questionably referred to as 'pump-head') include hypoperfusion of brain tissue, effect of anaesthetic agent used, post-operative medications such as narcotics and sedatives, and length of admission to the relatively disorientating intensive care unit (ICU) environment. Perhaps the mechanism most likely to be responsible is the effect of emboli showering the brain after either being dislodged from atherosclerotic arterial walls, or as a result of imperfections in the extra-corporeal circulatory system.

The reported incidence of short-term cognitive changes ranges from 33 to 83% (Selnes and McKhann, 2001). The variation appears to be a result of differences in testing instruments used, as well as patient variables such as age, sex and presence of pre-operative cognitive impairment. In some cases patients report that their memory or concentration has deteriorated following surgery. This observation was investigated by Newman et al (1989), who assessed patients' cognition pre-operatively and 1 year after surgery. While the study revealed high degrees of reported, perceived cognitive change, no significant correlations were found between these complaints and any objectively measured cognitive domains. This appears to be consistent with the accepted notion that depressed patients subjectively report cognitive difficulties more often than those who are not depressed.

A more recent study of 261 patients looking at longer-term cognitive changes following CABG procedures revealed a decline in cognitive performance (defined as 1 standard deviation below baseline) in 53% at discharge, 36% 6 weeks post-surgery, 24% after 6 months and 42% at 5 years (Newman et al, 2001). An explanation could be that these patients are more likely to develop cognitive changes due to emergent dementia, especially given the recently described association between cardiac risk factors and Alzheimer's disease (Kivipelto et al, 2001). The study of Newman et al like many others, is limited in its methodology, but what is clear from this and other studies is the significance and frequency of cognitive change following this type of surgery. Further studies, particularly looking at the very long-term outcome, are needed. The increased use of standardized instruments for measuring cognitive change, careful selection and exclusion of subjects, together with higher patient numbers and lengthier follow-up will shed more light on this important area.

Aetiology of mood disorders associated with cardiac surgery

As mentioned, the heart conjures up feelings and thoughts of life and mortality like no other organ in the body. This subject is concisely reviewed by Blacher (1987). In this section, we examine aetiological factors that may be linked with cardiac surgery and associated depression.

There are a number of compelling reasons why patients undergoing cardiac surgery might become depressed or anxious. First, when faced with a mortality rate of, say, 1%, an objective cardiac surgeon will impart this information to a patient as a 1 in 100 chance of dying. For the patient, given the gravity of the situation, the prognosis may be seen as only one of two outcomes: 'I either live, or I die!' Thus a more subjective 50:50 scenario may be envisaged.

This subjective view can lead to other encountered 'fantasies' of cardiac surgery and possible triggers for affective change. Denial and an inability to take in threatening information also play a part. It has been shown that patients remember less than 30% of what is explained to them about their surgical procedure (Nichols, 1984). Indeed, Blacher (1971) found that 20% of patients due for mitral valve surgery requiring the intra-operative use of a heart–lung machine believed that their heart and lungs would be surgically removed and placed upon this machine for the duration of the operation! Some did not acknowledge that their hearts needed to be opened for the procedure to go ahead. All this was found despite a controlled, structured information session with their surgeon beforehand. This goes some way to illustrate the psychological mechanisms that can be brought to bear when such surgery is contemplated.

Other explanations of depression associated with cardiac surgery rest with more unconscious, dynamic processes. Take, for example, a patient who is to undergo surgery during which the heart will be temporarily stopped and later re-started. During the time the heart does not beat, the patient is, in a sense 'dead'. The act of resuscitation brings the patient back from this state where they have been, in some part, re-united with lost 'objects' such as deceased relatives and friends. The process of separation once again from these objects and the return to the land of the living may re-kindle primitive feelings of loss and abandonment, causing intra-psychic anxiety that may manifest externally as depression.

Another explanation put forward for depression following cardiac surgery is something approaching 'survivor guilt'. This is seen in cases of post-traumatic stress disorder, or when subjects have lived through an event during which others have died. Here, the patient wakes up and realizes that the worst is over and they have survived, when they perhaps had prepared themselves for death. This scenario re-awakens primitive death-wishes towards ambivalently viewed objects such as deceased parents or siblings. So, an unconscious 'I have survived and you did not' victory over a lost object is manifested as feelings of anxiety and depression due to its blatantly unacceptable nature. This hypothesis has been invoked to explain the depression felt by soldiers who manage to avoid death during combat whilst their comrade is killed, or among death camp survivors (Blacher, 1987).

How accurate these psychodynamic ideas of depression associated with cardiac surgery are is debatable. They depend upon concepts that are by their very nature unconscious. They do, however, offer a model which may permit some empathic understanding of the experience of the cardiac surgery patient.

In addition to postulated psychodynamic models of depression in cardiac surgery, a large number of factors have been found to be associated with increased rates of subsequent affective disorders.

One of the strongest risk factors for post-operative depression is pre-operative depression. Many studies confirm this relationship (McKhann et al, 1997; Timberlake et al, 1997; Pirraglia et al, 1999). Other studies mention personality traits including non-dominant, passive and dependent attitudes as markers that put subjects at higher risk (Boll et al, 1990), or higher scores on measures of pessimism, cautiousness or trait anxiety (Timberlake et al, 1997). Patients who perceive heart surgery as a mere 'technical event', thus avoiding emotional involvement, tend to be more depressed and to have less mental stability following the operation (Langosch and Schmoll-Flockerzier, 1992).

Social risk factors appear to include, in keeping with risk factors for depression unrelated to surgery, a deficient social support network (Pirraglia et al, 1999). An excess of life stressors also has been shown to be evident in patients who go on to develop post-CABG depression (Pirraglia et al, 1999). However, in one study looking at age and its relationship to post-surgical depression using measures including the Beck Depression Inventory (BDI), Rosenburg Self-Esteem Scale and a variety of physical health outcome measures, age did not appear to carry any altered risk of post-operative depression (Trygar Artinian et al, 1993).

Medical factors have also been identified as being associated with higher risk of post-operative depression. These include severity of somatic symptoms (Blacher, 1987) and length of stay in an ICU following surgery (Pirraglia et al, 1999). Contrary to what one might expect, in a study of 121 patients undergoing CABG, Timberlake et al (1997) found that shorter operations and lower numbers of individual artery grafts were associated with greater rates of post-operative depression. The authors suggest possible reasons for this unexpected finding. It may be that patients with relatively severe coronary artery disease requiring multiple bypasses would stand to gain the most from such a major procedure. Moreover, patients with milder coronary symptoms, who have perhaps one artery bypassed and hence a shorter operation, might have less to gain from the intervention. Both groups would awaken in

ICU, with painful thoracotomy scars and requiring a prolonged cardiac rehabilitation programme. While the aftermath in both groups may be similar, the difference in severity of symptoms before the procedure might explain this finding. This outcome makes empirical sense, especially when viewed with the as yet unpublished anecdotal finding that a shorter time from symptom onset (e.g. acute myocardial infarction) to intervention (e.g. CABG) often results in worse outcomes in both physical and psychological rehabilitation. The presumed explanation is that a critical period of time to adjust to the surgery beforehand is needed. Studies looking at this issue in cardiac surgery have yet to be carried out (N. Strathmore, personal communication).

In summary, post-operative depression seems to depend on predictable factors relating to the surgery itself or to psychological elements that create an increased vulnerability to a stressful life event, which, of course, is exactly what life-saving cardiac surgery is!

Frequency of depression before and after surgery

Studies that have assessed the frequency and intensity of depression before and after open heart surgery have tended to focus on symptoms rather than explicit diagnoses fulfilling agreed criteria. The essential details of these studies are set out in the Table 5.1.

In an influential study by McKhann et al (1997), 124 patients about to undergo CABG were subjected to psychiatric examination at three intervals: pre-surgery; 1 month; and 1 year after surgery. In addition to a variety of cognitive tests, depressive symptomatology was evaluated using the Center for Epidemiological Study of Depression (CES-D) scale. This is a 20-item self-report questionnaire developed for the study of depression in the general population. The scores can range from 0 to 60, a score of 16 being regarded as indicative of a depressed mood. Twenty-seven percent of subjects were 'depressed' prior to surgery, 24% at 1 month and 19% at 1 year. In the subgroup that was depressed prior to surgery, over half (53%) were still depressed after 1 month and 47% continued to be depressed at 1 year. This led the authors to suggest that pre-operative depression is a significant risk factor for post-operative depression – a conclusion also drawn by many other studies.

Timberlake et al (1997) surveyed 121 CABG patients before their operation, as well as at 8 days, 8 weeks and 1 year post-operatively, using the Beck Depression Inventory (BDI). Pre-operative depression levels were 37%, compared to post-operative levels of 50%, 24% and 23% at the three post-operative intervals, respectively. Those depressed beforehand had significantly higher rates of depression at all post-operative times, when compared to those not depressed prior to surgery. This study also looked at patterns of depression as well as simple frequencies. It identified several discrete trends. In 30% of patients, depression persisted at all times. Thirty-nine percent of

Table 5.1 Studies of depression before and after cardiac surgery.

Year	Author(s)	Number of patients pre-/ post-operatively	Instrument or diagnostic criteria used	Depressive symptoms (S) or diagnosis? (D)	Percentage meeting criteria for pre-operative depression	Percentage meeting criteria for post-operative depression	Time to follow up
1984	Horgan et al	77/68	Carroll self-rating	S	62%	32%	1 year
1987	Magni	57/57	Zung self-rating	S	61%	26%	1 year
1997	McKhann et al	127/124	CES-D	S	27%	19%	1 year
1997	Timberlake et al	121/?	BDI	S	37%	23%	1 year
1999	Pirraglia et al	237/218	CES-D	S	43%	23%	6 months
2000	Junior et al	50/48	DSM-III-R Depressive syndrome diagnosed after CIS interview	D	22% (8% MD)	21% (8% MD)	Hospital discharge
2000	Andrew et al	147/147	DASS	S	16%	19%	6 days
2001	Baker et al	158/NA	DASS	S	15%	-	No follow-up

Notes
CES-D   =   Center for Epidemiological Studies of Depression Scale
BDI   =   Beck Depression Inventory
DSM-III-R =   Diagnostic and Statistical Manual of Mental Disorders, 3rd edn (revised)
CIS   =   Clinical interview schedule
DASS   =   Depression, Anxiety and Stress Scale
MD   =   Major depression

patients were depressed before and shortly afterwards but this lifted by 1 year. Six percent of patients were depressed before surgery, but never were again, and 5% were depressed before, recovered somewhat in the immediate period following surgery, before becoming depressed again by 1 year.

The McKhann and Timberlake studies are typical of the model of research that exists on the association between cardiac surgery and depression. A variety of studies have quoted a range of pre-operative depression from 16 to 47% (Pirraglia et al, 1999; Andrew et al, 2000) whilst post-operative depression rates vary between 19 and 61% (Pirraglia et al, 1999), albeit at differing times following surgery.

A major factor involved in the wide range of pre- and post-operative rates is the different scales and instruments used, both self-administered and observer-rated. These include, in addition to the CES-D and BDI already mentioned, the Depression, Anxiety and Stress Scale (DASS) (Andrew et al, 2000), the Zung Self Rating Depression Scale (Magni, 1987), the Hamilton Rating Scale for Depression and Clinical Interview Schedule (Junior et al, 2000) and the Carroll Rating Scale for Depression (Horgan et al, 1984), to mention just a few. Symptom scales such as these give a useful indication of the mental state of the patient, but they do not allow precise diagnoses to be made. In such scales, certain levels of depressive symptomatology are regarded as being 'suggestive' or 'indicative' of depression whereas diagnostic criteria such as those of the Diagnostic and Statistical Manual of Mental Disorders version III-Revised (DSM-III-R) (Junior et al, 2000) allow actual cases to be identified, thereby strengthening the methodology of the investigation. Junior et al (2000) found relatively low rates of major depression pre- (8%) and post-operatively (8%) compared to the high percentage of patients classed as depressed by symptom scales alone. Other forms of depression were more common than major depression in this sample (dysthymic disorder 6% pre-operatively and 4% post-operatively, adjustment disorder with depressed mood 6% and 8%, 'non-specific' depression 2% and 0%). The paper is contradictory on the topic of anxiety. Either 0% or 4% had a pre-operative anxiety disorder, while 4% had an anxiety disorder after surgery (Junior et al, 2000).

The use of different instruments – some that have been validated in the physically ill, others that have not, some that give a quantitative indication of depressive symptomatology, others that give a categorical diagnosis – has contributed to a set of highly variable prevalence and incidence rates. This theme is discussed in a South Australian paper by Baker et al (2000), which draws attention to the need for more realistic, comparative studies and highlights their apparent dearth in the current literature. What does seem to be clear is that pre-operative rates of depression in cardiac surgery patients far exceed those of the general population; an accepted rate of around 20% is regularly quoted (Blacher, 1987; Cassens et al, 1990). Also, following surgery, rates are somewhat higher than their pre-operative levels in the short term, falling back to below or equivalent to pre-operative rates in due course.

Why is depression important?

As has been stated, pre-operative depression appears to be a significant predictor of post-operative depression. Depression at any stage of life is undesirable, but the added burden of life-saving surgery makes this doubly so. As with depression not associated with surgery, it brings about suffering, both on the part of the individual and also for those around him or her. In addition it has costs to society as a whole. Attempts to treat depression, thereby diminishing this suffering and expense, constitute a worthwhile goal.

Over and above the psychological morbidity that post-surgical depression carries with it, there are risks to the patients' physical health. This can be seen in longer rehabilitation times and raised levels of cardiac symptoms. As reported in a recent paper, Baker et al (2000) studied 158 patients undergoing CABG and demonstrated a six-fold increase in mortality associated with significant post-operative depressive symptomatology. This is concordant with the accepted view that depression, unrelated to surgery, is associated with higher cardiac morbidity and mortality.

Summary and implications for management

Four of the major cardiac surgical interventions have been outlined. A review of the relevant literature reveals that the majority of studies on this topic concentrate on depression associated with CABG patients. This is, presumably, because the numbers of procedures are higher than for some of the other techniques. This would in turn lead to greater patient numbers to study. However, it is noticeable that despite similar numbers, post-angioplasty depression studies appear to be absent from the published literature. The reason for this is not clear, although these procedures are somewhat less involved, do not need bypass, and do not share the same mortality.

Most of the current literature is *descriptive* regarding the nature of depression associated with cardiac surgery. That is to say we have a range of depressive symptomatology rates and a host of aetiological factors associated with such surgery. What is lacking are data on specific interventions for this patient group.

Given this relative lack of evidence, it would be prudent to suggest that the management of a patient who is depressed following cardiac surgery should be modelled on that of a non-surgical depressed subject. First there must be an appreciation that cardiac surgery carries with it an increased risk of affective symptomatology, and that post-surgical depression is associated with increased mortality and physical morbidity. When prescribing antidepressant medication, it would seem reasonable to opt for newer preparations such as selective serotonin re-uptake inhibitors or serotonin/noradrenaline re-uptake inhibitors. These products carry less cardiac risk than older preparations such as tricyclic antidepressants, although no psychotropic medication is side-effects or interaction free. In dealing with this vulnerable population, extra vigilance to these effects would be advisable (Evans et al, 1997).

Psychological well-being might be enhanced by pre-planned, well-organized and well-attended rehabilitation programmes. This is supported by the literature that lists the benefits of such programmes and the positive effects of psychological interventions, such as cognitive behavioural therapy (CBT), seen in other surgical specialties (Gardner and Worwood, 1997). If there were a need for such specific psychological work, this would have to acknowledge the potential presence of cognitive deficits post-surgery. Allowances in the structure and content of the therapy may need to be incorporated into the programme. There would appear to be no reason why a therapy such as CBT should not be effective in cognitively intact members of this group as a focused, short-term intervention.

Finally, in any developing branch of medicine and research, there are significant areas that remain understudied. What is lacking in the field of cardiac surgery and affective disorders are studies focusing on specific interventions for these patients (both pharmacological and psychological). Also, differences in depressive symptomatology between different cardiac procedures remain to be elucidated. Are those undergoing heart transplantation more depressed than those undergoing CABG, for example? If so, what does that tell us and how might we manage such patients in the future? Liaison psychiatrists are already involved in many cardiac surgical units across the world. It remains to be seen how much further research will contribute to this field of medicine.

Acknowledgement

Neil Strathmore gave much helpful advice about the content of this chapter.

References

American Heart Association (2001) www.americanheart.org

Andrew MJ, Baker RA, Kneebone AC, Knight JL, Mood state as a predictor of neuropsychological deficits following cardiac surgery, *J Psychosom Res* (2000) **48**:537–46.

Baker RA, Andrew MJ, Schrader G, Knight JL, Preoperative depression and mortality in coronary artery bypass surgery: preliminary findings, *Aust NZ J Surgery* (2001) **71**:139–42.

Bedford PD, Adverse cerebral effects of anaesthesia on old people, *Lancet* (1955) **ii**:259–63.

Blacher RS, Open heart surgery the patient's point of view, *Mount Sinai J Med* (1971) **38**(1): 74–8.

Blacher RS, Heart Surgery: the patient's experience. In: Blacher RS, ed, *The Psychological Experience of Surgery* (New York: John Wiley and Sons 1987).

Boll A, Dahme B, Meffert HJ, Spiedel H, Psychological adaptation of patients 3 to 5 years after heart surgery. In: Willner AE, Rodewald G, eds, *Impact of Cardiac Surgery on the Quality of Life* (New York: Plenum Press 1990).

British Heart Foundation (2001) www.bhf.org.uk

Cassens G, Wolfe L, Zola M, The neuropsychology of depressions, *J Neuropsychiatry Clin Neurosci* (1990) **2**:202–13.

Evans M, Hammond M, Wilson K, Copeland J, Placebo-controlled treatment trial of depression in elderly physically ill patients, *Int J Geriatr Psychiatry* (1997) **12**:817–24.

Gardner FV, Worwood EV, Psychological effects of cardiac surgery: a review of the literature, *JR Soc Health* (1997) **117**:245–9.

Horgan D, Davies B, Hunt D, Westlake GW, Mullerworth M, Psychiatric aspects of coronary artery surgery, *Med J Aust* (1984) **141**:587–90.

Hunt S, A fair way of donating hearts for transplantation, *BMJ* (2000) **321**:526.

Isles LJ, Orrel MW, Secondary mania after open-heart surgery, *Br J Psychiatry* (1991) **159**:280–2.

Junior RF, Ramadan ZBA, Pereira ANE, Wajngarten M, Depression with irritability in patients undergoing coronary artery bypass graft surgery: the cardiologist's role, *Gen Hosp Psychiatry* (2000) **22**:365–74.

Kivipelto M, Helkala E-L, Laasko MP et al, Midlife vascular risk factors and Alzheimer's disease in later life: longitudinal population based study, *BMJ* (2001) **322**:1447–51.

Langosch W, Schmoll-Flockerzier H, Psychological reactions to open heart surgery: results of a quantitative and qualitative analysis of the recovery process. In: Walter PJ, ed, *Quality of Life After Open Heart Surgery* (Dordrecht: Kluwer, 1992) 193–203.

Magni G, Depressive symptoms before and one year after heart surgery, *Psychol Rep* (1987) **61**:173–4.

McKhann GM, Borowicz LM, Goldsborough MA, Enger C, Selnes OA, Depression and cognitive decline after coronary artery bypass grafting, *Lancet* (1997) **349**:1282–4.

National Heart Foundation of Australia (2001) www.heartfoundation.com.au

Newman M, Kirchner JL, Phillips-Brute B et al, Longitudinal assessment of neuro-cognitive function after coronary artery bypass surgery, *N Engl J Med* (2001) **344**:395–402.

Newman S, Klinger L, Venn G et al, Subjective reports of cognition in relation to assessed cognitive performance following coronary artery bypass surgery, *J Psychosom Res* (1989) **33**:227–33.

Nichols KA, *Psychological Care in Physical Illness* (Philadelphia: The Charles Press, 1984).

Pirraglia PA, Peterson JC, Williams-Russo P, Gorkin L, Charleson ME, Depressive symptomatology in coronary artery bypass graft surgery patients, *Int J Geriatr Psychiatry* (1999) **14**:668–80.

Selnes OA, McKhann GM, Coronary artery bypass surgery and the brain, *N Engl J Med* (2001) **344**:451–2.

Shaw PJ, Bates D, Cartlidge NEF et al, Early neurological complications of coronary artery bypass surgery, *BMJ* (1985) **291**:1384–6.

Timberlake N, Klinger L, Smith P, Venn G, Treasure T et al, Incidence and patterns of depression following coronary artery bypass graft surgery, *J Psychosom Res* (1997) **43**:197–207.

Trygar Artinian N, Duggan C, Miller P, Age differences in patient recovery patterns following coronary artery bypass surgery, *Am J Crit Care* (1993) **6**:453–61.

6

Cardiovascular disease, affective disorders and impaired fatty acid and phospholipid metabolism

David F Horrobin

Introduction

There is a steadily increasing stream of articles which describe a strong association between depression and cardiovascular disease. The publication of this book is an indication of the rising interest in this subject. The association is thoroughly described in other chapters and so will not be documented in detail here. The first reports tended, quite reasonably, to describe depression as a logical consequence of a life-threatening event. The cardiovascular disease was thought to cause the depression. While such an event sequence may occur, it cannot be the only explanation for the association. Several prospective studies have now clearly demonstrated that depression occurring years before there is any evidence of cardiovascular disease is predictive of later cardiac events (e.g. Pratt et al, 1996; Ford et al, 1998; Ferketich et al, 2000).

So there is some evidence that depression may precede cardiovascular disease, and some that cardiovascular disease may precede depression. Such time relationships may or may not indicate causation. They may mean that both the cardiovascular disease and the depression are caused by a third factor: the correlation between cardiovascular disease and depression could therefore be secondary, dependent on the fact that both are correlated with a third factor.

Epidemiological studies alone, and time sequence studies alone, cannot demonstrate causation. Causation can be established only if there is a plausible mechanism that links the two phenomena, and only if manipulation of that mechanism is able to change outcome.

There has therefore been a search for possible mechanisms. Many have been proposed (Carney et al, 1995; Nemeroff and O'Connor, 2000). The most plausible are that stress might cause biological changes which lead to both heart disease and depression (Rozanski et al, 1999; Stanford et al, 1999) or that changes in blood platelet reactivity (Musselman et al, 1996; Berk and Plein, 2000; Nemeroff and Musselman, 2000), in autonomic function and heart rate variability (Carney et al, 1988, 1995; Rechlin et al, 1994; Yeragani et al, 2001), or in vascular wall pathology (Agewall et al, 1996), all of which have been described in depression, might lead to adverse cardiovascular events. However, these are all physiological changes which must in turn have some underlying biochemical explanation.

The proposed hypothesis reviewed in this chapter is that defects in metabolism of omega-3 essential fatty acids are the underlying causative factors which predispose individuals to both cardiovascular disease and depression (Horrobin and Bennett, 1999a; Horrobin, 2001b). In brief the evidence is as follows:

1.   Similar defects of omega-3 fatty acid biochemistry are described in both depression and cardiovascular disease.
2.   These defects are well documented as being able to cause disturbances in neuronal signal transduction, and also abnormalities in heart rate and platelet function, and vascular pathology.
3.   Correction of these defects has been shown in randomized placebo-controlled trials to reduce mortality in patients with cardiovascular disease and to improve depression in those who are depressed.

The remainder of this chapter will document the evidence for these statements.

Biochemistry of essential fatty acids and phospholipids

The essential fatty acids (EFAs) are nutrients that cannot be synthesized de novo by the human body. There are two types, the omega-6 or n-6 derived from linoleic acid, and the omega-3 or n-3 derived from alpha-linolenic acid. EFAs within each type can be interconverted, but the two types cannot be converted to each other. The pathways of metabolism are shown in Figure 6.1.

Four of these fatty acids are of particular importance with regard to nervous system and cardiovascular function (Horrobin et al, 1994; Horrobin, 1995, 1998, 2001a; Horrobin and Bennett, 1999a). Two of them are of major structural importance. These are arachidonic acid (AA) of the omega-6 series and docosahexaenoic acid (DHA) of the omega-3 series, both of which are substantial components of the phospholipids of all cell membranes, being particularly attached to the Sn2 (middle) carbon atom of the phospholipid backbone: they make up about 15% of the dry weight of the brain. Three EFAs are of particular functional importance because they are precursors of large numbers of highly active eicosanoids. These are dihomogammalinolenic acid (DGLA), AA of the omega-6 series, and eicosapentaenoic acid (EPA) of the omega-3 series. Most neurotransmitters and cytokines employ AA, DGLA and EPA as components of their post-receptor signal transduction systems. Occupation of the receptor changes configuration of a G-protein which activates phospholipase A2-, C- and D-related systems which then directly or indirectly release AA, DGLA or EPA from the membrane phospholipids. The fatty acids themselves may then act

ESSENTIAL FATTY ACID (EFA) METABOLISM

n-6 series		*n-3 series*	
18:2n-6	LINOLEIC	ALPHA LINOLENIC	18:3n-3
	↓ Delta-6-desaturation	↓	
18:3n-6	GAMMA-LINOLENIC	STEARIDONIC	18:4n-3
	↓ *Elongation*	↓	
20:3n-6	DIHOMOGAMMALINOLENIC	EICOSATETRAENOIC (n-3)	20:4n-3
	↓ *Delta-5-desaturation*	↓	
20:4n-6	ARACHIDONIC	EICOSAPENTAENOIC	20:5n-3
	↓ *Elongation*	↓	
22:4n-6	ADRENIC	DOCOSAPENTAENOIC (n-3)	22:5n-3
	↓ *Delta-4-desaturation*	↓	
22:5n-6	DOCOSAPENTAENOIC (n-6)	DOCOSAHEXAENOIC	22:6n-3

Figure 6.1

An outline of the metabolic pathways of the omega-6 (n-6) and omega-3 (n-3) essential fatty acids. These are particularly incorporated into the Sn2 position of phospholipids in excitable tissues such as neurons, glia, endothelial cells, heart and muscle. Arachidonic acid and docosahexaenoic acid are important structural elements of such phospholipids, while arachidonic, dihomogammalinolenic and eicosapentaenoic acids play key roles in signal transduction processes following receptor activation by neurotransmitters, cytokines and growth factors.

as second messengers regulating enzymes or ion channels or genes directly, or may do so after being converted to eicosanoids by an array of cyclo-oxygenase, lipoxygenase, prostaglandin synthase and other enzymes.

Given the central importance of this fatty acid/eicosanoid signal transduction system in all excitable tissues, it would not be surprising if abnormalities in the system were to lead to both cardiovascular and psychiatric or neurological problems.

Abnormal eicosanoid production in depression

Overproduction of arachidonic acid-derived eicosanoids is one of the most consistently reported biochemical abnormalities in depression. Lieb et al (1983) were the first to report substantially elevated blood levels of thromboxane (TX) B2 and prostaglandin (PG) E2 levels in depressed patients. TXB2 is the stable metabolite of TXA2 which in the blood is derived mostly from platelets. This was therefore an early indication of platelet overactivity in depression.

Since then almost every investigation has reported elevated AA-derived eicosanoids in depressed patients. Calabrese et al (1986) reported high levels of blood PGE2 in depression, and Piccirillo et al (1994) also found high levels of PGE2. In saliva from depressed patients, Ohishi et al (1988) and Nishino et al (1989) reported high levels of three AA-derived eicosanoids, PGE2, PGD2 and PGF2 alpha. Linnoila et al (1983) reported high levels of PGE2 in cerebrospinal fluid of depressed, as compared to normal or schizophrenic, patients.

Severe depression is also associated with systemic mastosis, an illness in which AA-derived prostaglandin levels are very high (Lowinger, 1989). Lowering of these elevated levels with non-steroidal anti-inflammatory drugs (NSAIDs) relieves the depression (Lowinger, 1989; Lloyd, 1992). Infusion of prostaglandins for the management of peripheral vascular disease can cause depressed mood (Ansell et al, 1986).

Treatment with NSAIDs is not usually thought to relieve depressed mood. However, psychotropic effects of such drugs have rarely been looked for, and moreover most such drugs do not effectively penetrate the blood–brain barrier. In mastocytosis NSAIDs are clearly antidepressant and it has recently been reported that patients with cardiovascular disease taking the NSAID aspirin have a more positive mood than patients not taking aspirin (Stanford et al, 1999).

Antidepressant drugs as modulators of prostaglandin synthesis and action

The conventional view of antidepressant drug action is that it is related to modulation of catecholamine biochemistry. Almost all research and all marketing of such drugs emphasizes this aspect. However, Healey (1997) has pointed out that some effective antidepressants have relatively little effect on catecholamines while other drugs which have potent effects are not good antidepressants. Moreover, many other biochemical actions of antidepressants have been described which have been largely ignored.

One such action of tricyclic antidepressants is their ability to antagonize prostaglandin-related calcium movements (Manku and Horrobin, 1976a,b; Mtabaji et al, 1977; Horrobin, 1977; Horrobin et al, 1977). High doses of NSAIDs are able to inhibit both entry of calcium from the extracellular fluid and the release of calcium from intracellular stores in response to various stimuli. With the NSAID still present, normal calcium responses can be restored by the addition of exogenous PGE2. Tricyclic antidepressants are then able to inhibit the effects of PGE2 on calcium in a competitive, dose-dependent manner. Given the elevation of AA-derived eicosanoids in depression, it is possible that this calcium-related PG antagonism could play a major role in antidepressant action.

Another class of antidepressants, the monoamine oxidase inhibitors, are unlike the NSAIDs in that they penetrate the brain, but are like the NSAIDs in that they are potent inhibitors of prostaglandin synthesis from arachidonic acid (Lee, 1974; Fjalland, 1976; Bekemeier et al, 1977; Lambert and Jacquemin, 1980). Indeed, if their PG inhibitory activity had been discovered before their action on monoamine oxidase, they might have been given a different name and the whole history of the psychopharmacology of depression might have been different (Horrobin and Bennett, 1999a).

Abnormal essential fatty acid biochemistry in depression

The earlier reported abnormalities in AA-derived eicosanoid production in depression are now explicable in terms of recent findings relating to fatty acid biochemistry. Reports from Australia, Japan, Europe and North America are all consistent in reporting either an absolute deficit of omega-3 fatty acids in depression, or a relative deficit of omega-3 fatty acids in relation to normal, or elevated levels of arachidonic acid. Since omega-3 fatty acids inhibit the conversion of arachidonic acid to eicosanoids, these relative or absolute deficits could explain why AA-derived eicosanoid production is increased in depression (Horrobin and Bennett, 1999a).

Adams et al (1996) from Australia reported that the ratio of the omega-3 fatty acid eicosapentaenoic acid (EPA) to AA was reduced in red blood cells of depressed patients. Red cell EPA levels were inversely related to depression rating scores, whereas the red cell and plasma AA/EPA ratio was positively related to those scores. Levels of the structural omega-3 fatty acid docosahexaenoic acid (DHA) were not related to depression in either red cells or plasma. This suggests that EPA and AA are the key fatty acids involved.

Two studies from the same Belgian group (Maes et al, 1996; 1999) reported similar findings. They looked at both phospholipid and cholesteryl ester lipid fractions in plasma. In both studies, both absolute levels of EPA and the ratio of EPA to AA were significantly reduced in patients with major depression. Again in both studies, DHA levels were not significantly related to depression (Horrobin and Bennett, 1999a).

A Japanese investigator found similar results (Seko, 1997). EPA levels in blood cells were inversely related to depression whereas the AA/EPA ratio was positively related. DHA levels were unrelated to depression. Two UK/Canadian studies also obtained similar findings in both plasma and red cells (Edwards et al, 1998; Peet et al, 1998), although in these investigations both EPA and DHA were reduced in the depressed patients. Of great interest is the fact that in the study by Edwards et al, there was an inverse relationship between dietary intake of omega-3 fatty acids and depression scores on the Beck Depression Inventory.

Thus the biochemical studies on fatty acids and eicosanoids show an unusual degree of consistency between investigations performed at different locations and by different research groups. There are elevations of the AA-derived eicosanoids, notably PGE2 and TXB2, which can readily be explained by the elevated ratios of AA to EPA in various lipid fractions.

Do the fatty acid/eicosanoid abnormalities play a causal role in depression?

The idea that the observed abnormalities in fatty acid and eicosanoid metabolism may play a causal role in depression is not implausible on biochemical and pharmacological grounds (Hibbeln and Salem, 1995; Hibbeln, 1998; Hibbeln et al, 1998a; Horrobin and Bennett, 1999a; Horrobin, 2001b). The phospholipids of nerve endings and synaptic vesicles are rich in essential fatty acids: their precise composition determines the fluidity and flexibility of membranes and therefore modulates the quaternary structure of membrane-associated proteins. All neurotransmitter, cytokine and growth factor receptors that have been investigated lead to the release of arachidonic acid and other fatty acids and the formation of eicosanoids as a result of various phospholipase-activated processes. The fatty acids and eicosanoids modulate ion channels, calcium movements, neurotransmitter metabolism, various enzymes and genes. Thus it would not be surprising if changes in fatty acid/eicosanoid/phospholipid metabolism were to lead to the functional changes observed in depression (Horrobin and Bennett, 1999a).

There are many animal and cell culture studies reviewed and documented in the above articles. Human studies are just beginning. In normal volunteers, Hibbeln et al (1998a) noted that there were significant positive correlations between long chain omega-6 and omega-3 fatty acids and cerebrospinal fluid (CSF) levels of both the serotonin metabolite 5-HIAA and the dopamine metabolite homovanillic acid (HVA). In another study, in normal individuals there was a positive correlation between plasma DHA levels and CSF 5-HIAA, whereas in depressed individuals this correlation was reversed (Hibbeln et al, 1998b). These studies suggest that fatty acids may modulate neurotransmitter metabolism in humans although no studies have yet been reported in depressed patients.

The basic science is consistent with a potential effect of fatty acid metabolism on nerve function and hence on depression. However, much more direct evidence is now available which points to the idea that in humans mood state may be modulated by essential fatty acid metabolism. The evidence comes in three forms: epidemiological studies that compare the prevalence of depression between different populations; studies that compare mood in individuals with different fatty acid intakes; and intervention studies that attempt to change mood by changing fatty acid intake.

Population studies

Hibbeln and colleagues have been responsible for three studies on the prevalence of depression in relation to intake of fish and seafood. This is of interest because fish and seafood are the main sources in the diet of the long chain omega-3 fatty acids EPA and DHA. The annual prevalence of major depression shows a nearly 60-fold variation between countries with good data and is strongly and highly significantly inversely related to annual fish consumption in these countries (R = -0.84, P < 0.005) (Hibbeln, 1998). Very similar observations have been made for post-partum depression (R = -0.63, P < 0.01) (Hibbeln, 1999) and for bipolar disorders (bipolar 1, R = -0.63, P < 0.04: bipolar II, R = -0.89, P < 0.004) (Noaghiul et al, 2001).

Correlations are not causations. However, whereas it is not difficult to see how fish or seafood consumption might influence depression, it is almost impossible to construct a plausible mechanism whereby the national prevalence of depression might influence the consumption of fish and seafood. For all three conditions, the data suggest that there is a sharp rise in depression prevalence when fish or seafood consumption falls below the range of 20–30 kg/person/year. Because the EPA and DHA contents of fish and seafood are highly variable, it is not possible precisely to convert total consumption into daily intakes of EPA and DHA. However, 20–30 kg/year converts into daily intakes of the order of 60–90 g of fish/seafood. Since on average EPA + DHA are likely to make up around 0.5–1% of the total weight of a mixed range of fish and seafood, this translates into a daily EPA + DHA intake of around 300–900 mg/day as compared to the average intake per day in Europe and North America in the range of 50–200 mg/day. If the epidemiological evidence does indicate a causal relationship, then relatively low doses of EPA or DHA may be required to improve the condition of most depressed individuals.

Fish, seafood or omega-3 dietary intake in relation to depression

Only one study to date has carefully evaluated actual dietary intake of fatty acids in individuals in relation to severity of depression. Edwards et al (1998) collected information on all food intake for 7 days in a group of depressed subjects and found a significant inverse correlation between the intake of omega-3 fatty acids and severity of depression on the Beck Depression Inventory.

Data compatible with this finding have been obtained from studies in which self-rated assessment of fish consumption was associated with mood or suicide tendency. In a study of 265 000 Japanese subjects followed for 17 years, regular fish consumption was associated with a reduced risk of suicide (Hirayama, 1990). In a study of 3000 randomly selected individuals from a general population in Finland, regular fish consumption was associated with a significantly reduced risk of depression and of suicidal ideation as indicated by the self-rated Beck Depression Inventory (Tanskanen et al, 2001).

Thus it seems that the evidence of an inverse relation between fish and seafood intake between populations is supported by equivalent evidence from individuals within populations.

Treatment of depression with omega-3 fatty acids

Proof that a causal relationship exists between omega-3 fatty acid intake in fish and seafood and depression requires placebo-controlled intervention studies. Several such studies have now been carried out.

In patients with bipolar disorder, Stoll et al (1999) demonstrated a significantly reduced risk of relapse in patients given treatment with over 9 g/day of mixed ethyl esters of EPA and DHA as compared to placebo olive oil. There was also a significant beneficial effect specifically on depressed mood in these patients. However, this trial could not distinguish between the effects of EPA and DHA, and the high dose used may be difficult in practice to follow for long periods.

Edwards (unpublished work) compared a placebo with a high DHA (Docanol) and a high EPA (Kirunal) triglyceride oil in treatment of depression. Docanol provided about 2 g/day of DHA while Kirunal provided about 2 g/day of EPA. EPA but not DHA was significantly better than placebo in improving depression. Marangell et al (2000) compared 4 g/day of pure DHA and of placebo in treating depression. There were no significant differences between the groups, but if anything the DHA group tended to do worse. Similarly in attention deficit hyperactivity disorder, Voigt et al (2001) compared DHA with placebo. Again the DHA group did consistently worse, sometimes significantly so.

These observations suggest that, with respect to depression, it is the EPA rather than the DHA which is beneficial. There are hints that DHA-treated patients may actually do worse. Since DHA and EPA are relatively similar in structure and may compete with one another for binding sites, mixed EPA/DHA formulations may exhibit weaker effects than pure EPA preparations delivering the same absolute amount of EPA.

An open-label study in a single late adolescent male with severe and completely treatment-unresponsive depression was conducted by Puri et al (2001a,b). This individual had been severely depressed for 6 years and was thought to be at high risk of suicide. No drug had been effective. MRI scans suggested ventricular enlargement. Treatment with 2 g/day ultra-pure ethyl-EPA (LAX-101) led to rapid improvement and normalization of mood which has now persisted for over a year. Repeat MRI scans also suggested normalization of ventricular size.

Two trials have now been conducted in which ultra-pure ethyl-EPA (LAX-101) was compared with placebo. Horrobin and Peet (2001) investigated 70 patients who had failed to respond to standard antidepressant therapy with tricyclic or SSRI drugs. They were randomly assigned to receive placebo or 1 g/day, 2 g/day or 4 g/day on a double-blind basis. The 1 g/day dose was significantly better than placebo on all three rating scales used, the Hamilton, the Montgomery–Åsberg and the Beck. All aspects of the syndrome improved, including depression, anxiety, sleep, suicidal ideation and lassitude and active treatment was better than placebo on every item of all three rating scales (Peet and Horrobin, 2002). The effect was detectable at the first assessment point at 4 weeks and became progressively greater to the last assessment point at 12 weeks. Higher doses of ethyl-EPA were also better than placebo but less strikingly so than the 1 g/day dose. A similar bell-shaped dose–response curve, with higher doses being less effective, has been noted in schizophrenia (Horrobin et al, 2001).

Belmaker's group (Nemers et al, 2001) also conducted a placebo-controlled trial, this time of 2 g/day ethyl EPA (LAX-101) for 4 weeks in 20 patients with depression who had relapsed while on continuing standard drug therapy. Six of 10 patients on EPA but only one of 10 on placebo achieved a 50% improvement in symptoms within 4 weeks. The difference in change in score on the Hamilton depression rating scale was very highly significant.

Conclusions: omega-3 fatty acids and depression

The basic science, the evidence of abnormal eicosanoid and fatty acid biochemistry, the between-country and within-individual epidemiological studies, and the clinical intervention trials are all consistent. Deficits of omega-3 essential fatty acids, and particularly of EPA, are associated with depression. The intervention and epidemiological studies strongly suggest that the association reflects a causal relationship.

Omega-3 fatty acids and cardiovascular disease

There are remarkable parallels in the relationships between omega-3 fatty acids and depression and between those same fatty acids and cardiovascular disease (Hibbeln and Salem, 1995; Peet and Edwards, 1997; Horrobin and Bennett, 1999a; Horrobin, 2001). There is a very large literature in this field. In addition to the above references, substantial reviews of the whole subject can be found in Leaf and Kang (1998), Horrobin (1995) and Simopoulos (1999a,b). The main findings can be summarized as follows:

1. In cardiovascular disease, as in depression, there is evidence of platelet activation with over-production of arachidonic-acid-derived eicosanoids, including thromboxane. This platelet overactivity is the basis for the treatment and prevention of cardiovascular disease with aspirin, which even at low doses inhibits conversion of arachidonic acid to thromboxane in platelets.
2. In cardiovascular disease, as in depression, the heart rate is unusually stable, a condition which seems to predispose to a high risk of cardiac arrhythmia and sudden death (Carney et al, 1995; Krittayaphong et al, 1997; Carney, 1998).
3. In cardiovascular disease, as in depression, patients have low levels of omega-3 fatty acids in the blood and those low levels are predictive of future cardiovascular events.

4.   In cardiovascular disease, as in depression, there are inverse relationships between fish and seafood consumption and risk of adverse outcomes both on a between-population and on a within-population basis.

As in depression, the question arises as to whether these relationships reflect cause or simply correlation. The answer can only come from randomized intervention studies. Four such studies have shown strikingly beneficial effects from intake of omega-3 fatty acids as compared to placebo. In Wales oily fish or fish oils containing EPA and DHA significantly reduced cardiac mortality (Burr et al, 1989). In India fish oil had a similar effect (Singh et al, 1997). An 11 000 patient study in Italy showed that 1 g/day of mixed ethyl-EPA and ethyl-DHA significantly reduced cardiovascular mortality (Gruppo Italiano per lo Studio della Streptochinasi nell'Infarto Miocardico [GISSI], 1999). In France, treatment with alpha-linolenic acid, the parent compound of EPA and DHA, also significantly reduced mortality (de Lorgeril et al, 1994). In all four studies the effects were observed with low doses of omega-3 fatty acids. In all three the initial evidence of benefit appeared rapidly, suggesting a primary effect on an acute phenomenon such as platelet aggregation or cardiac arrhythmias.

The concept of an effect on cardiac rhythm is strongly supported by the direct evidence that omega-3 fatty acids regulate the behaviour of cardiac ion channels and can block the development of arrhythmias in various animal models (Leaf and Kang, 1998). In patients who had survived a myocardial infarction, a randomized placebo-controlled trial showed that treatment with EPA and DHA could normalize heart rate variability (Christensen et al, 1996). These effects on the excitable tissue of cardiac muscle are consistent with the concept of equivalent effects on neurons and glial cells.

Of particular interest is the fact that as with depression and schizophrenia, intervention with higher doses of omega-3 fatty acids seems to have less thera-peutic effect than intervention with lower doses (Horrobin, 1995). One possible basis for this is that whereas high levels of arachidonic acid, and the uncontrolled conversion of AA to some eicosanoids, may be harmful, normal levels of arachi-donic acid are essential for the functioning of all tissues. AA plays a key role both in membrane structure and in signal transduction processes. If AA is reduced too far, as may happen as a consequence of high intakes of omega-3 fatty acids, then some of the beneficial effects of EPA or DHA may be lost (Horrobin, 1995). The diminished efficacy of higher doses of omega-3 fatty acids in both depres-sion and cardiovascular disease is consistent with this concept.

The relationship between depression, cardiovascular disease and omega-3 fatty acids

The evidence reviewed so far suggests that deficits of omega-3 fatty acids, and particularly of EPA, play causal roles in the development of both cardio-vascular disease and depression. In each case there are plausible mechanisms derived from basic science, there is epidemiological evidence based both on between-country and within-country studies, there is biochemical evidence based on comparing fatty acid and eicosanoid levels in affected patients and controls, and there is intervention evidence from placebo-controlled studies showing that treatment with omega-3 fatty acids can improve outcome in both depression and cardiovascular disease.

The hypothesis proposed here, therefore, is that abnormal omega-3 metabolism is a primary event which can lead to depression and also to cardiovascular disease. The many associations between mood state and cardiovascular disease which are documented in this volume occur because both clinical conditions are caused by the same underlying biochemical abnormality.

Much research needs to be done to explore further the origins of the abnormalities in omega-3 metabolism. Multiple mechanisms are likely to be involved, some of which are discussed below.

The influence of diet

The epidemiological and intervention studies suggest that a low dietary intake of omega-3 fatty acids, and particularly of EPA and DHA from fish and seafood, has a major impact on mood. There is evidence that the absolute intakes of omega-3 fatty acids and the intakes relative to omega-6 and saturated fatty acids have fallen dramatically over the last 100 years (Simopoulos, 1999b). These changes have coincided with substantial increases in the prevalence of both depression and cardiovascular disease in industrialized countries over the same period. The increase in depression has been particularly striking in the past 50 years. It may be significant that whereas in the first half of the 20th century treatment of children with cod liver oil was near universal, in the second half of the 20th century this practice virtually ceased. Cod liver oil was given primarily because it was regarded as a rich source of vitamins A and D. However, it was also a rich source of EPA and DHA. It is an interesting possibility that the rapid rise in childhood and adolescent psychiatric disorders may be partly attributable to sharp falls in the consumption of cod liver oils and oily fish.

Saturated fats, as well as competing with omega-3 fatty acids for incorporation into complex lipids, may have another effect by inducing the synthesis of cyclo-oxygenase 2 which will enhance the conversion of arachidonic acid to eicosanoids. This is related to their activation of the lipopolysaccharide receptor, toll-like receptor 4 (Lee et al, 2001). This mechanism may be related to the actions of cytokines in depression (see below).

Stress

There is enormous interest in the role of stress in depression and one of the new potential modalities of treatment involves antagonists of corticotrophin-releasing-hormone (CRH).

It is not generally known in the psychiatric research community that stress-related hormones such as glucocorticoids and catecholamines have profound effects on the metabolism of essential fatty acids (Brenner, 1981; Mills, 1991; Horrobin, 1992). They are able to inhibit the desaturase enzymes which convert the main dietary essential fatty acids, linoleic acid and alpha-linolenic acid, to their long chain metabolites which are important in excitable tissues (Figure 6.1). Stress will therefore reduce the endogenous formation of EPA and DHA which could predispose to depression, especially in those with low dietary intakes of these fatty acids.

Cytokines

The cytokine concept of depression was first proposed by Smith and then extensively developed by Maes, Leonard and their colleagues (Smith, 1991; Maes et al, 1992, 1996; Connor and Leonard, 1998; Song et al, 1998). This was based on the fact that treatment with various cytokines can induce severe depression and that in depression there is extensive evidence of activation of immunological and inflammatory mechanisms which are associated with overproduction of cytokines. Many of these mechanisms can be imitated in animals by the administration of lipopolysaccharide which activates both cytokine release and induction of eicosanoid synthesis via the toll-like receptor 4 (Lee et al, 2001).

There is now substantial evidence that cytokine production and various inflammatory diseases such as rheumatoid arthritis and inflammatory bowel disease can be modulated by omega-3 fatty acids. The literature in this field is now very extensive and leaves little doubt that realistic doses of EPA and DHA can reduce both clinical inflammation and the cytokine release (Endres et al, 1989; Meydani et al, 1991; Cooper et al, 1993; Blok et al, 1996; Caughey et al, 1996; Hughes et al, 1996; Calder, 1997; Purasiri et al, 1997).

Thus the overproduction of cytokines, which is now well-documented in depression, may be enhanced by deficits of omega-3 fatty acids and suppressed by increased intake of EPA and DHA.

Genetic and environmentally induced variation in omega-3 fatty acid metabolism

Although diet plays an important role in the supply of omega-3 fatty acids, it is far from being the only factor involved in the formation of EPA and DHA, their incorporation into membranes, their turnover and their roles in signal transduction. Very large numbers of carrier proteins and enzymes are involved in these processes and each one could be a candidate for a role in psychiatric disorders (Horrobin and Bennett, 1999a,b; Bennett and Horrobin, 2000). These proteins include fatty acid binding and transport proteins, enzymes involved in the transfer of fatty acids between complex lipid fractions, enzymes involved in phospholipid synthesis and breakdown, and the many phospholipases, G proteins, protein kinases and acyl-CoA synthetases involved in signal transduction. This is not the appropriate place for an extensive discussion of all the potential candidates, but attention should be drawn to three important possibilities.

Enzymes involved in the metabolism of dietary alpha-linolenic acid to EPA and DHA are possible candidates for a role in depression. These enzymes can be inhibited by stress-related hormones and show impaired function in both diabetes and in atopic disorders (Brenner, 1981; Horrobin, 1992). Stress is undoubtedly related to depression and there is good epidemiological evidence of an increased risk of depression in diabetes (Winocour et al, 1990; Lustman et al, 1992; Gavard et al, 1993; Carney, 1998) and in atopic disorders (Nasr et al, 1981; Marshall, 1993; Hashiro and Okumura, 1998). Stressed individuals, and those with diabetes or with atopy, might thus be expected to be particularly susceptible to depression if dietary omega-3 fatty acid intake is low.

Depression is associated with increased formation of eicosanoids from arachidonic acid. Such increased formation depends on cyclo-oxygenase 1 and 2 and these enzymes also must be candidates for a role in depression. Their activity in relation to arachidonic acid can be competitively inhibited by EPA and DHA.

Release of eicosanoids in response to cytokines and lipopolysaccharide is dependent on the transfer of arachidonic acid in the cell into a compartment which is accessible to the relevant signal transduction system. Such transfer may be competitively inhibited by omega-3 fatty acids. The key enzyme in this situation is coenzyme-A-independent transacylase (CoAIT) (Horrobin, 2001b). This too may be a candidate, therefore, for a role in the overactive immunological and immune responses seen in depression.

There are many other possible candidates which might contribute to abnormal omega-3 metabolism in depression but space is too restricted to discuss them here.

Conclusions

There is now a substantial body of evidence that links deficits in omega-3 fatty acids, and especially in EPA, to both depression and cardiovascular disease. These deficits may be important biochemical bases for both disorders and may explain many of the observed links between the two as well as the observed physiological abnormalities in platelet function and heart rate regulation.

The intervention studies in both disorders suggest that EPA offers an entirely novel treatment modality in both types of disorder. Apart from its novelty, this treatment approach is exciting because it may be correcting a fundamental defect in biochemistry in depression. Depressed patients are not suffering from deficits of tricyclic compounds or SSRIs but they are suffering from deficits of EPA. Thus treatment may provide a more physiological correction of the underlying state than is possible with existing drugs. The implications of this are as follows:

1. Existing drugs do nothing to correct the documented abnormalities in fatty acid and phospholipid metabolism. This may provide part of the explanation for the common phenomenon of treatment failure. All three trials to date in major depression have shown that EPA is effective in patients who have failed to respond to standard treatment.
2. No trials to date have been conducted in treatment-naïve depressed patients and so the therapeutic effect in this situation is unknown. However, the between-country and within-country epidemiological evidence relating omega-3 intake to prevalence and risk of depression suggests that EPA is likely to be effective in treatment-naïve patients. However, this can be assessed only on the basis of randomized trials.
3. A major concern in the management of depression is the management of side effects. High proportions of patients using both tricyclic antidepressants and SSRIs discontinue treatment because of side effects, which may seem mild to the physician but which are unacceptable to the patient. EPA when used in ultra-pure form at a dose of 1-2 g/day is free of side effects other than mild and transient gastro-intestinal disturbances which occur in about 5% of patients. Almost never do these disturbances require cessation of treatment. This freedom from side effects is to be expected given the fact that EPA is a normal intermediate in human metabolism and is being used at dose levels which are commonly met by those who regularly eat oily marine fish.
4. The side effects of antidepressants are of particular concern in patients who have cardiovascular disease or who are at risk of such disease (Meier et al, 2001). There is reasonable evidence that the tricyclic compounds increase the risk of adverse outcomes. While the selective serotonin reuptake inhibitors (SSRIs) pose less risk, they are certainly not actively beneficial with respect to cardiovascular actions. In contrast, not only is EPA safe but in the form of fish oil or mixed EPA/DHA preparations it has actually been found to reduce mortality in patients with cardiovascular disease, probably by modulating abnormal platelet aggregation and cardiac rhythm. Thus, if EPA is used to manage depression in patients with cardiovascular problems, it is likely to improve the outcome of the cardiovascular disease also. Again randomized studies are required in patients with both depression and cardiovascular disease to confirm the results which have already been demonstrated separately in depressed patients and in cardiovascular patients.
5. Three other groups for which there is particular concern about the potential adverse effects of antidepressants are pregnant and lactating women, children and the elderly. In the first two groups there is concern not only about immediate side effects but about possible long-term effects on

neurodevelopment. In the last group there is concern about the considerably increased risk of adverse effects. As Freeman (2000) has pointed out, omega-3 fatty acids are positively required for normal fetal and infant development and therefore may represent a particularly appropriate form of management of depression in pregnant and lactating women. As with cardiovascular problems, there are several positive effects of omega-3 fatty acids in pregnancy (Allen and Harris, 2001; McGregor et al 2001) including facilitation of brain development, attenuation of pre-eclampsia and prevention of premature labour. The freedom from side effects of ultra-pure ethyl-EPA (LAX-101) and the beneficial cardiovascular actions, make this also an attractive treatment option for the elderly.

In conclusion, the understanding of the role of omega-3 fatty acids in both depression and cardiovascular disease offers a novel explanation for the links between these two conditions. The use of ultra-pure ethyl-EPA to manage depression offers a new, physiologically-based treatment modality which has particular advantages for those who fail to respond to standard treatment, for those with or at risk of cardiovascular disease, for the elderly, for pregnant and lactating women, and for infants and children.

References

Adams PB, Lawson S, Sanigorski A, Sinclair AJ, Arachidonic acid to eicosapentaenoic acid ratio in blood correlates positively with clinical symptoms of depression, *Lipids* (1996) **31**: S157–61.

Agewall S, Wikstrand J, Dahlof C, Fagerberg B, Negative feelings (discontent) predict progress of intima-media thickness of the common carotid artery in treated hypertensive men at high cardiovascular risk, *Am J Hypertens* (1996) **9**: 545–50.

Allen KG, Harris MA, The role of n-3 fatty acids in gestation and parturition, *Exp Biol Med* (2001) **226**: 498–506.

Ansell D, Belch JJ, Forbes, CD, Depression and prostacyclin infusion, *Lancet* (1986) **2**: 509.

Bekemeier H, Giessler AJ, Vogel E, Influence of MAO-inhibitors, neuroleptics, morphine, mescaline, divascan, aconitine, and pyrogenes on prostaglandin-biosynthesis, *Pharmacol Res Commun* (1977) **9**: 587–98.

Bennett CN, Horrobin DF, Gene targets related to phospholipid and fatty acid metabolism in schizophrenia and other psychiatric disorders: an update, *Prostaglandins Leukot Essent Fatty Acids* (2000) **63**: 47–59.

Berk M, Plein H, Platelet supersensitivity to thrombin stimulation in depression: A possible mechanism for the association with cardiovascular mortality, *Clin Neuropharmacol* (2000) **23**: 182–5.

Blok WL, Katan MB, van der Meer JWM, Modulation of inflammation and cytokine production by dietary (n-3) fatty acids, *J Nutr* (1996) **126**: 1515–33.

Brenner RR, Nutritional and hormonal factors influencing desaturation of essential fatty acids, *Prog Lipid Res* (1981) **20**: 41–8.

Burr ML, Fehily AM, Gilbert JF et al, Effects of changes in fat, fish, and fibre intakes on death and myocardial reinfarction: diet and reinfarction trial (DART) *Lancet* (1989) **ii**: 757–61.

Calabrese JR, Skwerer RG, Barna B et al, Depression, immunocompetence, and prostaglandins of the E series, *Psychiatry Res* (1986) **17**: 41–7.

Calder PC, N-3 polyunsaturated fatty acids and cytokine production in health and disease, *Ann Nutr Metab* (1997) **41**: 203–34.

Carney C, Diabetes mellitus and major depressive disorder: an overview of prevalence, complications, and treatment, *Depres Anxiety* (1998) **7**: 149–57.

Carney RM, Rich MW, teVelde A et al, The relationship between heart rate, heart rate variability and depression in patients with coronary artery disease, *J Psychosom Res* (1988) **32**: 159–64.

Carney RM, Freedland KE, Rich MW, Jaffe AS, Depression as a risk factor for cardiac events in established coronary heart disease: a review of possible mechanisms, *Ann Behav Med* (1995) **17**: 142–9.

Caughey GE, Mantzioris E, Gibson RA, Cleland LG, James MJ, The effect on human tumor necrosis factor alpha and interleukin 1 beta production of diets enriched in n-3 fatty acids from vegetable oil or fish oil, *Am J Clin Nutr* (1996) **63**: 116–22.

Christensen JH, Gustenhoff P, Korup E, Aaroe J, Toft E et al, Effect of fish oil on heart rate variability in survivors of myocardial infarction: a double blind randomised controlled trial, *BMJ* (1996) **312**: 677–8.

Connor TJ, Leonard BE, Depression, stress and immunological activation: the role of cytokines in depressive disorders, *Life Sci* (1998) **62**: 583–606.

Cooper AL, Gibbons L, Horan, MA, Little RA, Rothwell NJ, Effect of dietary fish oil supplementation on fever and cytokine production in human volunteers, *Clin Nutr* (1993) **12:** 321–8.

de Lorgeril M, Renaud S, Mamelle N et al, Mediterranean alpha-linolenic acid-rich diet in secondary prevention of coronary heart disease, *Lancet* (1994) **343**: 1454–9.

Edwards R, Peet M, Shay J, Horrobin D, Omega-3 polyunsaturated fatty acid levels in the diet and in red blood cell membranes of depressed patients, *J Affect Disord* (1998) **48**: 149–55.

Endres S, Ghorbani R, Kelley VE et al, The effect of dietary supplementation with n-3 polyunsaturated fatty acids on the synthesis of interleukin-1 and tumor necrosis factor by mononuclear cells, *N Engl J Med* (1989) **320**: 265–71.

Ferketich AK, Schwartzbaum JA, Frid DJ, Moeschberger ML, Depression as an antecedent to heart disease among women and men in the NHANES I study, *Arch Intern Med* (2000) **160**: 1261–8.

Fjalland B, Influence of various substances on prostaglandin biosynthesis by guinea-pig chopped lung, *J Pharm Pharmacol* (1976) **28**: 683–6.

Ford DE, Mead LA, Chang PP et al, Depression is a risk factor for coronary artery disease in men: the precursors study, *Arch Intern Med* (1998) **158**: 1422–6.

Freeman MP, Omega-3 fatty acids in psychiatry: a review, *Ann Clin Psychiatry* (2000) **12**: 159–65.

Gavard JA, Lustman PJ, Clouse RE, Prevalence of depression in adults with diabetes. An epidemiological evaluation, *Diabet Care* (1993) **16**: 1167–78.

Gruppo Italiano per lo Studio della Streptochinasi nell'Infarto Miocardico (GISSI), Dietary supplementation with n-3 polyunsaturated fatty acids and vitamin E after myocardial infarction: results of the GISSI-Prevenzione trial, *Lancet* (1999) **354**: 447–55.

Hashiro M, Okumura M, The relationship between the psychological and immunological state in patients with atopic dermatitis, *J Dermatol Sci* (1998) **16**: 231–5.

Healy D, *The Antidepressant Era* (Harvard University Press: Cambridge, 1997).

Hibbeln JR, Fish consumption and major depression, *Lancet* (1998) **351**: 1213.

Hibbeln JR, Long-chain polyunsaturated fatty acids in depression and related conditions. In: *Phospholipid Spectrum Disorder in Psychiatry,* Peet M, Glen I, Horrobin DF, eds, (Marius Press: Carnforth, UK, 1999) 195–210.

Hibbeln JR, Salem N Jr, Dietary polyunsaturated fatty acids and depression: when cholesterol does not satisfy, *Am J Clin Nutr* (1995) **62**: 1–9.

Hibbeln JR, Linnoila M, Umhau JC, Essential fatty acids predict metabolites of serotonin and dopamine in cerebrospinal fluid among healthy control subjects, and early- and late-onset alcoholics, *Biol Psychiatry* (1998a) **44**: 235–42.

Hibbeln JR, Umhau JC, Linnoila M et al, A replication study of violent and nonviolent subjects: Cerebrospinal fluid metabolites of serotonin and dopamine are predicted by plasma essential fatty acids, *Biol Psychiatry* (1998b) **44:** 243–9.

Hirayama T, *Life-Style and Mortality: A Large Census-Based Cohort Study in Japan* (Karger: Basel, 1990).

Horrobin DF, The roles of prostaglandins and prolactin in depression, mania and schizophrenia, *Postgrad Med J* (1977) (Suppl 4) **53**: 160–5.

Horrobin DF, Nutritional and medical importance of gamma-linolenic acid, *Prog Lipid Res* (1992) **31**: 163–94.

Horrobin DF, Abnormal membrane concentrations of 20 and 22-carbon essential fatty acids: a common link between risk factors and coronary and peripheral vascular disease? *Prostaglandins Leukot Essent Fatty Acids* (1995) **53**: 385–96.

Horrobin DF, The membrane phospholipid hypothesis as a biochemical basis for the neurodevelopmental concept of schizophrenia, *Schizophr Res* (1998) **30**: 193–208.

Horrobin DF, Disorders of phospholipid metabolism in schizophrenia, affective disorders and neurodegenerative disorders. In: *Fatty Acids: Physiological and Behavioral Functions*, Mostofsky DI,

Yehuda S and Salem N, eds, (Humana Press: Totowa, NJ, (2001a) 331–44.

Horrobin DF, Phospholipid metabolism and depression: the possible roles of phospholipase A2 and coenzyme A-independent transacylase, *Hum Psychopharmacol* (2001b) **16**: 45–52.

Horrobin DF, Bennett CN, Depression and bipolar disorder: relationships to impaired fatty acid and phospholipid metabolism and to diabetes, cardiovascular disease, immunological abnormalities, cancer, aging and osteoporosis: possible candidate genes, *Prostaglandins Leukot Essent Fatty Acids* (1999a) **60**: 217–34.

Horrobin DF, Bennett CN, New gene targets related to schizophrenia and other psychiatric disorders: enzymes, binding proteins and transport proteins involved in phospholipid and fatty acid metabolism, *Prostaglandins Leukot Essent Fatty Acids* (1999b) **60**: 111–67.

Horrobin DF, Bennett CN, Peet, M, Correlation between clinical improvement and red cell fatty acid changes when treating schizophrenia with eicosapentaenoic acid, *Schizophr Res* (2001) **49**: 232.

Horrobin DF, Manku MS, Mtabaji JP, A new mechanism of tricyclic antidepressant action. Blockade of prostaglandin-dependent calcium movements, *Postgrad Med J* (1977) (Suppl 4) **53**: 19–23.

Horrobin DF, Glen AI, Vaddadi K, The membrane hypothesis of schizophrenia, *Schizophr Res* (1994) **13**: 195–207.

Horrobin DF, Peet M, A dose-ranging study of ethyl-eicosapentaenoate in treatment-unresponsive depression, *Biol Psychiatry* (2001) **49**: 37S.

Hughes DA, Pinder AC, Piper Z, Johnson IT, Lund EK, Fish oil supplementation inhibits the expression of major histocompatibility complex class II molecules and adhesion molecules on human monocytes, *Am J Clin Nutr* (1996) **63**: 267–72.

Krittayaphong R, Cascio WE, Light KC et al, Heart rate variability in patients with coronary artery disease: differences in patients with higher and lower depression scores, *Psychosom Med* (1997) **59**: 231–5.

Lambert B, Jacquemin C, Synergic effect of insulin and prostaglandin E1 on stimulated lipolysis, *Prostagland Med* (1980) **5**: 375–82.

Leaf A, Kang JX, Omega 3 fatty acids and cardiovascular disease, *World Rev Nutr Diet* (1998) **83**: 24–37.

Lee JY, Sohn KH, Rhee SH, Hwang D, Saturated fatty acids, but not unsaturated fatty acids, induce the expression of cyclooxygenase-2 mediated through Toll-like receptor 4, *J Biol Chem* (2001) **276**: 16683–9.

Lee RE, The influence of psychotropic drugs on prostaglandin biosynthesis, *Prostaglandins* (1974) **5**: 63–8.

Lieb J, Karmali R, Horrobin DF, Elevated levels of prostaglandin E2 and thromboxane B2 in depression, *Prostaglandins Leukot Med* (1983) **10**: 361–7.

Linnoila M, Whorton AR, Rubinow DR et al, CSF prostaglandin levels in depressed and schizophrenic patients, *Arch Gen Psychiatry* (1983) **40**: 405–6.

Lloyd DB, Depression on withdrawal of indomethacin, *Brit J Rheum* (1992) **31**: 211.

Lowinger P, Prostaglandins and organic affective syndrome, *Am J Psychiatry* (1989) **146**: 1646–7.

Lustman PJ, Griffith LS, Gavard JA, Clouse RE, Depression in adults with diabetes, *Diabetes Care* (1992) **15**: 1631–9.

Maes M, Scharpe S, Bosmans E et al, Disturbances in acute phase plasma proteins during melancholia: Additional evidence for the presence of an inflammatory process during that illness, *Prog Psychopharmacol Biol Psychiatry* (1992) **16**: 501–15.

Maes M, Smith R, Christophe A et al, Fatty acid composition in major depression: decreased omega 3 fractions in cholesteryl esters and increased C20:4 omega 6/C20:5 omega 3 ratio in cholesteryl esters and phosopholipids, *J Affective Disord* (1996) **38**: 35–46.

Maes M, Christophe A, Delanghe J et al, Lowered omega-3 polyunsaturated fatty acids in serum phospholipids and cholesteryl esters of depressed patients, *Psychiatry Res* (1999) **85**: 275–91.

Manku MS, Horrobin DF, Chloroquine, quinine, procaine, quinidine and clomipramine are prostaglandin agonists and antagonists, *Prostaglandins* (1976a) **12**: 789–801.

Manku MS, Horrobin DF, Chloroquine, quinine, procaine, quinidine, tricyclic antidepressants, and methylxanthines as prostaglandin agonists and antagonists, *Lancet* (1976b) **ii**: 1115–7.

Marangell LB, Zboyan HA, Cress KK et al, A double blind, placebo-controlled study of docosahexaenoic acid in the treatment of depression, *Inform* (2000) **11**: S78.

Marshall PS, Allergy and depression: a neurochemical threshold model of the relation between the illnesses, *Psychol Bull* (1993) **113**: 23–43.

McGregor JA, Allen KG, Harris MA et al, The omega-3 story: nutritional prevention of preterm birth and other adverse pregnancy outcomes, *Obstet Gynecol Surv* (2001) **56**: S1–13.

Meier CR, Schlienger RG, Jick H, Use of selective serotonin reuptake inhibitors and risk of developing first-time acute myocardial infarction, *Br J Clin Pharmacol* (2001) **52**: 179–84.

Meydani SN, Endres S, Woods MM et al, Oral (n-3) fatty acid supplementation suppresses cytokine production and lymphocyte proliferation: comparison between young and older women, *J Nutr* (1991) **121**: 547–55.

Mills DE, Dietary omega 3 and omega 6 fatty acids and cardiovascular responses to pressor and depressor stimuli, *World Rev Nutr Diet* (1991) **66**: 349–57.

Mtabaji JP, Manku MS, Horrobin DF, Actions of the tricyclic antidepressant clomipramine on responses to pressor agents. Interactions with prostaglandin E2, *Prostaglandins* (1977) **14**: 125–32.

Musselman DL, Tomer A, Manatunga AK et al, Exaggerated platelet reactivity in major depression, *Am J Psychiatry* (1996) **153**: 1313–7.

Nasr S, Altman EG, Meltzer HY, Concordance of atopic and affective disorders, *J Affect Disord* (1981) **3**: 291–6.

Nemeroff CB, Musselman DL, Are platelets the link between depression and ischemic heart disease? *Am Heart J* (2000) **140**: 557–62.

Nemets B, Stahl Z, Belmaker R, Omega-3 fatty acid treatment of depressive breakthrough during unipolar maintenance, *Am J Psychiatry* (2001) in press.

Nemeroff CB, O'Connor CM, Depression as a risk factor for cardiovascular and cerebrovascular disease: Emerging data and clinical perspectives – introduction, *Am Heart J* (2000) **140**: 555–6.

Nishino S, Ueno R, Ohishi K, Sakai T, Hayaishi O, Salivary prostaglandin concentrations: possible state indicators for major depression, *Am J Psychiatry* (1989) **146**: 365–8.

Noaghiul SF, Hibbeln JR, Weissman MM, Seafood consumption and cross-national prevalence rates of bipolar disorders and schizophrenia, *Biol Psychiatry* (2001) **49**: 110S

Ohishi K, Ueno R, Nishino S, Sakai T, Hayaishi O, Increased level of salivary prostaglandins in patients with major depression, *Biol Psychiatry* (1988) **23**: 326–34.

Peet M, Edwards RW, Lipids, depression and physical diseases, *Curr Opinon Psychiatry* (1997) **10**: 477–80.

Peet M, Horrobin DF, A dose-ranging study of the effects of ethyl eicosapentanoate in patients with ongoing depression in spite of apparently adequate treatment with standard drugs, *Arch Gen Psychiatry* (2002) in press.

Peet M, Murphy B, Shay J, Horrobin D, Depletion of omega-3 fatty acid levels in red blood cell membranes of depressive patients, *Biol Psychiatry* (1998) **43**: 315–9.

Piccirillo G, Fimognari FL, Infantino V et al, High plasma concentrations of cortisol and thromboxane B2 in patients with depression, *Am J Med Sci* (1994) **307**: 228–32.

Pratt L, Ford DE, Crum RM et al, Depression, psychotropic medication, and risk of myocardial infarction: prospective date from the Baltimore ECA follow-up, *Circulation* (1996) **94**: 3123–9.

Purasiri P, McKechnie A, Heys SD, Eremin O, Modulation in vitro of human natural cytotoxicity, lymphocyte proliferative response to mitogens and cytokine production by essential fatty acids, *Immunology* (1997) **92**: 166–72.

Puri BK, Counsell SJ, Hamilton G, Richardson AJ, Horrobin DF, Eicosapentaenoic acid (EPA) in treatment-resistant depression associated with symptom remission, structural brain changes and reduced neuronal phospholipid turnover, *Int J Clin Pract* (2001a) **55**: 560–63.

Puri BK, Counsell SJ, Richardson AJ, Horrobin DF, Eicosapentaenoic acid in treatment-resistant depression, *Arch Gen Psychiatry* (2001b) **59**: 91–2

Rechlin T, Weis M, Spitzer A, Kaschka WP, Are affective disorders associated with alterations of heart rate variability? *J Affect Disord* (1994) **32**: 271–5.

Rozanski A, Blumenthal JA, Kaplan J, Impact of psychological factors on the pathogenesis of cardiovascular disease and implications for therapy, *Circulation* (1999) **99**: 2192–217.

Seko C, Relationship between fatty acid composition in blood and depressive symptoms in the elderly, *Jpn J Hyg* (1997) **52**: 539.

Simopoulos AP, Essential fatty acids in health and chronic disease, *Am J Clin Nutr* (1999a) **70**: 560S–9S.

Simopoulos AP, Evolutionary aspects of omega-3 fatty acids in the food supply,

Prostaglandins Leukot Essent Fatty Acids (1999b) **60**: 421–9.

Singh RB, Niaz MA, Sharma JP et al, Randomized, double-blind, placebo-controlled trial of fish oil and mustard oil in patients with suspected acute myocardial infarction: the Indian experiment of infarct survival—4, *Cardiovasc Drugs Ther* (1997) **11**: 485–91.

Smith RS, The macrophage theory of depression, *Med Hypotheses* (1991) **35**: 298-306.

Song C, Lin A, Bonaccorso S et al, The inflammatory response system and the availability of plasma tryptophan in patients with primary sleep disorders and major depression, *J Affect Disord* (1998) **49**: 211–9.

Stanford SC, Salmon P, Mikhail G et al, Plasma catecholamines, pharmacotherapy and mood of subjects with cardiovascular disorder, *J Psychopharmacol* (1999) **13**: 255–60.

Stoll AL, Severus WE, Freeman MP et al, Omega 3 fatty acids in bipolar disorder – A preliminary double-blind, placebo-controlled trial, *Arch Gen Psychiatry* (1999) **56**: 407–12.

Tanskanen A, Hibbeln JR, Hintikka J et al, Fish consumption, depression, and suicidality in a general population, *Arch Gen Psychiatry* (2001) **58**: 512–3.

Voigt RG, Llorente AM, Jensen CL et al, A randomized, double-blind, placebo-controlled trial of docosahexaenoic acid supplementation in children with attention-deficit/hyperactivity disorder, *J Pediatr* (2001) **139**: 189–96.

Winocour PH, Main CJ, Medlicott G, Anderson DC, A psychometric evaluation of adult patients with type 1 (insulin-dependent) diabetes mellitus: prevalence of psychological dysfunction and relationship to demographic variables, metabolic control and complications, *Diabetes Res* (1990) **14**: 171–6.

Yeragani VK, Rao KA, Pohl R, Jampala VC, Balon R, Heart rate and QT variability in children with anxiety disorders: a preliminary report, *Depress Anxiety* (2001) **13**: 72–7.

7
Treatment of affective disorders in cardiovascular disease

Greg Swanwick and Brian A Lawlor

Introduction

The treatment of patients with affective disorders and co-morbid cardio-vascular disease is a complex, and not uncommon, clinical problem. The co-morbidity of these disorders is not simply due to chance but rather reflects complex interactions causing physiological effects in both directions. These relationships have a direct relevance to treatment. They raise the tantalizing, but as yet unproven, possibility that optimum treatment of mood could improve outcome in cardiovascular disease (CaVD) while treatment of vascular disease and vascular risk factors could have a direct impact on 'vascular depression', a form of mood disorder due to cerebrovascular disease. The tolerability, safety and efficacy of various management options and their appropriateness to specific clinical situations will influence the clinician's choice of treatment, or indeed the decision whether to treat at all. Where possible, such decisions should be evidence-based and the purpose of this chapter is to present the available evidence, review current clinical guidelines, and highlight research needs where evidence is lacking.

General principles

History and examination

A thorough physical history and examination are essential to the management of affective disorders. This is particularly the case for the elderly who are at higher risk of virtually all common cardiac pathologies. Cardiovascular disease may not have been previously recognized and further assessment and investigation may be appropriate. Where cardiovascular disease is established, the nature of the problem must be determined with particular attention to current pharmacotherapy.

Polypharmacy and drug interactions

Ideally, polypharmacy with psychotropic drugs should always be avoided but this is particularly important with co-morbid cardiovascular disease. For example, attention should be paid to interactions with drugs that produce alterations in heart rate, electrolyte balance, or that influence the cytochrome P450 system.

Direct effects of psychotropic drugs on the cardiovascular system

The direct effects of psychotropic drugs on the cardiovascular system are many and varied and will be discussed in more detail in the section on specific drugs. Clinically important effects include orthostatic hypotension, hypertension, cardiac muscle depressant effects, tachycardia, bradycardia, arrhythmias, electrocardiograph (ECG) changes, and fluid retention.

Indirect effects

While the more acute direct effects of psychotropics are well recognized, much less is known about the impact of longer-term adverse effects on the cardiovascular system. For example, consideration should be given to the potential of some drugs to induce weight gain or diabetes mellitus. On the other hand, effective management of affective disorders may improve compliance with cardiovascular treatments or smoking cessation.

Effects of cardiovascular drugs on mental state

Whenever psychological symptoms are found in a medical or surgical patient the possibility that they have been induced by medication should be considered. Antihypertensive drugs and corticosteroids, for example, have been implicated in mood disorders (for review see McClelland, 1981; Patten and Love, 1997). Drug classes associated with mood change and mood disorders are shown in Table 7.1.

Start low, go slow

Pharmacokinetic changes associated with cardiovascular disease and ageing must be taken into consideration. There is an age-related increase in the fat : muscle ratio. This results in a greater volume of distribution for lipid-soluble drugs. There is a correlation between increasing age and decreasing renal drug or metabolite clearance. This will assume even greater importance where renal function is compromised by cardiovascular disease. In contrast, there is no clear correlation between ageing and hepatic drug metabolism (although total liver mass and blood flow decrease with age, co-administered drugs and concomitant diseases including heart failure have a much more significant effect). High initial doses and rapid escalation of drug doses should therefore be avoided in established cardiac disease.

Table 7.1.   Drug groups implicated in drug-induced mood change.

Effect	Drug groups implicated
Linked to depression (e.g. Patten and Love, 1997; Rathman et al, 1999)	Steroids, clonidine, calcium channel blockers, and digoxin
Possible link* to depression (e.g. Patten and Love, 1997; Rathman et al, 1999)	Statins, beta blockers, and angiotensin-converting enzyme inhibitors
Possible link* to increased suicide risk (e.g. Lindberg et al, 1998; Toft et al, 2001)	Beta blockers and calcium channel blockers

*Possible link refers to case reports or where data are inconsistent (e.g. for beta blockers and depression, (Patten and Love, 1997) or where there is conflicting evidence [e.g. Lindberg et al (1998) report a link between calcium channel blockers and suicide but Gasse et al (2000) report no link]. Although studies may demonstrate that cardiovascular drugs are associated with an increased risk of depression, interpretation is often confounded by the effect of the cardiovascular morbidity itself.

Specific clinical situations

Myocardial infarction

Among survivors of acute myocardial infarction (MI) both major depression and subsyndromal depressive symptoms are associated with increased mortality independently of other risk factors (Ballenger et al, 2001). On the other hand, there are as yet no data to support a beneficial effect of antidepressant pharmacotherapy on cardiovascular mortality. Inevitably, in the absence of an adequate evidence base there is some variation in published guidelines, but there is a degree of consistency. For example, The Maudsley 2001 Prescribing Guidelines (Taylor et al, 2001) point out that depressive illness 'adversely affects the mortality post-MI and should therefore be actively treated'. They go on to recommend that clinicians should 'avoid all antidepressants if possible for 2 months after MI'! With regard to United Kingdom licensed restrictions post-MI, tricyclic antidepressants (TCAs) and lofepramine are listed as contraindicated in patients with recent MI; moclobemide and sertraline have no restrictions; while other antidepressants carry a range of cautions (Taylor et al, 2001). The International Consensus Group on Depression and Anxiety in a consensus statement on depression, anxiety, and cardiovascular disease (Ballenger et al, 2001) include the following clinical guidelines for primary care: '... risk–benefit analysis suggests that there is no reason not to treat cardiac patients with a safe drug... Intervention is particularly important in the myocardial infarction survivor...'.

(The consensus statement arose from a consensus meeting supported by an unrestricted educational grant from SmithKline Beecham Pharmaceuticals). The authors suggest that the selective serotonin reuptake inhibitors (SSRIs) have a benign cardiovascular profile relative to the TCAs and in support of this cite a comparison of paroxetine and nortriptyline in patients with significant but stable ischaemic heart disease (Roose et al, 1998). Perhaps with greater relevance to acute MI, the Sertraline Antidepressant Heart Attack Trial included patients 5–30 days after acute myocardial infarction and preliminary data did not demonstrate any significant effect on blood pressure or heart rate (Shapiro et al, 1999). A full randomized controlled trial (the Sertraline Antidepressant Heart Attack Recovery Trial, SADHART) will soon report its findings (Ballenger et al, 2001).

Further important data on the potential risks relating to TCA use in the acute MI patient comes from the Cardiac Arrhythmia Suppression Trial (CAST) (The Cardiac Arrhythmia Suppression Trial II Investigators, 1992). CAST was designed to determine whether antiarrhythmic agents would be of benefit in controlling ventricular irritability and arrhythmias post-acute MI. In contrast to expectations there was a significant increase in mortality in those treated with the class 1A compound moricizine (or with type 1Ca agents) compared to placebo. TCAs also have the electrophysiological characteristics of type 1A antiarrhythmics and in the absence of any evidence to the contrary should be assumed to carry a similar risk.

Associated psychotic symptoms are relatively common in late-life depression (a group in which cardiovascular morbidity is also high). These may present as delusions of guilt, nihilistic delusions, hypochondriacal delusions, or tormenting hallucinations. One option is to prescribe an antipsychotic. (Given that psychotic depression is frequently associated with suicidal ideation or a failure to maintain hydration, emergency treatment may be required and electroconvulsive therapy may be a preferable option outside the immediate post-MI period – see below.) Post-MI, damaged myocardial muscle will be more susceptible to the direct cardiac muscle depressant effects of antipsychotics. In addition orthostatic hypotension and tachycardia may cause significant problems. However, the Maudsley guidelines suggest that olanzapine may be a relatively safe choice in the acute post-MI patient as it only rarely causes hypotension (Taylor, 2001).

Psychotherapy, particularly cognitive–behavioural approaches, have been included in post-MI cardiac rehabilitation programmes. As yet there is an insufficient evidence base to make clear recommendations and the results of the ongoing National Institutes of Health sponsored study (Enhanced Recovery in Coronary Heart Disease ENRICHD) are awaited (Ballenger, 20001).

Electroconvulsive therapy (ECT) is relatively containdicated within 3 months of an acute MI, with the greatest risk in the first 10 days (Wilkinson, 1997) – see below.

Angina

The general principle with regard to the pharmacological management of depression co-morbid with angina is to avoid drugs that are known to cause orthostatic hypotension. This is because hypotension may result in rebound tachycardia and thereby exacerbate the angina. Nortriptyline is the least likely of the TCAs to cause orthostatic hypotension (Roose et al, 1981). As already noted antipsychotic drugs can also cause tachycardia and therefore should be used with caution.

Hypertension

Although hypertension is one of the most common cardiovascular conditions there are few studies on the impact of antidepressant therapy on blood pressure control. The majority of antidepressants including the TCAs have little effect on lying systolic or diastolic blood pressure (Roose and Dalack, 1992). An exception is venlafaxine which may result in hypertension at higher doses. However, the choice of antidepressant is important in the treatment of the hypertensive patient. In general this impact lies with the potential for drug interactions. For example, antidepressants that cause orthostatic hypotension may be more problematic in hypertensive patients treated with diuretics, and mirtazepine has been reported to block the anti-hypertensive effect of clonidine.

Arrhythmias and conduction disease

As already discussed, TCAs have properties that are characteristic of type 1A antiarrhythmic compounds. In addition TCAs slow cardiac conduction at therapeutic doses and commonly result in atrioventricular block in overdose. In patients with conduction disease below the atrioventricular node, therapeutic doses of TCAs may cause 2:1 atrioventricular block (Roose and Dalack, 1992). Consequently, other classes such as the SSRIs are preferable in patients with bundle branch block. The potential for antipsychotics to induce arrhythmias is discussed below.

Heart failure

Current evidence suggests that TCAs do not have a negative effect on left ventricular function (Roose and Dalack, 1992). Much more important is the potential indirect effect of psychotropics to cause orthostatic hypotension. Of note, venlafaxine can cause hypertension which may also have a negative effect in cardiac failure. Treatment with lithium can be particularly problematic in patients with heart failure, especially when changes in diuretic therapy are required.

Stroke

Stroke is a common condition, and depression is the most commonly reported post-stroke psychiatric condition (reported rates range from 18 to 61%). In 1984, the first double-blind, placebo-controlled treatment study of post-stroke depression was published by the Robinson group (Lipsey et al, 1984). In a study of 39 patients the nortriptyline group (N=17) had significantly greater reductions in depression rating scores. Since that time, at least four other double-blind randomized studies of treatment of post-stroke depression have been reported. Reding et al (1986) reported that an abnormal dexamethasone suppression test result was associated with significant improvement in the Barthel ADL scores of patients receiving trazodone. Lauritzen et al (1994) reported that imipramine (mean dose 75 mg daily) plus mianserin (mean dose 25 mg daily) was superior to desipramine (mean dose 66 mg daily) plus mianserin (27 mg daily). However, in line with the general principle of avoiding polypharmacy, combination antidepressant therapy should not be considered a first-line approach. Andersen et al (1994) reported significantly greater improvement in patients treated with citalopram (10–40 mg daily) for 3 and 6 weeks vs placebo. Finally, 16 years after the first trial the Robinson group (Robinson et al, 2000) published the first comparison of a TCA with an SSRI. They reported a significantly higher response rate in treating post-stroke depression (PSD) for nortriptyine compared to fluoxetine or placebo.

More controversial is the effect of antidepressant treatment on rehabilitation post stroke. PSD is associated with an increased 10-year mortality, impaired recovery of activities of daily living, greater severity of cognitive impairment, and more impairment of social functioning. However, studies of the effect of successful treatment of PSD on recovery from stroke have been inconsistent. Demonstrating such an effect may depend on the selection of specific subgroups of patients and optimizing the timing of treatment.

Of course patients with stroke are at increased risk of the other cardiovascular conditions already discussed. Hence the results of the treatment studies for PSD must be considered in the context of the guidelines available for those conditions (see above).

Anticoagulation

Patients with depression complicating vascular disease often require anticoagulation, particularly patients with post-stroke depression. Antidepressants can interact with warfarin either by displacing it from plasma proteins or interfering with metabolism at the CYP2D system. The most important mechanism for antidepressant drug interaction with warfarin is via the P450 system; hence this aspect of adverse drug interaction between antidepressants and warfarin is predictable and therefore potentially avoidable. Nefazodone, sertraline, and citalopram have relatively low potential drug interaction with warfarin, whereas fluoxetine and fluvoxamine, paroxetine and moclobemide have a high risk (Duncan et al, 1998; Sayal et al, 2000). In general, it is good practice to check articoagulation control within 7 days of initiating or changing the dose of any antidepressant.

Specific drug groups

In general, the most readily available treatment option for depression is antidepressant medication. Clinicians are less likely to diagnose depression in the physically ill if they do not believe that an effective and safe treatment is available to them (Gill and Hatcher, 2001). Therefore, it is important to examine the evidence as to whether or not antidepressants are effective and safe in the depressed patient with cardiovascular disease.

Antidepressants (see Table 7.2)

Tricyclic antidepressants (TCAs)
Cardiovascular effects of the TCAs include orthostatic hypotension, slowing of cardiac conduction, and electrophysiological properties of type 1A antiarrhythmic agents. TCAs have no significant effect on left ventricular function. Nortriptyline is less likely to cause postural hypotension than other TCAs but has the same effect on cardiac conduction (Roose and Dalack, 1992). Lofepramine is a TCA in structure but both in vitro studies and clinical trials demonstrate that it has a relative lack of anticholinergic side effects (Katona, 1997).

Tetracyclic antidepressant – mianserin
Limited data to date would suggest that mianserin has relatively low cardiotoxicity (Bazire, 1999). However, there is a recognized risk of bone marrow depression and blood tests are recommended every 4 weeks during the first 3 months of therapy and in those who develop infection.

Selective serotonin reuptake inhibitors (SSRIs)
Current evidence indicates that the SSRIs have a safer cardiovascular profile in comparison to the TCAs. However, adverse effects of the SSRIs that may be relatively more common or more problematic in older patients with cardiovascular disease include bradycardia and hyponatraemia (Lebowitz et al, 1997). The syndrome of inappropriate antidiuretic hormone secretion (SIADH) is thought to be an important mechanism underlying the development of hyponatraemia associated with SSRI use. However, in many cases the pathophysiology has not been fully elucidated. All of the SSRIs (and venlafaxine) have been implicated, but it remains unclear whether any specific SSRI is more strongly associated with hyponatraemia. It is also possible that the relationship between older antidepressant drugs and hyponatraemia has been underestimated. Risk factors for the development of SSRI-associated hyponatraemia include increasing age, female gender, and the concomitant

Table 7.2 Summary of major points regarding antidepressant therapy in cardiovascular disease.

Antidepressant	Important cardiac effects	Acute MI	Angina	Heart failure	Post-stroke depression	Other comments
Tricyclics	Increased heart rate, orthostatic hypotension, slowing of cardiac conduction, type 1A antiarrhythmic activity	Avoid	May be best avoided due to potential for hypotension resulting in rebound tachycardia	May be best avoided due to potential for hypotension	Randomized controlled trial evidence supporting use of nortriptyline	Nortriptyline is less likely to cause postural hypotension. Lofepramine has a relative lack of anticholinergic side effects
SSRIs	Limited data to date would suggest that SSRIs are relatively safe but consider hyponatraemia and bradycardia				Randomized controlled trial evidence supporting use of citalopram	
Buproprion	Limited data to date would suggest that it is relatively safe					
MAOIs	Decreased heart rate, orthostatic hypotension, risk of hypertensive crisis, may cause arrhythmias and reduced left ventricular function	May be best avoided due to range of potential cardiac effects	May be best avoided due to range of potential cardiac effects	May be best avoided due to range of potential cardiac effects		Interactions – always carry MAOI card
Moclobemide	Limited data to date would suggest that it is relatively safe					
Mianserin	Limited data to date would suggest that it is relatively safe					Risk of bone marrow depression – blood tests recommended every 4 weeks during first 3 months and in those who develop infection
Mirtazepine	Limited data to date would suggest that it is relatively safe					
Nefazodone	Limited data to date would suggest that it is relatively safe					Rarely blood dyscrasias
Reboxetine	Increased heart rate, orthostatic hypotension at higher doses, rhythm abnormalities and ectopic beats may occur					
Trazodone	Can cause significant postural hypotension and may be arrhythmogenic in those with co-morbid heart disease		Very limited data but need to consider potential impact of important cardiac effects listed in 1st column	Very limited data but need to consider potential impact of important cardiac effects listed in 1st column		
Venlafaxine	Limited data to date would suggest that it is relatively safe but need to monitor BP [especially at higher doses]. Reports of hyponatraemia			Can cause hypertension which may have a negative effect		

use of medications known to cause hyponatraemia (Kirby and Ames, 2001). In the context of cardiovascular disease the concomitant use of SSRIs and thiazide diuretics should be considered a risk factor for hyponatraemia (see Kirby and Ames, 2001 for a review of this topic). Another important consideration is the potential for drug interactions via the cytochrome P450 system. Cardiovascular drugs metabolized by the 2D6 system include beta blockers and antiarrhythmics. Some of the SSRIs can inhibit this enzyme in vitro. The most powerful inhibitor is paroxetine, followed by fluoxetine, sertraline has an intermediate effect, while citalopram and fluvoxamine are the weakest inhibitors (Taylor and Lader, 1996). Substrates for the 3A family include antiarrhythmics and calcium channel blockers. Some of the SSRIs also have an in vitro effect on this enzyme but it is not likely to be clinically relevant.

With regard to safety in overdose, the SSRIs are safer in overdose than the TCAs (Henry et al, 1995). However, it has been suggested that fluvoxamine and citalopram may be more cardiotoxic than the other SSRIs in overdose. Öström et al (1996) reported six deaths following overdoses of citalopram, raising the possibility that this drug could be more intrinsically toxic in overdose than the other SSRIs. However, in all but one of these cases other sedative anxiolytics were taken in combination with citalopram. The fatality involving citalopram taken alone followed ingestion of 4000 mg, giving concentrations which resembled those reported for the only well-documented death from an overdose of fluoxetine taken alone (Glassman, 1997). Furthermore these six deaths may be viewed in the context of the extremely small number of successful suicides associated with citalopram overdose (Isacsson and Bergman, 1996). Personne et al (1997a) reported widened QRS complexes in the ECG and/or convulsions in about a third of patients who had taken 600–1800 mg of citalopram and in all of those who had taken more than 1900 mg. However, they have concluded that clinically significant arrhythmias are very rare (Personne et al, 1997b). Fluvoxamine has also been associated with limited ECG changes (Taylor et al, 2001). Overdoses of the other SSRIs have not been associated with convulsions or clinically significant ECG abnormalities (Dechant and Clissold, 1991; Henry, 1991; Borys et al, 1992; Klein-Schwartz and Anderson, 1996) although the amounts ingested may have been lower than those involved in the citalopram fatalities (Glassman, 1997).

Other antidepressants

Bupropion: One small study (N=36) of co-morbid depression and cardiac disease did not detect any significant effect on heart rate, conduction, or left ventricular function. Neither was there any significant orthostatic hypotension or antiarrhythmic activity (Roose et al, 1991).

Mirtazepine: Minimal changes in heart rate and blood pressure have been noted (Smith et al, 1990). Limited data to date would suggest that it is relatively safe (Bazire, 1999).

Moclobemide: There are a number of case reports of hypertension associated with moclobemide.

Monoamine oxidase inhibitors (MAOIs): This group of drugs should be used with caution as there is a risk of postural hypotension and of hypertensive crisis. In addition they may cause arrhythmias and impair left ventricular function.

Nefazodone: Postural hypotension may occur. In vitro nefazodone inhibits cytochrome P450 3A4.

Reboxetine: Significant increases in heart rate have been noted. Also, significant orthostatic hypotension occurs at higher doses.

Trazodone: The best-known cardiac effect is that it can cause significant postural hypotension. However, there are also case reports of arrhythmias; it has a variable effect on heart rate; it can prolong the QTc interval; and it may be arrhythmogenic in patients with co-morbid cardiovascular disease.

Venlafaxine: The best-known cardiac effect is hypertension at higher doses. However, it also may cause hyponatraemia, postural hypotension, and a marginal increase in heart rate. There are reports of cardiac arrhythmias, conduction abnormalities, and possible QTc prolongation in overdose.

Antipsychotics

The conventional or 'typical' antipsychotics are associated with significant autonomic and cardiovascular effects. These cardiac effects may be either direct or secondary to hypotension and anticholinergic-induced tachycardia. The most serious direct effects are the quinidine-like changes that can be observed on ECG. These include QT prolongation, altered T-wave morphology, and widening of the QRS complex. Patients receiving some antipsychotic drugs are at particular risk for torsade de pointes arrhythmia (Arana, 2000). This describes the ventricular arrhythmia that results in the progressive twisting of the QRS axis around an imaginary baseline associated with a prolonged QT interval in the last sinus beat preceding the onset of the arrhythmia. Corrected QT interval (QTc) prolongation is a frequent occurrence with many antipsychotics and its true clinical significance is not completely clear. However, the balance of cardiological opinion suggests that the longer the QTc interval the higher the risk of an arrhythmia occurring. Co-incident cardiac damage, other drugs (prescribed and illicit), and electrolyte disturbance may all contribute to the problem. With regard to pimozide, the UK Committee on the Safety of Medicines has had over 40 reports, including 16 fatalities, of serious cardiac events secondary to pimozide and guidance is that pimozide is contra-indicated in the presence of known cardiac disease (Bazire, 1999). Similarly, droperidol has been withdrawn and the indications for thioridazine have been restricted to second-line treatment in adult schizophrenia due to concerns regarding sudden deaths and QTc change. However, not all conventional antipsychotics have been implicated and the FDA is quoted as saying '...we have an abundance of data from multiple independent development programs showing no difference between haloperidol [at doses up to 15 mg / day] and placebo on QTc.' (FDA, 2000a)

With the exception of sertindole and possibly ziprasidone there is less evidence to suggest that atypical neuroleptics significantly alter the QTc interval in patients treated for psychotic depression. Sertindole, an atypical antipsychotic, was voluntarily suspended in the European Union in 1998 following regulatory concerns over reports of serious cardiac dysrhythmias and sudden unexpected deaths. The Pfizer Study 54 (FDA, 2000b) compared the effects of thioridazine, haloperidol, and four atypical antipsychotics (olanzapine, risperidone, quetiapine, and ziprasidone) on QTc. The study demonstrated no significant difference in mean QTc change between the haloperidol, olanzapine, risperidone, and quetiapine groups (Figure 7.1).

The effect of clozapine on QTc appears to be similar to that of risperidone, quetiapine, and olanzapine (Gury et al, 2000). However, clozapine is associated with other potentially significant cardiovascular effects, including tachycardia and hypotension (Buckley and Sanders, 2000), severe cardiorespiratory dysregulation when used in combination with benzodiazepines (Grohmann et al, 1989), and it may also be associated with potentially fatal myocarditis and cardiomyopathy in physically healthy young adults with schizophrenia (Killian et al, 1999; Buckley and Sanders, 2000). No significant cardiovascular changes have been reported in short- and long-term studies of amisulpiride (Agelink et al, 2001).

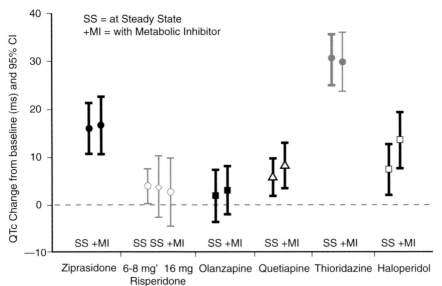

Figure 7.1

Pfizer Study 54: Mean QTc change from baseline in the absence and presence of metabolic inhibitor.

Of course it is possible that the adverse cardiac effects of the newer atypical antipsychotics may become apparent after a longer period of use in a broader population of patients including those at an increased risk of cardiac toxicity. It must also be remembered that in the management of psychosis associated with mood disorder it is likely that antipsychotics may be used in combination with other psychotropics. In such circumstances the potential for significant cardiac effects will be increased.

Mood stabilizers

Lithium

The potential effects of lithium include T-wave flattening, T-wave inversion, ventricular ectopics, congestive myopathy, bradycardia, and conduction changes. T-wave changes may be benign and can disappear with continued therapy (Taylor et al, 2001). Although licensed restrictions list cardiovascular disease as a contraindication, Ahrens et al (1995) have suggested that the excess cardiovascular and suicide mortality of affective disorders may actually be reduced by lithium prophylaxis. The Maudsley guidelines state that lithium is contraindicated in cardiac failure and sick sinus syndrome and that it should be used with caution in patients with pre-existing conduction abnormalities (Taylor et al, 2001). In clinical practice drug interactions may pose the greatest difficulties. In particular changes in diuretic therapy will alter lithium clearance. Baseline ECG with regular follow-up monitoring would seem a sensible precaution in patients with cardiovascular risk factors.

Carbamazepine

Cardiovascular effects of carbamazepine are uncommon but well recognized. A number of case reports of conduction changes have been published and one review of these suggested that there may be two distinct forms of carbamazepine-associated cardiac dysfunction: one patient group exhibits sinus tachycardias in the setting of carbamazepine overdose; the second group consists primarily of elderly women who develop potentially life-threatening bradyarrhythmias or atrioventricular conduction delay associated with either therapeutic or modestly elevated carbamazepine serum levels (Kasarskis et al, 1992). Carbamazepine therapy may also be complicated by hyponatraemia.

Sodium valproate

The most important consideration is the possibility of drug interactions. For example, sodium valproate potentiates the activity of aspirin and warfarin.

Verapamil (Nimodipine)

Potentially serious or fatal cardiovascular side effects include hypotension, bradycardia, atrioventricular block, and interaction with other hypotensives, antiarrhythmics, digoxin, and beta blockers.

Anxiolytics / hypnotics

Benzodiazepines

Benzodiazepines are relatively safe but are contraindicated in acute pulmonary insufficiency that may be associated with cardiovascular disease. One study of temazepam in 12 elderly patients reported a fall in systolic blood pressure and an increase in heart rate (Ford et al, 1990). Another study of temazepam in healthy males demonstrated orthostatic reflex changes, but these did not impair the maintenance of arterial blood pressure in these healthy subjects (Patrick et al, 1987). In a study of seven healthy volunteers Vogel et al (1996) demonstrated significant heart rate increase and heart period variability decreases consistent with a vagolytic effect of lorazepam during 24 h of normal physiological activity.

Buspirone

The occurrence of hypertension in patients receiving both buspirone and MAOIs (phenelzine and tranylcypramine) has been reported.

Non-benzodiazepine hypnotics

Zaleplon, zolpidem, and zopiclone are safe from a cardiovascular point of view as sedative hypnotics. In a study of the cardiovascular and respiratory effects of chlormethiazole on patients and volunteers, Scott (1986) reported that the only significant effect was an increase in heart rate. However, chlormethiazole is contraindicated in acute pulmonary insufficiency and should be used with caution in patients with chronic pulmonary insufficiency (Bazire, 1999).

Other treatments

Psychotherapy

As indicated in a recent review by Musselman et al (1998), stress management and behavioural counselling programmes have had mixed results in patients with cardiovascular disease. Some have been associated with reduced risk of recurrent cardiovascular events (Friedman et al, 1986) and increased rates of long-term (5-year) survival (Frasure-Smith and Prince, 1985; Frasure-Smith, 1991; Frasure-Smith et al, 1992). However, more recent studies have reported no benefit to patients (Jones and West, 1996; Taylor et al, 1997) and even a worse outcome for women in comparison with usual care (Frasure-Smith et al, 1997). As pointed out by Frasure-Smith et al (1997), it should not be forgotten that psychosocial and psychotherapeutic treatment can have adverse psychological effects for some patients. Despite their intuitive appeal, these types of intervention may not be completely benign, as also demonstrated in the Gospel Oak Study (Blanchard et al, 1995). In this study of the effect of a primary care nurse intervention upon older people screened as depressed, requests for interventions to increase patient's social networks were found to be difficult to implement due to patient's refusal to attend clubs or day centres (Blanchard et al, 1995). Frasure-Smith et al (1997) conclude that their results do not warrant the routine implementation of psychological-distress screening and home nursing intervention for post-MI patients. As noted in the International Consensus Group on Depression and Anxiety consensus statement, cognitive–behavioural interventions are potentially of great interest. However, the results of the ENRICHD or other similar studies are required before clear recommendations can be made (Ballenger et al, 2001). The ENRICHD study is a multicentre, randomized, controlled clinical trial of a cognitive–behavioural treatment for depression and low social support in post-MI patients (ENRICHD investigators, 2001). A total of 2481 patients have been recruited to this 4- – 5-year follow-up study. Key features of the intervention include the integration of cognitive–behavioural and social learning approaches to the management of depression and of problems that can contribute to low social support. The study aims to provide rapid initiation of treatment after MI using a combination of individual and group modalities. If the initial cognitive–behavioural approach is ineffective or if patients relapse the study makes provision for drug treatment.

Electroconvulsive therapy (ECT)

Indications for ECT include the need for a rapid response, cases where the risks of other treatments outweigh the risks of ECT, resistance to or intolerance of medication, a past history of a good response to ECT, and patient preference for ECT. Points to remember are that in the absence of continuation therapy following ECT, the vast majority of patients will relapse within 6 months. Therefore, pharmacotherapy to prevent relapse needs to take account of medication resistance or intolerance where these have been the indication for ECT in the first instance.

There appears to be a general consensus of opinion that there are no absolute contraindications to ECT. However, cardiovascular events are the leading cause of morbidity and mortality post-ECT and patients with known cardiac disease do have an increased risk of cardiac complications during ECT. Hence the situation is one of assessing the relative risk of complications vs the morbidity and mortality of untreated depression itself. ECT has been used safely in patients with impaired cardiac output (ejection fraction 20–25%) (Stern et al, 1997), with cardiac aneurysm (Gardner et al, 1997), post-stroke depression (Murray et al, 1986), with aortic aneurysm (Attar-Levy et al, 1995), with aortic stenosis (Rasmussen, 1997), in those with atrial fibrillation and on anticoagulant therapy (Petrides and Fink, 1996), and in those with implanted cardiac pacemakers (Alexopoulos and Frances, 1980).

Nevertheless precautions are advisable in the elderly and in those with known cardiovascular disease. The cardiovascular status should be assessed prior to ECT by an experienced physician, staff trained in cardiopulmonary resuscitation and the emergency treatment of arrhythmias should be available, and ECG monitoring before, during, and for at least 15 min post-ECT should be considered. Various techniques can be used to modify the cardiovascular response and post-ECT elevations in blood pressure and heart rate (e.g. Stoudemire et al, 1990; Stern et al, 1997). Recent MI (within 3 months) and aortic aneurysm are relative contraindications, and wherever possible ECT should be avoided with cerebral aneurysm or a history of cerebral haemorrhage (Royal College of Psychiatrists, 1995). Full muscular relaxation is important in a patient with an abdominal aortic aneurysm. Patients with pacemakers should have them checked prior to treatment for breaks in wires or faulty insulation. During ECT the patient and monitoring equipment should be completely insulated from the ground.

Research questions

The nature of depression in cardiovascular disease – lack of randomized clinical trials

'Clinicians often withhold potentially effective antidepressant drugs because they assume that the medical illness caused the depression, or they consider the medical illness to be a contraindication to antidepressant drug treatment' (Song et al, 1993). There is continuing debate regarding the status of affective disorders in patients with symptomatic cardiac disease. In turn this leads to uncertainty as to whether such symptoms are 'understandable' in the context of the individual's physical ill-health or whether they reflect a 'real' mental disorder. In clinical practice it is often impossible to be certain about the status of anxiety or depressive symptoms in an individual patient with cardiovascular disease or other physical illness. In the end, clinical practice often comes down to a decision whether a patient with significant heart disease and persistent affective symptoms should receive a trial of treatment. Unfortunately, in such situations there is considerable uncertainty about optimum management of affective disorders. This is due, at least in part, to the fact that most treatment trials of depression exclude the physically ill.

Against this background a recent Cochrane review (Gill and Hatcher, 2000) addressed the issue of antidepressant treatment in the physically ill, including those with cardiovascular disease. The review concluded that treating the depressed physically ill with antidepressants was effective. Furthermore, there was no difference between placebo and antidepressants in the number of people who dropped out of studies. However, it is notable that only one study specifically addressing heart disease (Veith et al, 1982) met the inclusion / exclusion criteria for the meta-analysis. Hence, there is a clear need for randomized, placebo-controlled clinical trials in this area. It is of some comfort that the SADHART and ENRICHD trials are ongoing, but these will address only some of the unanswered research needs.

Vascular depression

A related issue is the uncertainty regarding the optimum management of 'vascular depression'. For a significant percentage of patients with late-life depression cerebrovascular disease may be an important aetiological factor (Alexopoulos et al, 1997). This concept of 'vascular depression' is supported by the high rate of depression associated with hypertension, diabetes, and heart disease; the high prevalence of depression following stroke; the frequent findings on neuroimaging of silent vascular lesions in late-life depression; and the infrequent family history of affective disorder in those with depression and silent vascular lesions. However, with regard to course, management, and outcome, the results of studies to date have been contradictory and no firm conclusions can be drawn (Krishnan, 1999).

Long-term effects

There are virtually no medium- or long-term clinical trial data on which to base recommendations regarding safety and effectiveness of drug therapies for the long-term maintenance or prophylaxis of affective disorders in cardiac patients. Compared to adverse event data from acute treatment trials, much less is known about the impact of longer-term adverse effects on the cardiovascular system. In particular, consideration should be given to the long-term impact of some of the more 'minor' or indirect effects such as mild increases in heart rate or the potential of some drugs to induce weight gain or diabetes mellitus. On the other hand, effective management of affective disorders may improve compliance with cardiovascular treatments or smoking cessation.

Promising questions for future research

The most pressing needs include the development of treatment algorithms, identification of the most useful approaches in dealing with patients who have complex co-morbidity, development of psychotherapeutic approaches tailored to the physical illness / disability status of the patient, assessment of the long-term efficacy / safety of continuation and maintenance therapies, and the clarification of the interaction between vascular disease and other factors in the aetiology and pathophysiology of affective disorders.

Conclusions

Despite the lack of an adequate evidence base, there is a degree of consistency across published guidelines with regard to the management of affective disorders in patients with cardiovascular disease. There is no reason not to treat cardiac patients with safe treatments. There are limited, well-controlled data to support the use of some agents (particularly the SSRIs). There is a general consensus that ECT can be used when clinically indicated. Consequently, there are grounds for clinicians to believe that management of psychiatric morbidity in cardiac patients is both worthwhile and safe. Patients with cardiovascular disease should therefore be routinely screened for affective disorders.

References

Agelink MW, Majewski T, Wurthmann C et al, Effects of newer atypical antipsychotics on autonomic neurocardiac function: a comparison between amisulpride, olanzapine, sertindole, and clozapine, *J Clin Psychopharmacol* (2001) **21**:8–13.

Ahrens B, Muller-Oerlinghausen B, Schou M et al, Excess cardiovascular and suicide mortality of affective disorders may be reduced by lithium prophylaxis, *J Affect Disord* (1995) **33**: 67–75.

Alexopoulos GS, Frances RJ, ECT and cardiac patients with pacemakers, *Am J Psychiatry* (1980) **137**: 1111–2.

Alexopoulos GS, Meyers BS, Young RC et al, 'Vascular depression' hypothesis, *Arch Gen Psychiatry* (1997) **54**:915–22.

Andersen G, Vestergaard K, Lauritzen L, Effective treatment of poststroke depression with the selective serotonin reuptake inhibitor citalopram, *Stroke* (1994) **25**:1099–104.

Arana GW, An overview of side effects caused by typical antipsychotics, *J Clin Psychiatry* (2000) **61** Suppl 8: 5–11.

Attar-Levy D, Fidelle G, Brochier P, Van Steenbruge L, Loo H, [Electroconvulsive therapy and aortic aneurysm: apropos of a case.] [Article in French] *Encephale* (1995) **21**:473–6.

Ballenger JC, Davidson JR, Lecrubier Y et al, Consensus statement on transcultural issues in depression and anxiety from the International Consensus Group on Depression and Anxiety, *J Clin Psychiatry* (2001) **62** (Suppl) 13:47–55.

Bazire S, *Psychotropic Drug Directory 1999* (Quay Books Division Mark Allen Publishing Ltd: Dinton, 1999).

Blanchard MR, Waterreus A, Mann AH, The effect of primary care nurse intervention upon older people screened as depressed, *Int J Geriatric Psychiatry* (1995) **10**: 289–98.

Borys DJ, Setzer SC, Ling LJ et al, Acute fluoxetine overdose: a report of 234 cases, *Am J Emerg Med* (1992) **10**:115–20.

Buckley NA, Sanders P, Cardiovascular adverse effects of antipsychotic drugs, *Drug Saf* (2000) **23**:215–28.

Cardiac Arrhythmia Suppression Trial II Investigators, Effect of the antiarrhythmic agent moricizine on survival after myocardial infarction, *N Engl J Med* (1992) **327**:227–33.

Dechant KL, Clissold SP, Paroxetine. A review of its pharmacodynamic and pharmacokinetic properties, and therapeutic potential in depressive illness, *Drugs* (1991) **4**:225–53.

Duncan D, Sayal K, McConnell H, Taylor D, Antidepressant interactions with warfarin, *Int Clin Psychopharmacol* (1998) **13**:87–94.

ENRICHD Investigators, Enhancing Recovery in Coronary Heart Disease (ENRICHD) study intervention: rationale and design, *Psychosom Med* (2001) **63**:747–55.

FDA, (2000a) FDA background on Zeldox™ (ziprasidone hydrochloride capsules) Pfizer, Inc. http://www.fda.gov/ohrms/dockets/ac/00/backgrd/3619b1a.pdf

FDA (2000b) FDA background on Zeldox™ (ziprasidone hydrochloride capsules) Pfizer, Inc. http://www.fda.gov/ohrms/dockets/ac/00/backgrd/3619b1b.pdf

Ford GA, Hoffman BB, Blaschke TF, Effect of temazepam on blood pressure regulation in healthy elderly subjects, *Br J Clin Pharmacol* (1990) **29**:61–7.

Frasure-Smith N, Prince R, The ischemic heart disease life stress monitoring program: impact on mortality, *Psychosom Med* (1985) **47**:431–45.

Frasure-Smith N, In-hospital symptoms of psychological stress as predictors of long-term outcome after acute myocardial infarction in men, *Am J Cardiol* (1991) **67**:121–7.

Frasure-Smith N, Lesperance F, Juneau M, Differential long-term impact of in-hospital symptoms of psychological stress after non-Q-wave and Q-wave acute myocardial infarction, *Am J Cardiol* (1992) **69**:1128–34.

Frasure-Smith N, Lesperance F, Prince RH et al, Randomised trial of home-based psychosocial nursing intervention for patients recovering from myocardial infarction, *Lancet* (1997) **350**:473–9.

Friedman M, Thoresen CE, Gill JJ et al, Alteration of type A behavior and its effect on cardiac recurrences in post myocardial infarction patients: summary results of the recurrent coronary prevention project, *Am Heart J* (1986) **112**:653–65.

Gardner MW, Kellner CH, Hood DE, Hendrix GH, Safe administration of ECT in a patient with a cardiac aneurysm and multiple cardiac risk factors, *Convuls Ther* (1997) **13**:200–3.

Gasse C, Derby LE, Vasilakis C, Jick H, Risk of suicide among users of calcium channel blockers: population based, nested case-control study, *BMJ* (2000) **320**:1251.

Gill D, Hatcher S, Antidepressants for depression in people with physical illness. [Systematic Review] Cochrane Depression Anxiety and Neurosis Group Cochrane Database of Systematic Reviews (2001) Issue 2.

Glassman AH, Citalopram toxicity, *Lancet* (1997) **350**:818.

Grohmann R, Ruther E, Sassim N, Schmidt LG, Adverse effects of clozapine, *Psychopharmacology* (Berl) (1989) **99**: Suppl:S101–4.

Gury C, Canceil O, Iaria P, [Antipsychotic drugs and cardiovascular safety: current studies of prolonged QT interval and risk of ventricular arrhythmia] [Article in French] *Encephale* (2000) **26**:62–72.

Henry JA, Overdose and safety with fluroxamine, *Int Clin Psychopharmacol* (1991) **6**(Suppl 3): 41–5.

Henry JA, Alexander CA, Sener EK, Relative mortality from overdose of antidepressants, *BMJ* (1995) **310**:221–4.

Isacsson G, Bergman U, Risks with citalopram in perspective, *Lancet* (1996) **348**:1033.

Jones DA, West RR, Psychological rehabilitation after myocardial infarction: multicentre randomised controlled trial, *BMJ* (1996) **313**:1517–21.

Kasarskis EJ, Kuo CS, Berger R, Nelson KR, Carbamazepine-induced cardiac dysfunction. Characterization of two distinct clinical syndromes, *Arch Intern Med* (1992) **52**:186–91.

Katona CLE, New antidepressants in the elderly. In: Holmes C, Howard R, eds, *Advances in Old Age Psychiatry Chromosomes to Community Care* (Wrightson Biomedical Publishing Ltd: Petersfield, UK, 1997)) 143–60.

Killian JG, Kerr K, Lawrence C, Celermajer DS, Myocarditis and cardiomyopathy associated with clozapine, *Lancet* (1999) **354**:1841–5

Kirby D, Ames D, Hyponatraemia and selective serotonin re-uptake inhibitors in elderly patients, *Int J Geriatr Psychiatry* (2001) **16**:484–93.

Klein-Schwartz W, Anderson B, Analysis of sertraline-only overdoses, *Am J Emerg Med* (1996) **14**:456–8.

Krishnan R, Depression and vascular disease. Presented at the 9th Congress of the International Psychogeriatric

Association, Vancouver, 15–20 Aug 1999.

Lauritzen L, Bendsen BB, Vilmar T et al, Post-stroke depression: combined treatment with imipramine or desipramine and mianserin. A controlled clinical study, *Psychopharmacology* (1994) **114**:119–22.

Lebowitz BD, Pearson JL, Schneider LS et al, Diagnosis and treatment of depression in late life, consensus statement update, *JAMA* (1997) **278**:1186–90.

Lindberg G, Bingefors K, Ranstam J, Rastam L, Melander A, Use of calcium channel blockers and risk of suicide: ecological findings confirmed in population based cohort study, *BMJ* (1998) **316**:741–5.

Lipsey JR, Robinson RG, Pearlson GD, Rao K, Price TR, Nortriptyline treatment of post-stroke depression: a double blind treatment trial, *Lancet* (1984) **i**:297–300.

McClelland HA, Psychiatric disorders. In: Davies DM, ed, *Textbook of Adverse Drug Reactions, 2nd edn* (Oxford University Press: Oxford, 1981)

Murray GB, Shea V, Conn DK, Electroconvulsive therapy for poststroke depression, *J Clin Psychiatry* (1996) **47**:258–60.

Musselman DL, Evans DL, Nemeroff CB, The relationship of depression to cardiovascular disease: epidemiology, biology, and treatment, *Arch Gen Psychiatry* (1998) **55**:580–92.

Öström M, Eriksson A, Thorson J, Spigset O, Fatal overdose with citalopram, *Lancet* (1996) **348**:339–40.

Patten SB, Love EJ, Drug-induced depression, *Psychother Psychosom* (1997) **66**:63–73.

Patrick JM, Dikshit MB, Macdonald IA, Fentem PH, Human orthostatic reflexes after taking temazepam at night, *Br J Clin Pharmacol* (1987) **24**:799–807.

Personne M, Sjoberg G, Persson H, Citalopram overdose—review of cases treated in Swedish hospitals, *J Toxicol Clin Toxicol* (1997a) **35:**237–40.

Personne M, Persson H, Sjoberg E, Citalopram toxicity, *Lancet* (1997b) **350**:518–9.

Petrides G, Fink M, Atrial fibrillation, anticoagulation, and electroconvulsive therapy, *Convuls Ther* (1996) **12**:91–8.

Rasmussen KG, Electroconvulsive therapy in patients with aortic stenosis, *Convuls Ther* (1997) **13**:196–9.

Rathmann W, Haastert B, Roseman JM, Giani G, Cardiovascular drug prescriptions and risk of depression in diabetic patients, *J Clin Epidemiol* (1999) **52**:1103–9.

Reding MJ, Orto LA, Winter SW et al, Antidepressant therapy after stroke. A double-blind trial, *Arch Neurol* (1986) **43**:763–5.

Robinson RG, Schultz SK, Castillo C et al, Nortriptyline versus fluoxetine in the treatment of depression and in short term recovery after stroke: a placebo-controlled, double-blind study, *Am J Psychiatry* (2000) **157**:351–9.

Roose SP, Dalack GW, Treating the depressed patient with cardiovascular problems, *J Clin Psychiatry* (1992) **53** Suppl:25–31.

Roose SP, Glassman AH, Siris SG et al, Comparison of imipramine- and nortriptyline-induced orthostatic hypotension: a meaningful difference, *J Clin Psychopharmacol* (1981) **1**:316–9.

Roose SP, Dalack GW, Glassman AH et al, Cardiovascular effects of bupropion in depressed patients with heart disease, *Am J Psychiatry* (1991) **148**:512–6.

Roose SP, Laghrissi-Thode F, Kennedy JS et al, Comparison of paroxetine and nortriptyline in depressed patients with ischemic heart disease, *JAMA* (1998) **279**:287–91.

Royal College of Psychiatrists, *The ECT Handbook (Second Report of the Royal College of Psychiatrists' Special Committee on ECT) Council Report CR39* (Royal College of Psychiatrists: London, 1995).

Sayal KS, Duncan-McConnell DA, McConnell HW, Taylor DM, Psychotropic interactions with warfarin, *Acta Psychiatr Scand* (2000) **102**:250–5.

Scott DB, Circulatory and respiratory effects of chlormethiazole, *Acta Psychiatr Scand* (1986) **329** Suppl: 28–31.

Shapiro PA, Lesperance F, Frasure-Smith N et al, An open-label preliminary trial of sertraline for treatment of major depression after acute myocardial infarction. Sertraline Anti-Depressant Heart Attack Trial (SADHAT). *Am Heart J* (1999) **137**:1100–6.

Smith WT, Glaudin V, Panagides J, Gilvary E, Mirtazapine vs. amitriptyline vs. placebo in the treatment of major depressive disorder, *Psychopharmacol Bull* (1990) **26**:191–6.

Song F, Freemantle N, Sheldon TA et al, Selective serotonin reuptake inhibitors: meta-analysis of efficacy and acceptability, *BMJ* (1993) **306:**683–7.

Stern L, Hirschmann S, Grunhaus L, ECT in patients with major depressive disorder and low cardiac output, *Convuls Ther* (1997) **13**:68–73.

Stoudemire A, Knos G, Gladson M et al, Labetalol in the control of cardiovascular responses to electroconvulsive therapy in high-risk depressed medical patients, *J Clin Psychiatry* (1990) **51**:508–12.

Taylor CB, Miller NH, Smith PM, DeBusk RF, The effect of a home-based, case-managed, multifactorial risk-reduction program on reducing psychological distress in patients with cardiovascular disease, *J Cardiopulm Rehabil* (1997) **17**:157–62.

Taylor D, Lader M, Cytochromes and psychotropic drug interactions, *Br J Psychiatry* (1996) **168**:529–32.

Taylor D, McConnell H, McConnell D, Kerwin R, *The Maudsley 2001 Prescribing Guidelines* (Martin Dunitz: London, 2001).

Toft Sorensen H, Mellemkjaer L, Olsen JH, Risk of suicide in users of beta-adrenoceptor blockers, calcium channel blockers and angiotensin converting enzyme inhibitors, *Br J Clin Pharmacol* (2001) **52**:313–8.

Veith RC, Raskind MA, Caldwell JH et al, Cardiovasculareffects of tricyclic antidepressants in depressed patients with chronic heart disease, *N Engl J Med* (1982) **306**:954–9.

Vogel LR, Muskin PR, Collins ED, Sloan RP, Lorazepam reduces cardiac vagal modulation in normal subjects, *J Clin Psychopharmacol* (1996) **16**:449–53.

Wilkinson D, ECT in the elderly. In: Holmes C, Howard R, eds, *Advances in Old Age Psychiatry Chromosomes to Community Care* (Wrightson Biomedical Publishing Ltd: Petersfield, UK, 1997) 161–71.

Cerebrovascular Disease and Affective Disorders

8
Methodology of studying affective disorders in cerebrovascular disease

Carol J Schramke

Why study vascular disease and depression?

In spite of advancements in the prevention of stroke and a declining prevalence over the last 30 years, it is estimated that 500 000 Americans are affected by stroke annually and it is believed that these rates are similar or even higher in other parts of the world (Adams et al, 1998). Although there is normally some degree of recovery of physical and cognitive functioning following stroke, there is little to be done to repair or replace lost neurons. As a result, much of the damage from stroke is irreparable. Depression is recognized as a fairly common problem following stroke, with incidence estimates typically ranging from 20 to 50% (Morris et al, 1990), although Spencer et al (1997), in their review of the literature, found reported prevalence rates from 3 to 68%. Post-stroke depression (PSD), unlike many of the other symptoms and sequelae of stroke, may be treated and cured.

Vascular dementia is thought to be the second most common form of dementia, after senile dementia of the Alzheimer's type, and depression appears to be more common in vascular dementia than Alzheimer's (Metter and Wilson, 1993). The exact prevalence rate is not clear, with reported prevalence estimates for depression in patients with vascular dementia ranging from 0 to 71%, with a mean of approximately 30% (McPherson and Cummings, 1997). Similarly, although there is little to offer patients with regards to ameliorating the cognitive and motor deficits that are caused by vascular dementia, behaviour and quality of life may improve substantially with treatment of depression. Research aimed at improving our ability to identify and understand these affective disorders and problems with mood will help us to take advantage of this opportunity for meaningful intervention.

Most of the detailed research dealing with vascular disease and depression has focused on PSD. A Medline search for articles between 1960 and 2001 referencing stroke and depression yielded 1378 articles, compared to 812 articles referencing Alzheimer's and depression and 155 referencing multi-infarct dementia and depression. The primary questions that have been explored in the study of stroke and depression, and about which there continues to be significant disagreement, include: 1) what is the incidence of depression in patients with stroke and what factors influence the prevalence of stroke?

2) what is the natural course of depression following stroke – what symptoms do these patients show, what happens to patients who are not treated with regards to spontaneous remission and development of other problems? 3) how does depression affect mortality, recovery in other domains, and overall level of functioning? and 4) what treatments are appropriate and effective for PSD? Although there has been some research completed in all these areas, there has been considerable variability in results between studies and relatively little research on some of the issues that are most important for patient care (e.g. treatment). There is also considerable variability in how exacting this research has been with regards to controlling the multiple factors that may greatly influence the results of these investigations.

Issues with studying patients with vascular disease

At least some of the variability between studies can be attributed to differences in the populations sampled. Stroke is not a uniform disorder and research in this area can be further complicated by the fact that patients with stroke frequently have multiple other health problems, many of which may also affect the brain, physical abilities, cognitive functioning, and other variables of interest. Factors that have been found to influence the prevalence of depression following stroke include time since stroke, the type of stroke (e.g. haemorrhagic or ischaemic), lesion size, lesion location (e.g. right or left hemisphere or bilateral, anterior or posterior, and cortical or subcortical), gender, age, psychiatric history of the patient prior to stroke, and family history of affective disorder. It is reasonable to expect that socioeconomic variables (e.g. income level and psychosocial support), which have been shown to influence the incidence of depression in other populations, would influence the development of mood disorders in this population as well. Nonetheless, these variables have not been systematically studied or routinely assessed in the PSD literature.

In order to understand better PSD and the factors that influence the occurrence and course of this disorder, we need to attend to population characteristics that can alter the findings. There are likely to be systematic differences, related to differences in type, location, and severity of stroke, between patients who are or are not admitted to hospital for stroke, sent to a rehabilitation facility, or referred to a neurologist. Studies sampling only patients admitted to hospital or including only patients who are acutely hospitalized for a sufficient period to be assessed for depression are likely to sample a different subset of post-stroke patients compared to studies recruiting from outpatient samples presenting to a neurologist or studies that recruit only patients who are impaired enough to require intensive rehabilitation services.

Investigators must also contend with sample bias due to factors, clearly related to stroke, that can influence the likelihood that patients will agree to participate in research studies. Patients who have problems with ambulation or speech, as well as patients who are depressed, can be expected to be less likely to volunteer or consent to a study that requires them to walk or talk for lengthy time periods. Although not systematically studied in the PSD litera-ture, based on research examining depression in older adults it appears that individuals who are of lower socioeconomic status, who are more physically ill, and who have a lower level of social integration are less likely to volunteer for research projects (Thompson et al, 1994). This may result in samples that are not representative of the population of interest. These same variables may have a profound influence on the incidence and character of the affective problems identified and addressed in a post-stroke sample.

As suggested by Adams et al (1998), another complication is that thinking of stroke as an isolated cerebrovascular accident is misleading, since stroke occurs secondary to diseases of the cerebrovascular system. They further note that multiple diseases often cause or contribute to occlusions or haem-orrhage in the brain. These other conditions may profoundly influence a number of areas of interest when studying PSD.

Researchers attempting to attend to the physiological variables believed to influence PSD face considerable challenges quantifying these variables. For example, lesion size can be challenging to measure and can itself be influ-enced by a number of factors. Imaging procedures can vary greatly in sensitivity to vascular lesions (e.g. CT compared to MRI) and estimation of lesion size; even using the same scanner, can yield different results depend-ing on how soon after the stroke a patient undergoes imaging. Additional error variance will be introduced in lesion size if participants are not scanned on the same machine and at the same time following stroke or at the same time relative to the time of the evaluation. The significance of lesion size may vary over time (e.g. lesion size immediately post-stroke may be less predic-tive of sequelae than lesion size at 1 month, but more predictive than at 3 years), and important relationships may be missed or discounted if not examined systematically. Deciding exactly how to define the lesion and quantify lesion size (e.g. percentage of brain volume, absolute lesion size, or more gross classification such as small, medium, or large) may also dramat-ically influence findings.

The study of vascular dementia and depression has received much less attention than depression in stroke and Alzheimer's disease, but many of the same concerns outlined above would still apply and there are additional dif-ficulties. Although vascular dementia may be the second most common type of dementia, the multiple challenges that are inherent in studying this disorder probably contribute substantially to the comparative paucity of research on depression and vascular dementia. The study of vascular dementia is com-plicated by disagreement in the diagnostic criteria (Metter and Wilson, 1993), difficulties distinguishing it from Alzheimer's, and the possibility of multiple types of the disorder (McPherson and Cummings, 1997). It has only been since 1994 that there has been relatively well-recognized published clinical criteria for defining this disorder (Erkinjunnti, 1994), and these criteria have helped in ensuring consistency across studies in defining the population of interest. The incidence and character of affective disturbances is likely to vary depending on how vascular dementia is defined, whether patients also have Alzheimer's disease, how severe the Alzheimer's pathology is, and the type of vascular dementia the patient has.

Issues related to the study of affective disorders

Depression may not be easy to define, and this issue is particularly problematic for studies interested in PSD and in vascular dementia and depression. Numerous authors have noted the overlap between affective symptoms and normal ageing, and similar concerns arise when examining any neurological population for symptoms of depression. Patients with stroke and other forms of vascular disease may be unable to engage successfully in previously pleasurable activities, may develop sleep disturbance due to pain problems, or may experience a change in body image due to hemiplegia. Patients with stroke are more likely to have other health problems, since illnesses such as hypertension, cardiovascular disease, and diabetes increase the risk of stroke, and since the risk of stroke and the risk of many other health problems increases substantially with age. Chronic pain and other physical discomfort caused by these medical illnesses (e.g. pain due to arthritis) may in itself increase the risk of a patient developing depression. Depression may also be a side effect of medications given for co-morbid conditions (e.g. antihypertensives) or be more likely because of the side effects caused by these medications (e.g. impotence).

Researchers must balance the risk of over- and under-diagnosing depression. Including symptoms that are the result of the neurological disease or other medical conditions may result in inaccurately labelling patients as depressed; excluding symptoms that may reflect affective disturbance but are dismissed in context of medical illness may result in under-diagnosing affective disorders. In addition, depression may not be a single entity that can be answered with a simple 'yes' or 'no', or as present or absent. Furthermore, the incidence, course, and response to treatment may be different for stroke patients who present with symptoms more suggestive of major depressive disorder, minor depression, or an adjustment reaction with depressed mood, and may vary based on the severity of the mood disturbance.

Although the Diagnostic and Statistical Manual IV (American Psychiatric Association, 1994), or DSM-IV, suggests that physical causes of symptoms should be excluded from consideration when diagnosing an affective disorder, in the clinic and in research there may be considerable overlap between symptoms of stroke and symptoms of depression. It can be difficult to disentangle the degree to which a particular symptom is due solely to the stroke, normal ageing, or other medical conditions as opposed to a patient's reaction to changes and problems they now have and/or a mood disorder.

Eliminating all the somatic symptoms would reduce the risk of inappropriately attributing physical problems to a mood disturbance, but this could also make it more likely that mood disturbance, symptoms are overlooked, particularly since older adults may be more comfortable admitting to physical rather than psychological symptoms. Patients may also misattribute symptoms of depression to physical problems or fail to report depression symptoms because they believe these symptoms are normal (Slater and Katz, 1995). Excluding these symptoms, as recommended by the DSM-IV, is problematic if it is believed that the patient's depression is masked by their physical problems (Slater and Katz, 1995).

Another source of concern, which is more complicated when examining PSD, involves how depression symptoms are rated. Affective symptoms are largely conveyed by what the patient says and the majority of well-known and well-replicated scales rely on the patient verbally sharing their symptoms. Including patients with aphasia can be problematic since these patients may be less able to respond to questions regarding mood state and symptoms since they may have comprehension and/or expressive language problems. Language problems are fairly common in these populations, and excluding patients with language problems may make the sample unrepresentative. However, including these patients will limit the scales that can be used and/or may increase the amount of error because their ability to report on their symptoms may be less reliable.

Having an observer, such as a care-provider or spouse, make a rating of the patient's mood may allow the inclusion of patients with language problems. This does not, unfortunately, alter the fact that even the observer has less data, and possibly less reliable data, on which to base their rating of the patient's mood. There is also some evidence that observer ratings, at least when done by spouses, may correlate more strongly with the rater's mood rather than the patient's mood, as determined by independent observers (Teri and Truax, 1994). Additionally, family members frequently assume and report a patient feels a certain way because the family believes this is a normal response to being in this situation and having to cope with these infirmities and frustrations, despite little or no objective evidence of this emotional response from the patient. Differentiating depression from dementia is well recognized as a challenging endeavour for even experienced clinicians (Kaszniak and Ditraglia Christenson, 1994).

Choosing a specific scale to measure depression is difficult. While there is a considerable amount of literature based on neurologically normal samples that suggests a very high degree of correlation between these scales, our comparison of a structured interview, examiner-rated scale, and self-report measures of anxiety and depression found strong correlations in the neurologically normal portion of our sample but did not find this same degree of correlation in the stroke population (Schramke et al, 1998). This suggests that the choice of a measurement instrument may have a significant impact on diagnosis or classification in a neurologically impaired sample but not in a neurologically normal sample. In addition, the various scales designed to specifically measure depression or anxiety may not, in fact, have the desired degree of specificity. This same study was consistent with the suggestion of Fechner-Bates et al (1994), who examined neurologically normal participants, that self-report ratings of depression and anxiety may reflect the individual's level of distress more than symptoms specific to an anxiety or affective disorder. We found that while participants who met DSM-IV criteria for an anxiety or affective disorder were more likely to have a higher score on the rating scales, elevations on these scales were not specific to the particular disorders. Researchers should be aware of the overlap between symptoms of anxiety and symptoms of depression. While the effects of anxiety and affective problems following stroke may be similar, and likewise there may be considerable overlap in designing appropriate interventions once psychopathology is identified in this population, it would not be unexpected to find considerable differences between patients depending on the degree to which they have problems related to anxiety vs depression.

Additional variables of interest

There are numerous other variables that are of interest but few standardized ways to measure many of these variables. Studies of PSD or vascular dementia may examine other variables that might influence an individual's level of risk for developing the disorder, such as the patient's history of psychiatric symptoms and family history of psychiatric disorders. Comparing results across studies is difficult given that there is no standard method of assessing a patient's history or family history of depression or anxiety.

Relatively few treatment studies have been completed in PSD and even fewer studies have focused on the treatment of depression in patients with vascular dementia. Many of the same problems that plague other treatment studies need to be addressed if one is interested in treatment response in these populations. Ethical concerns are raised about having control groups who do not receive treatment. Mood may vary across time, especially in PSD patients. Some studies have suggested that within 1–2 years after stroke most affective symptoms have resolved and relationships between depression and other variables are no longer significant (Parikh et al, 1988). Failure to include an appropriate control may result in incorrect attribution of improvement to treatment rather than recognition of the way in which depression symptoms may vary over time. Including patients who vary in their time since stroke could also greatly influence results, since depression may be more or less likely to spontaneously remit at different times. Patients who continue to have affective symptoms for some time following stroke may have more severe mood disturbances, and the aetiology and response to treatment could be dramatically different over time.

Cognitive impairment and changes in cognitive abilities are to be expected following stroke. The types of problems and severity of deficits can be expected to vary depending on lesion size and lesion location, and these deficits may influence a patient's ability to recognize and share their symptoms. Studies interested in cognitive dysfunction and depression must struggle with how to define and measure this dysfunction. Particularly in patients with focal lesions, conceptualizing cognitive abilities as a unitary domain may be misleading, while attempting to investigate the myriad of types of problems more finely will make it difficult to generalize findings to larger groups. Proponents of cognitive–behavioural psychotherapy have demonstrated that an individual's way of thinking influences the likelihood of depression, and that changing how and what one thinks, and what one does, is an effective treatment of depression. However, no research has specifically addressed whether one's ability to think and alter cognition plays a role in PSD or depression and vascular dementia.

Researchers interested in the behavioural aspects of ageing have long acknowledged the importance of methodology in determining what a study is likely to find. Ageing researchers have demonstrated, for example, that dramatically different results are found with cross-sectional vs longitudinal designs. Studies using a cross-sectional approach tend to find greater differences between younger and older adults when following participants over time relative to the less pronounced differences if the same participants are followed over time (Nesselroade and Lebouvie, 1985). Since researchers interested in stroke are primarily studying older adults and may examine how symptoms change over time, these methodological concerns need to be recognized. Patients who do poorly, psychologically or physically, may be more likely to drop out or be unavailable for follow-up in a longitudinal study, which could significantly influence findings and whether these findings can be generalized to the larger population.

Studies in this area may not collect data on pre-existing dementia. Patients with evidence of cognitive impairment prior to their stroke are more likely to be excluded from the study than to constitute a focus of interest. Studies that do not address this issue may find different results due to their failure to recognize that dementia may increase the risk of developing depression. In addition, depression that is labelled as a pre-existing condition may be the first sign of many neurological disorders, and depression can be present even before the onset of measurable cognitive impairment (Nussbaum et al, 1995). Including and excluding patients with pre-existing cognitive impairment each have drawbacks. Following patients over time and collecting data on this variable would be helpful in determining whether there are systematic influences of pre-existing cognitive impairment. Defining and recognizing pre-existing cognitive impairment is a challenge since patients, even with fairly significant cognitive impairment, may be unaware or unable to report on these deficits. Family members can also be unaware of subtle problems and can sometimes dismiss even obvious signs of dementia and impairment as normal ageing. Reviewing medical records prior to stroke may provide some additional information, but other health-care providers may not note or recognize these pre-existing conditions if the patient or their family does not complain about or report these changes.

Although there have been many studies examining how vascular dementia and Alzheimer's disease differ, there is an impressive degree of overlap between these two conditions. O'Brien (1994) suggests that 50% of patients diagnosed with vascular dementia also have evidence of Alzheimer's pathology at autopsy, and 30% of patients diagnosed with Alzheimer's also have significant vascular disease. When studying factors that increase the risk of developing PSD, it is important to consider how there can be overlap between risks for depression and dementia and for patients who have had stroke or vascular dementia. It may also be difficult to differentiate retrospectively between symptoms that were suggestive of depression vs dementia when deciding which patients to include and exclude.

Recommendations for future studies

At a minimum, researchers designing and implementing studies on PSD and the depression in vascular dementia need to be cognizant of the issues identified above. Recognizing the impact of the type of vascular problem, and other health problems that patients have, and systematically collecting data on the multitude of other health-related variables that can influence depression would be an important initial step. Whenever feasible, including patients from multiple sources, making personal contacts when recruiting participants, offering to test participants at home, and making greater efforts to increase the ease of participation should result in more representative samples. Developing more uniform and more easily replicated methods of lesion classification and attending more to how time since stroke may influence the relationships found also would be helpful.

More uniform criteria for identifying other factors thought to influence the incidence of depression would be helpful. Even studies not specifically interested in the effects of language and cognition on PSD would benefit from including at least some measure of the degree of language and cognitive impairment since these variables may profoundly influence many areas of interest as well as the reliability and validity of the measurement instruments used. Studies should also routinely collect and report on data that may confound or influence results, such as socioeconomic status, since this may help us understand the variability in this research. Even if these data are not analysed, reporting this descriptive data may make it easier to understand the discrepancies found between studies. Additional research needs to be completed on whether the scales and ways of assessing depression in neurological samples are reliable and valid, and consensus needs to be reached on how depression can or should be defined in neurological populations.

Studies that have suggested important relationships between lesion characteristics and depression may need to be replicated with samples that include other socioeconomic groups and patient samples at different times post-stroke. In addition, to understand better the degree to which these results can be generalized to other populations with PSD, researchers should track not only the patients who agree to participate but also collect at least minimal identifying information on the patients who decline to or are unable to participate in the study.

Although much research has already been completed in PSD, relatively little attention has been focused on vascular dementia and depression, which means there are even more opportunities for making significant contributions in understanding this disorder. Using consistent criteria for defining the disorder, appreciating the substantial overlap between vascular dementia and Alzheimer's disease, and exploring how cognitive impairment and preserved cognitive abilities influence the incidence and character of vascular dementia may all be important in helping us to understand this disorder better.

References

Adams HP, del Zoppo GJ, Von Kummer R, *Management of Stroke*, 1st edn (Professional Communications, Inc.: Caddo, 1998).

American Psychiatric Association, *Diagnostic and Statistical Manual of Mental Disorders* (American Psychiatric Association: Washington, DC, 1994).

Erkinjunnti T, Clinical criteria for vascular dementia: The NINDS-AIREN Criteria, *Dementia* (1994) 189–92.

Fechner-Bates S, Coyne J, Schwenk, The relationship of self-reported distress to depressive disorders and other psychopathology, *J Consult Clin Psychol* (1994) **62**:550–9.

Kaszniak AW, Ditraglia Christenson G, Differential diagnosis of dementia and depression. In: Storandt M, VandenBos G, eds, *Neuropsychological Assessment of Dementia and Depression in Older Adults: A Clinician's Guide*, 1st edn (American Psychological Association: Washington, DC, 1994) 81–91.

McPherson S, Cummings J, Vascular dementia: clinical assessment, neuropsychological features, and treatment. In: Nussbaum, P, ed, *Handbook of Neuropsychology and Aging* (Plenum Press: New York, 1997) 177–85.

Metter E, Wilson R, Vascular dementias. In: Parks R, Zec R, Wilson R, eds, *Neuropsychology of Alzheimer's Disease and Other Dementias* (Oxford University Press, Inc.: New York, 1993) 416–32.

Morris PL, Robinson RG, Rapheal B, Prevalance of depressive disorders in hospitalized stroke patients, *Int J Psychiatry Med* (1990) **20**:349–64.

Nesselroade JR, Labouvie EW, Experimental design in research on aging. In: Birren J, Schaie KW, eds, *Handbook of The Psychology of Aging*, 2nd edn (Van Nostrand Reinhold Company, Inc.: New York, 1985) 35–60.

Nussbaum PD, Kaszniak AW, Allender J, Rapcsak S, Depression and cognitive decline in the elderly: a follow-up study, *Neuropsychologist* (1995) **9**:101–11.

O'Brien M, How does cerebrovascular disease cause dementia, *Dementia* (1994) **5**:133–6.

Parikh RM, Lipsey JR, Robinson RG, Price TR, A two year longitudinal study of post stroke mood disorders: Prognostic factors related to one and two year outcome, *Int J Psychiatry Med* (1988) **18**:45–56.

Schramke CJ, Stowe RM, Ratcliff G, Goldstein G, Condray R, Post-stroke depression and anxiety: different assessment methods result in variations in incidence and severity estimates, *J Clin Exp Neuropsychol* (1998) **20**:723–37.

Slater SL, Katz IR, Prevalence of depression in the aged: formal calculations versus clinical facts. *JAGS* (1995) **43**:78–9.

Spencer K, Tompkins C, Schultz R, Assessment of depression in patients with brain pathology: The case of stroke, *Psychol Bulletin* (1997) **122**:132–52.

Teri L, Truax P, Assessment of depression in dementia patients: association of caregiver mood with depression ratings, *Gerontologist* (1994) **34**:231–4.

Thompson M, Heller K, Rody C, Recruitment challenges in studying late-life depression: do community samples adequately represent depressed older adults? *Psychol Aging* (1994) **9**:121–5.

9
Depressive disorders and cerebrovascular disease

Helen Lavretsky and Anand Kumar

Introduction

The link between depressive disorders and cerebrovascular disease has been recognized since the mid-19th century. Post (1962) noted that Durand-Fardel reported irritability and depression to be common acute sequelae of strokes in 1843 and that Guilarovsky suggested in 1926 that in the elderly, the predominance of affective symptoms was due to cerebro-arteriosclerotic changes. Mayer-Gross et al (1960) mentioned that sustained depressive symptoms occurred in patients with atherosclerosis more often than just by chance alone. Bumke (1948) suggested that a reason for the unfavourable outcome of some affective psychoses lay in the development of cerebral arteriosclerosis. There has been a recent increase in the number of studies examining the relationship between depression and cerebrovascular disease. Research on the contribution of cerebrovascular disease to late-life depression received a recent boost as structural brain imaging that can show the location and extent of vascular lesions became more widely available (Krishnan et al, 1988; Hickie et al, 1997; Simpson et al, 1997; O'Brien et al, 1998, 2000; Kumar et al, 2000).

Official nomenclature of stroke usually ignores non-physical symptoms and is primarily focused on neuropathology. The two major classifications used in the USA, the Stroke Data Bank (Gross et al, 1986) and the National Institute of Neurological Diseases and Stroke (NINDS, 1990), recognize asymptomatic stroke, also named 'silent' (Kempster et al, 1988) despite the fact that this produces subtle neurological signs and symptoms, as well as psychiatric symptoms, of which depression is the most frequent (Birkett, 1996).

Studies of the relation between cerebrovascular disease and depression fall into three distinct categories, investigating: depression following established stroke, or post-stroke depression (PSD); clinically significant depression occurring in patients with existing cerebrovascular factors or 'silent' strokes; and depression in patients with vascular or mixed dementias (Rao, 2000).

Several lines of evidence support a link between cerebrovascular disease (CVD) and depression. Depression is highly prevalent in patients with CVD. Approximately 30–50% of patients had depressive disorders at the initial evaluation after stroke (Robinson and Starkstein, 1990). Conversely, CVD is frequently observed in late-onset depression. Patients with vascular diseases such as hypertension, coronary artery disease, diabetes and vascular dementia often have depressive disorders (Rabkin et al, 1983; Carney et al, 1987). The relationship between depression and CVD has been explained in four ways:

1. Depression is an understandable psychological response to multiple neurological deficits associated with serious CVD, such as stroke.
2. Depression is a direct consequence of ischaemic brain damage or focal neurological lesions.
3. Depression as a risk factor for stroke or vascular risk factors.
4. Both conditions coexist (Ramasubbu, 2000).

This chapter will review the existing approaches to the diagnosis and classification of subtypes of depression, as well as the differential diagnosis of late-life depression, which occurs in the context of clinical stroke or subclinical CVD. It will also discuss biological and other mechanisms that may have pathophysiological implications for depression in patients with cerebrovascular compromise. The management and treatment approaches to depression are reviewed elsewhere in this volume (Chapters 7 and 16).

Clinical diagnosis of geriatric depression: syndromal 'threshold' and the concept of comorbidity

Although the clinical characteristics of depressive disorders associated with CVD have been discussed in the literature, the description is usually focused either on isolated symptoms (e.g. depressive symptoms, apathy, or emotionalism) (Marin et al, 1995; Levy et al, 1998) or on the *Diagnostic and Statistical Manual* (DSM-IV) (American Psychiatric Association, 1994) diagnostic categories. These categories include major or minor depression, and mood disorder due to a general medical condition. In general, subsyndromal mood symptoms are more prevalent in patients with central nervous system disorders, including CVD, than major depression (Akiskal et al, 1996; Lavretsky and Kumar, 2001). Patients with non-major depression associated with CVD are usually diagnosed with the DSM categories of depressive disorder due to a general medical condition, adjustment disorder with depressed mood, or depression not otherwise specified (NOS).

The concept of comorbidity referring to co-existing disorders is helpful in understanding the relation of depression and CVD for several reasons. First, it combines overlapping or co-existing symptoms, syndromes, or diagnostic categories on Axis I, II and III of the DSM diagnosis. Most commonly in psychiatric practice, comorbidity refers to co-existing psychiatric conditions (e.g. mood disorders and substance abuse, or mood disorder and a personality disorder). However, this concept may also be extended to co-existing medical and psychiatric disorders, especially when they are likely to be aetiologically connected. Second, the concept of comorbidity may help integrate co-existing disorders that do not meet the threshold for a syndrome. Examples of these phenomena include subthreshold clinically significant depression or symptoms of anxiety in patients with stroke. Patients with CVD may also experience vegetative symptoms. These phenomena include anergia and changes in appetite, sleep and libido, as a result of medical illnesses or medications in the absence of depressed mood, which could contribute to the differential diagnosis of depression (Ramasubbu, 2000). In other words, comorbid conditions are treated as co-existing dimensions of symptoms and syndromes above and below threshold, rather than as mutually exclusive supra-threshold categories (Lavretsky and Kumar, 2001).

Post-stroke depression (PSD)

Depression following vascular injury to the cerebral hemispheres is now a well-recognized clinical entity. PSD may present as minor or major depression and occur within 12–24 months following the cerebrovascular accident (Kumar and Cummings, 2001). Depression occurs in 20–50% of patients in the first year post-stroke (Robinson et al, 1987; House et al, 1991). The DSM-IV categorized PSD as 'mood disorder due to a general medical condition' (i.e. stroke) with the specifiers of a) depressive features, b) major depressive-like episodes, c) manic features, or d) mixed features. It is obvious even from this classification that PSD is a heterogeneous phenomenon, which can occur in patients of different ages, but mainly in middle-aged and older adults. According to recent studies of the subtypes of PSD (Eastwood et al, 1989; Chemerinski and Robinson, 2000) the prevalence of major depression ranges from 0 to 25%; and minor depression occurs in 10–30% of patients following stroke (Robinson, 1997). However, after a comprehensive review of the literature, Primeau (1988) concluded that depression may be as common in patients with stroke as in the elderly with other physical illnesses.

Phenomenology and course

Despite its high prevalence, depression following a stroke is yet to be explained as there is an unresolved debate about the causality of such depression. This debate involves complex relationships between focal neurological deficits, cognitive impairment, disability, and comorbid psychiatric and physical conditions (Kauhanen et al, 1999).

The phenomenology of post-stroke major depression is very similar to that of 'functional' major depression (Robinson, 1997). A number of studies have assessed the duration of PSD (Lipsey et al, 1986; Morris et al, 1990). The majority of patients with major depression following a stroke experience remission within the first year. However, in a minority of patients depression becomes chronic and persists for more than 3 years following the stroke (Astrom et al, 1993). On the other hand, minor depression appears to be more variable, with both short-term and long-term depression occurring in post-stroke patients (Robinson, 1997). The clinical correlates of PSD include younger age, greater functional impairment, social impairment, premorbid personality neuroticism and prior personal or family history of psychiatric disorders (Robinson et al, 1983; Morris and Robinson, 1995). The neurological correlates include non-fluent aphasia, cognitive impairment and enlarged ventricle-to-brain ratio. The available data concerning the phenomenology of depression following stroke suggest that the presence of more than one vegetative symptom or association of dysphoric mood with sleep disturbance could be considered indicators of underlying depression in stroke patients (Fedoroff et al, 1991; Stern and Bachman, 1991). In a 12-month prospective study depression was diagnosed in 53% of patients at 3 months post-stroke and was associated with impairment in memory, non-verbal problem solving and attention and psychomotor speed. The presence of dysphasia also increased the risk of major depression (Kauhanen et al, 1999).

A few studies have examined the effect of PSD on outcome following stroke. Most such studies demonstrate greater functional impairment in depressed patients compared with their non-depressed counterparts (Parikh et al, 1990). In a 12-month follow-up of 106 patients, those who were depressed showed greater dependence in activities of daily living (ADLs) and more severe impairment and handicap than the non-depressed patients. In a study of 10-year mortality after an acute stroke, the likelihood of dying during the follow-up period was 3.5 times higher for depressed than for non-depressed patients even after controlling for demographic characteristics, comorbid physical illness, prior stroke, medication, physical and cognitive impairment and lesion parameters (Morris et al, 1993).

There is growing indirect evidence that syndromal and subsyndromal depression may also affect brain vasculature (Ramasubbu, 2000) and increase vascular risk factors. Simonsick et al (1995) reported that patients with high depressive symptoms defined as the Center for Epidemiologic Studies-Depression (CES-D) Scale scores of 15 and greater in a large cohort of elderly subjects with diagnosed hypertension were 2.3 –2.7 times more likely to suffer from stroke than non-depressed hypertensive patients, supporting the hypothesis that the presence of depression increases the likelihood of stroke in patients with vascular risk factors or disease (Ramasubbu, 2000). In a population-based 29-year follow-up study, depressive symptoms were associated with increased risk of stroke mortality in a cohort of 6676 stroke-free adults (Everson et al, 1998). Increased propensity for blood platelets to aggregate (Musselman et al, 1996) and high levels of cholesterol and high-density lipoproteins in depressed patients may also increase their risk of developing cardio- and cerebrovascular disease. In a prospective follow-up of 4538 subjects aged 60 and older with isolated hypertension, those who were depressed had more than twice the risk of heart failure as non-depressed patients which was not mediated by the infarction (Musselman et al, 1996).

Cerebrovascular lesion location and depressive subtypes

Two factors have been identified that influence the natural course of PSD (Robinson, 1997). One is active treatment with antidepressants. The second and better-studied factor is location of the stroke lesion, with subcortical basal ganglia lesions and brainstem lesions associated with significantly shorter-duration depressions than cortical lesions (Starkstein et al, 1987). Lesion location has been the correlate of depression attracting most attention. Several studies have replicated the relationship between lesion location and PSD (Robinson and Price, 1982; Robinson et al, 1987). Robinson and Szetela (1981) found an inverse correlation between severity of depression and the distance of the lesion from the left frontal pole in patients with sub-acute stroke. Major depression was significantly more frequent among patients with left anterior lesions than lesions in any other location.

However, there is some disagreement about the role of laterality in the development of depression. Bolla-Wilson et al (1989) found no relationship between left anterior lesions and depression. They attributed this discrepancy to the fact that their study excluded patients with any language disorder. Herrmann et al (1995) studied a group of German stroke patients selected as having a single demarcated unilateral infarct. They found no significant difference in depression rating scores between patients with right and left hemisphere infarcts, and no correlation between severity of depression and the anterior location of infarct. Starkstein et al (1989) suggested that the aetiology of depression may differ in right vs left hemisphere stroke.

Major depressive disorder is also commonly associated with subcortical infarcts. A study by Starkstein and colleagues (1988) indicated that lesions of the left basal ganglia resulted in significantly greater depression than lesions of the right basal ganglia or of the left or right thalamus. Manic-like symptoms appear to be associated more frequently with right-sided lesions (Starkstein et al, 1990b; 1991). Mendez et al (1989) reported 12 cases with unilateral lacunar infarcts of the caudate head, suggesting that concomitant cortical ischaemia was not a factor in these cases. Emotional changes were dependent on location of the infarct within the caudate head. Lesions of the dorsolateral caudate head resulted in apathy with decreased spontaneous verbal and motor behaviour. This area of the caudate head is involved in a cortico-striato-pallido-thalamic loop that terminates in the dorsolateral frontal cortex (Alexander et al, 1986), thus causing the resemblance to behaviour accompanying orbitofrontal lesions. Lesions involving most of the caudate head plus surrounding white matter produced affective symptoms with psychotic features. These effects did not depend on lateralization. Other studies, however, have failed to replicate findings suggesting that lesion location is important (Sharpe et al, 1990; Gass and Lawhorn, 1991). Table 9.1 describes the hypothesized relationship between depressive disorders and lesion location according to research so far conducted.

Table 9.1   Depression and related neuropsychiatric syndromes in relation to cerebrovascular lesion location.*

Syndrome	Prevalence	Associated lesion location
Major depression	20%	Left frontal lobe and left basal ganglia
Minor depression	10–40%	Right or left posterior parietal or occipital lobes
Anxiety	27%	Left cortical lesions, usually dorsal lateral frontal lobe
Apathy without depression	22%	Posterior internal capsule
Apathy with depression	11%	Posterior internal capsule
Pathological crying	20%	Bilateral hemispheric, almost any location

*Adapted from Robinson (1997).

Although important in the pathophysiology of depression, the location of stroke lesions may not be an exclusive aetiological factor. Personal vulnerability, psychosocial factors, life events preceding stroke, and physical and social impairment due to post-stroke neurological deficits may also contribute to the development of depression following stroke (Bush, 1999). In addition, PSD is commonly associated with a previous history of depression, and PSD patients with right-sided lesions often have a family history of depression (Robinson and Starkstein, 1990). Further, the observed lateralized changes in 5-hydroxytryptamine 2 receptors (Mayberg et al, 1991), and the influence of lateralized lesions on prolactin responsivity to d-fenfluramine challenge in depressed stroke patients (Ramasubbu et al, 1999) support the notion that different serotonin mechanisms might be responsible for depressive illness associated with right-sided lesions compared to that of left-sided lesions. Damage closer to the frontal lobes is likely to affect catecholamine-mediated brain activity (Robinson and Szetela, 1981). This notion is also supported by experimental data using foetal brain lesions of the frontal cortex in rats with methylazoxymethanol acetate (MAM), which resulted in elevated concentration of the monoaminergic presynaptic markers in the dopaminergic, noradrenergic, and serotonergic, but not GABAergic and cholinergic, terminals throughout postnatal development (Beaulieu and Coyle, 1983).

Differential diagnosis

The purpose of differential diagnosis is to make clinically useful distinctions among patients with similarities in clinical presentation. There are a number of related neuropsychiatric disorders occurring after stroke, which may resemble or co-exist with depression, but may have different out-comes and require different management approaches. Such phenomena include apathy, anxiety, 'catastrophic reaction', and emotional lability (Starkstein et al, 1990a; 1993a,b). A comprehensive assessment is usually needed to distinguish among related disorders. A thorough assessment may be difficult to perform due to existing neurological deficits, such as aphasia or anosognosia, and may require additional input from the caregivers.

Another unresolved issue involves instruments for the assessment of PSD. The majority of currently existing scales measuring the severity of depression require that patients be able to communicate verbally. This approach has only limited use in patients with dementia or aphasia following stroke. Attempts have been made to eliminate self-report by devising scales that can be completed from objective observation (Sunderland et al, 1988). Stern et al (1990) developed scales to measure mood in patients with aphasia. The Center for Epidemiological Studies Depression Scale (CES-D) (Radloff, 1977) has been validated in populations of non-aphasic stroke patients (Shinar et al, 1986). The Hamilton Depression Rating Scale (Hamilton, 1960) remains the most widely used rating scale for depression in psychiatry. Some of the scale items assess physical symptoms and ability to provide self-care and are difficult to complete accurately for a medically ill patient with motor deficits (Birkett, 1996).

Apathy

Apathy is defined as diminished motivation not attributable to decreased lev-els of consciousness, cognitive impairment, or emotional distress (Levy et al, 1998). Apathy often occurs following stroke (Finset and Andersson, 2000) and its presence depends, to some degree, on lesion location (Marin, 1990; 1996, 1997; Cummings, 1993; Duffy and Kant, 1997; Okada et al, 1997; Finset and Andersson, 2000). Apathy may or may not co-exist with depres-sion. Contrary to common belief, apathy is not a 'depressive equivalent' (Marin et al, 1995; Levy et al, 1998). Like depression, apathy has validity as a symptom or a syndrome and a dimension of behaviour (Marin 1990, 1996, 1997). The diagnosis of apathy depends on detecting simultaneous diminu-tion in goal-related actions, thoughts, and emotional responses. Motivation denotes that aspect of behaviour concerned with the initiation, direction, and intensity of goal-directed behaviour (Marin 1990, 1996, 1997). Diminished motivation may affect motor (e.g. lack of initiative), cognitive (e.g. lack of interest), and emotional (e.g. flat affect, indifference) aspects of behaviour (Marin, 1990, 1996, 1997).

Differentiating the syndromes of apathy and depression is sometimes dif-ficult because of overlapping or co-existing clinical features. In addition, in the DSM definition of major depressive syndrome, anhedonia and lack of energy are two essential features of depression, which complicates the dif-ferential diagnosis even further. The essential difference between apathy and depression is that apathy is a syndrome of diminished motivation whereas depression is a disorder of mood (Marin, 1990, 1996, 1997). The emotional responses of depressed patients are mostly unpleasant, negative, and dysphoric, while apathetic patients show attenuated positive and negative responses (Marin, 1997). Psychomotor retardation and bradyphrenia may be features of the depressive or apathy syndrome and are frequently associated with basal ganglia dysfunction. Patients with structural damage to forebrain neural systems mediating motivation are particularly at risk for such profound deficits in activity. The motivational circuitry of the brain includes such important structures as the nucleus accumbens, ventral pallidum, and ventral tegmental area. These structures send to and receive projections from the amygdala, hippocampus, basal ganglia, motor cortex and anterior cingulate. These circuits provide different components of motivation, including motivational working memory, cognitive colouring, and reward memory. Any interruption within these circuits would produce disorders of motivation. In a study of post-stroke apathy in relation to the regional cerebral blood flow measured by the 133 Xe inhalation method, apathy was accompanied by lower scores on verbal intelligence and frontal function tests, and lower cerebral blood flow bilaterally compared to patients without apathy (Okada et al, 1997).

Dopamine (DA) is the principal neurotransmitter in both the nigrostriatal and mesocorticolimbic systems and serves to modulate the regulation of arousal, motivation, locomotor response and sensorimotor integration. Therefore, it is likely to be involved in apathy. Several other neurotransmitters can modify DA action. The excitatory amino acid N-methyl-D-aspartate (NMDA), AMPA, mu- and delta-opioid receptor antagonists, nicotinic acid receptors, neurotensin, and substance P can augment DA activity in the nucleus accumbens (Duffy and Kant, 1997). The cholinergic system also appears to exert a modulatory influence on the motivational circuitry. A neuromodulatory role for serotonin on mesolimbic dopaminergic function is supported by numerous behavioural and radioligand binding studies (Mylecharane, 1996). Newer designer drugs targeting all these potential mechanisms could help to improve the treatment of apathy.

Post-stroke anxiety disorder
Approximately 50% of subjects meeting lifetime criteria for major depression may experience comorbid generalized anxiety disorder (GAD) (Rieger and Burke, 1990). Several studies suggest a significant relationship between GAD and CVD (Coyle and Sterman, 1986; Mathew et al, 1987; Schulz et al, 1997). GAD after stroke is a common and long-lasting affliction that interferes substantially with social life and functional recovery. Cerebral atrophy was associated with anxiety disorder no earlier than 3 years after stroke (Astrom, 1996). At 1 year, only 23% of patients with GAD had recovered; those who did not recover at this follow-up were at risk of development of chronic anxiety disorder. Comorbidity with major depression was high and

seemed to worsen the prognosis of depression. At the acute stage after stroke, GAD plus depression was associated with left hemispheric lesions. Cerebral atrophy was associated with both depression and anxiety disorder some time, but not immediately, after a stroke. Dependence in activities of daily living and a reduced social network were associated with GAD at all follow-up periods at the acute stage. Anxiety disorder without depression may be associated with right posterior lesions in stroke patients (Castillo et al, 1993), and in general, anxiety appears to be more common with cortical rather than subcortical lesions (Starkstein et al, 1990b).

Pre-existing anxiety has been implicated as a risk factor for CVD (Adler et al, 1971), and some studies suggest that premorbid anger and aggression may also increase the risk for CVD (Matsumoto et al, 1983).

Emotional incontinence

Although emotional incontinence is a cause of such signs as crying and looking sad, it may not correctly represent a manifestation of depression. Many patients find their condition embarrassing, and attribute their inability to control emotions to their disorder, rather than to sadness. The ICD-10 (World Health Organization, 1992) describes a 'right hemispheric affective disorder' in which patients superficially appear to be depressed, but depression is not present. Ross (1981) felt that spontaneous weeping belongs to the category of 'aprosodias,' or inability to express emotion.

Anger, agitation, and 'catastrophic reaction'

Outbursts of apparent anger, periods of agitation, and aggression are common in stroke patients (Birkett, 1996). A range of negative emotions such as irritability, hostility, bitterness, frustration and rage may be present in stroke patients. The presence of dementia and aphasia, as well as disinhibition following frontal lobe injury, may facilitate agitated behaviours. Goldstein (1939) described a phenomenon termed the 'catastrophic reaction', a reaction provoked by progressively difficult tasks and expressed in frustration, outbursts of tears, anger and aggression toward the examiner, and refusal to continue the task, seen particularly in patients with left-hemisphere damage.

Several areas of the brain have been proposed as the ones facilitating aggression following injury; these include the amygdala, hypothalamus, cingulum, and temporal and frontal lobes (Birkett, 1996). Several neurotransmitters have been implicated in aggressive behaviours, including reductions in gamma-aminobutyric acid (GABA) and increases in acetylcholine and catecholamine. A strategically located infarct could disrupt pathways from the sites of serotonin production in the raphe nuclei to the limbic system and, hypothetically, facilitate aggressive behaviours (Birkett, 1996).

Clinical depression in the presence of 'subclinical' cerebrovascular disease

Depression in late life is often viewed as a natural consequence of the ageing process and is attributed to psychological reactions to medical illnesses, functional and cognitive decline and the loss of social support. However, the contribution of brain structural changes to late-life and late-onset depression has been established in numerous studies, and extensively explored in patients diagnosed with major depressive disorder using DSM criteria (Sackeim, 2001). Research is just beginning to examine the impact of structural brain abnormalities on functional deficits, phenomenology and clinical correlates, including subtypes of depression, and disease course and outcomes.

Vascular depression

There is a growing consensus that vascular factors contribute to depression in a subgroup of patients with late-life major depression. This thesis is supported by the following observations: data from CT and MRI neuroimaging studies which identify hyperintensities (HI) in such patients; the association of HI with age and cerebrovascular risk factors; and the pathophysiological evidence indicating that HI are associated with widespread diminution in cerebral perfusion (Sackeim, 2001). The neuropathological correlates of HI are diverse and represent ischaemic changes together with demyelination, oedema and gliosis (Kumar et al, 2000, 2001; Sackeim, 2001). However, the putative link between HI and vascular disease forms the basis of the vascular theory of depression. In a study of patients who met DSM-III-R criteria for depression, 'silent cerebral infarctions' were reported in 65% of patients (Fujikawa et al, 1996). In comparison to normal control subjects and other neuropsychiatric groups, high rates of abnormality have been consistently observed in MRI evaluations of elderly patients with major depressive disorder (Coffey et al, 1993; Fujikawa et al, 1996; Kumar et al, 2001). These abnormalities appear as areas of increased signal intensity bright regions in balanced (mixed T1- and T2-weighted), T2-weighted, and fluid-attenuated inversion recovery (FLAIR) images (Sackeim, 2001). Abnormalities can be classified into three types: 1. Periventricular hyperintensities (PVHs) are halos or rims adjacent to ventricles, in severe forms these invade surrounding deep white matter; 2. Single, patchy, or confluent foci may be observed in subcortical white matter or deep white matter hyperintensities (DWMHs); 3. Hyperintensities may also be found in deep grey structures, particularly the basal ganglia, thalamus and pons (Sackeim, 2001). Collectively these three types of abnormalities have been referred to as leukoareosis or encephalomalacia. The rate of these findings is higher in geriatric depression compared to normal controls (Coffey et al, 1993; Kumar et al, 2000), or Alzheimer's disease (Erkinjunitti et al, 1994) and may be comparable to that in multi-infarct dementia (Zubenko et al, 1990). However, cerbrovascular abnormalities are not restricted to old age or unipolar depression. MRI hyperintensities are commonly reported in middle-aged unipolar and young bipolar patients relative to controls, or in bipolar patients with familial bipolar disorder (Dupont et al, 1990; Figiel et al, 1991b). MRI hyperintensities found in late-onset unipolar depression and bipolar disorder have been attributed to CVD on the basis that these abnormalities are commonly associated with vascular risk factors (Krishnan et al, 1988; Coffey et al, 1989). More recent observations (Kumar et al, 2000, 2001) suggest that, in the elderly, smaller brain volumes and HI may provide complementary, albeit autonomous, pathways to late-life major depression. Vascular and non-vascular medical comorbidity contribute to high-intensity lesions, which in turn lead to major depressive disorder. Smaller frontal brain volumes represent the complementary path.

Alexopoulos et al (1997) and Krishnan et al (1997) proposed the concept of vascular depression on the premise that CVD may be aetiologically related to geriatric depressive syndromes. Patients with clinically defined vascular depression experience greater cognitive dysfunction, disability and retardation, but less agitation and guilt feelings, than patients with non-vascular depression. Krishnan et al (1997) examined the specific clinical and demographic characteristics of elderly patients with vascular depression as defined by the presence of vascular lesions in MRI. Elderly patients with MRI-defined vascular depression were older, had a later age of onset, more apathy, and a lower incident family history of depression than elderly patients with non-vascular depression.

MRI research has been generally focused on inpatients with severe symptoms, often referred for ECT. However, there is no indication of a difference in rate of severity of HI between psychotic and non-psychotic depression (Sackeim, 2001). Krishnan et al (1997) reported that patients with HI were less likely to have psychotic symptoms, though more likely to present with apathy and anhedonia. Future studies should examine the validity of this proposed subtype of depression, and its relationship to other depression subtypes.

Late-onset depression

A number of studies found an association between CVD and age of onset of depression. Lesser and colleagues (1991) reported an excess of large deep white matter hyperintensities (DWMH) in patients with late-onset (i.e. age 50 years or older) psychotic depression compared with psychiatrically and neurologically healthy subjects. Figiel and associates (1991a,b) found that late-onset major depression was associated with a higher rate of caudate HIs and large DWMHs compared with early-onset major depression in a small sample of unipolar patients. In a larger sample, Hickie et al (1995) found that late age at onset and negative family history of mood disorders were associated with more severe DWMH. In general, a large number of investigators have seen higher prevalence of severity of HI in late-onset depression than in early-onset depression, with few negative findings (Dupont et al, 1995; Greenwald et al, 1996).

Treatment resistance in the context of cerebrovascular risk factors and MRI hyperintensities

The impact of CVD on treatment response has become a focus of recent studies. Fujikawa and associates (1996) found that patients with severe silent infarction (subcortical and cortical) had longer hospital stays and poorer response to antidepressants than major depression patients without infarction.

Simpson and colleagues (1997) studied 58 treatment resistant older people with DSM-III-R depression. Lesions of the basal ganglia, diabetes, lower mean arterial pressure and hyperintensity of the pontine reticular formation predicted 96% of patients with poor outcome. In a study of 75 elderly people with DSM-III-R major depression, Simpson et al (1998) found that neuropsychological impairment suggestive of frontal/subcortical dysfunction was more common in the treatment-resistant group than in controls. Resistance to antidepressant monotherapy over 12 weeks was associated with a higher prevalence of deep white matter and basal ganglia lesions as well as frontal, extrapyramidal and pyramidal neurological signs. A study of 39 elderly people with severe depression by Hickie et al (1995) also found subcortical HI on MRI to be associated with a poorer response to treatment.

Severe DWMHIs are also known to influence long-term survival. O'Brien et al (1998) followed 60 major depression patients over 55 years of age for an average of 32 months. Time to relapse with depressive symptoms, cognitive decline or death was the outcome measure. Patients with severe white matter HI at baseline had a median survival time of only 136 days, in contrast to 315 days for those without severe HI. Therefore, chronicity appears to be more likely in patients with 'vascular' lesions. However, in a 6-month follow-up study of standard antidepressant treatment, Krishnan and colleagues (1998) did not find significant differences in MRI-established 'vascular depression' compared to patients without MRI lesions. Although, even in this group of patients, elderly patients and patients with onset of depression at or after age 40 who had MRI-defined vascular depression showed a trend for non-recovery. In another pooled analysis of two multi-centre trials of sertraline, patients with hypertension or cardiovascular disease demonstrated comparable response to and tolerability of sertraline (Krishnan et al, 2001). Future research should examine the impact on depressive phenomenology, disease course and treatment response.

Cognitive impairment and disability associated with cerebrovascular disease

Cognitive impairments associated with subclinical cerebrovascular disease may be observed in healthy control subjects with large volume of HI reaching a 'threshold effect' and include deficits in attention, motor speed, and executive function (Boone et al, 1992). Lesser et al (1996) compared patients with late-onset depression (defined as age 50 and older), early-onset (before age 35), and normal controls. The late-onset group had more DWMH than either of the other groups. Cognitive deficits were most marked in the late-onset group and pertained to non-verbal intelligence, non-verbal memory, constructional ability, executive function, and speed of processing. Patients with greater severity of DWMH had significantly poorer executive function. Simpson and associates (1997) conducted neuropsychological assessment following treatment of an elderly MD sample of patients with major depression. Hyperintensities in the pons were associated with reduced psychomotor speed, those in the basal ganglia were linked to impaired category production (executive function), and periventricular hyperintensities were associated with impaired delayed recall.

In a retrospective case note analysis of 38 patients with MRIs performed 3 years earlier (Baldwin et al, 2000) poor outcome was associated with lesions in the pons. Pontine raphe lesions and confluent periventricular lesions were associated with later dementia and with death from cardiovascular disorders. Males had more depressive recurrences and a reduced survival rate.

Alexopoulos (2001) underscored the importance of executive dysfunction in geriatric depression by coining the term 'depression-executive dysfunction syndrome of late-life'. He observed that at least a proportion of patients with geriatric depression experience executive dysfunction, including disturbances in planning, sequencing, organizing, abstracting, and poor retrieval with relative preservation of recognition memory, as well as prominent disability. Depression occurring in the context of vascular disease, a syndrome associated with striato-frontal impairment, presents with executive dysfunction, psychomotor retardation, apathy and reduced agitation, guilt and insight (Alexopoulos et al, 1997; Krishnan et al, 1997). In depressed elderly patients, executive dysfunction was the cognitive impairment most likely to result in disruption of instrumental activities of daily living (IADLs) (Alexopoulos et al, 1996, 2000; Kiosses et al, 2000). Moreover, depression was found to contribute to IADL impairment mainly in patients with executive dysfunction, whereas it had a non-significant effect in patients without impaired executive functioning (Kiosses et al, 2000). In addition, executive impairment predicted poor or delayed antidepressant response of geriatric major depression. Executive dysfunction and CVD have been reported in association with poor or delayed antidepressant response, relapse, and recurrence of depression. Unlike executive dysfunction, neither memory impairment, nor disability, medical burden, social support, or number of previous episodes have been shown to influence the course of geriatric depression (Alexopoulos, 2001). Thus, interventions targeting improvement in executive dysfunction may improve the overall outcomes of geriatric depression.

Clinical correlates of subclinical cerebrovascular disease in neurodegenerative and vascular dementias

Subclinical cerebrovascular disease or leukoareosis is common in dementia patients and in the normal elderly (Barber et al, 1999). The prevalence, severity, and distribution of MRI HIs seem to vary between different disorders and with age (O'Brien et al, 1996; Schmidt et al, 1997). However, there is an inconsistency in the results estimating the prevalence of MRI HIs in these populations, most likely due to differences in the scanning techniques, sample size and selection, and rating scales used (Barber et al, 1999). The clinical significance of leukoareosis in dementia has been under-investigated and is poorly understood.

There is growing evidence that changes in white matter are linked to depressive illness in late life (Steffens and Krishnan, 1998; Kumar et al, 2000, 2001), thus stimulating similar explorations in dementia patients (Sultzer et al, 1993; Starkstein et al, 1997; Barber et al, 1999). In a cross-sectional study of patients with dementia with Lewy bodies, Alzheimer's disease, vascular dementia and normal controls, periventricular hyperintensities were positively correlated with age and were more severe in all dementia groups than in controls (Barber et al, 1999). Total deep hyperintensities scores were significantly higher in all dementia groups than among controls, and higher in patients with vascular dementia than in those with dementia with Lewy bodies or Alzheimer's disease. In all dementia patients, frontal WMHs were associated with higher depression scores. In another study of consecutive patients with probable Alzheimer's disease, the presence of leukoareosis on MRI was associated with increased apathy and extrapyramidal signs, as well as bilateral hypoperfusion in the basal ganglia, thalamus, and frontal lobes than in Alzheimer patients without leukoareosis (Starkstein et al, 1997). However, there were no differences between groups in age, duration of illness, depression scores, severity of delusions, or deficits on neuropsychological tasks. In a MRI and PET study of 11 subjects without cortical lesions who were diagnosed with vascular depression, subcortical MRI lesions were associated with cortical metabolic dysfunction, increased anxiety, depression, and the overall severity of neuropsychiatric symptoms (Sultzer et al, 1993). Unfortunately, there has been a dearth of studies trying to integrate the impact of CVD on depression and other neuropsychiatric symptoms across dementia subtypes. HI in dementia may have different pathological correlates, and reflect periventricular 'leakage' of CSF secondary to flattening of ependymal cells due to ventricular dilatation (O'Brien et al, 1996).

Conclusion

The existing data on the diagnosis and classification of depressive subtypes in the presence of clinical and subclinical CVD have been reviewed. There are some similarities and differences in phenomenology of depressive subtypes in post-stroke depression, geriatric 'vascular' depression, and depression in patients with different types of dementia. The existing similarities include 'fronto-subcortical' impairment associated with depression, apathy, and fronto-executive dysfunction, which has a negative impact on treatment response, rehabilitation, and disease outcomes and may reflect shared pathophysiological mechanisms. Clearly, some areas of research remain insufficient and include clinical descriptive and longitudinal studies, combined structural and functional neuroimaging, and neuropsychological studies. Narrowing all characteristics to a common phenotype will be necessary to further our understanding of geriatric depression associated with CVD.

Acknowledgement

The work involved in writing this chapter was supported in part by the NARSAD Young Investigator Award and K23-MH01948 to Dr Lavretsky and grants: MH55115, MH61567 and K02-MH02043 (AK).

References

Adler R, MacRitchie K, Engel GL, Psychologic processes and ischemic stroke (occlusive cerebrovascular disease). I. Observations on 32 men with 35 strokes, *Psychosom Med* (1971) **33**: 1–29.

Akiskal HS, Bolis CL, Cazzullo C et al, Dysthymia in neurological disorders, *Mol Psychiatry* (1996) **1**: 478–91.

Alexander GE, DeLong MR, Strick PL, Parallel organization of functionally segregated circuits linking basal ganglia and cortex, *Annu Rev Neurosci* (1986) **9**: 357–81.

Alexopoulos GS, New concepts for prevention and treatment of late-life depression, *Am J Psychiatry* (2001) **158**: 835–8.

Alexopoulos GS, Meyers BS, Young RC et al, 'Vascular depression' hypothesis, *Arch Gen Psychiatry* (1997) **54**: 915–22.

Alexopoulos GS, Meyers BS, Young RC et al, Executive dysfunction and long-term outcomes of geriatric depression, *Arch Gen Psychiatry* (2000) **57**: 285–90.

Alexopoulos GS, Vrontou C, Kakuma T et al, Disability in geriatric depression, *Am J Psychiatry* (1996) **153**: 877–85.

American Psychiatric Association *Diagnostic and Statistical Manual of Mental Disorders: DSM-IV* (American Psychiatric Association: Washington, DC, 1994).

Astrom M, Generalized anxiety disorder in stroke patients: a 3–year longitudinal study, *Stroke* (1996) **27**: 270–5.

Astrom M, Adolfsson R, Asplund K, Major depression in stroke patients, A

3–year longitudinal study, *Stroke* (1993) **24**: 976–82.

Baldwin RC, Walker S, Simpson SW, Jackson A, Burns A, The prognostic significance of abnormalities seen on magnetic resonance imaging in late life depression: clinical outcome, mortality and progression to dementia at three years, *Int J Geriatr Psychiatry* (2000) **15**: 1097–104.

Barber R, Gholkar A, Scheltens P et al, Apolipoprotein E epsilon4 allele, temporal lobe atrophy, and white matter lesions in late-life dementias, *Arch Neurol* (1999) **56**: 961–5.

Beaulieu M, Coyle JT, Postnatal development of aminergic projections to frontal cortex: effects of cortical lesions, *J Neurosci Res* (1983) **10**: 351–61.

Birkett DP, *The Psychiatry of Stroke* (American Psychiatric Press: Washington, DC, 1996).

Bolla-Wilson K, Robinson RG, Starkstein SE, Boston J, Price TR, Lateralization of dementia of depression in stroke patients, *Am J Psychiatry* (1989) **146**: 627–34.

Boone KB, Miller BL, Lesser IM et al, Neuropsychological correlates of white-matter lesions in healthy elderly subjects: a threshold effect, *Arch Neurol* (1992) **49**: 549–54.

Bumke O, *Lehrbuch der Geistestkrankheiten* (J.F. Bergmann: München, 1948).

Bush BA, Major life events as risk factors for post-stroke depression, *Brain Inj* (1999) **13**: 131–7.

Carney RM, Rich MW, Tevelde A et al, Major depressive disorder in coronary artery disease, *Am J Cardiol* (1987) **60**: 1273–5.

Castillo CS, Starkstein SE, Fedoroff JP, Price TR, Robinson RG, Generalized anxiety disorder after stroke, *J Nerv Ment Dis* (1993) **181**: 100–6.

Chemerinski E, Robinson R, The neuropsychiatry of stroke, *Psychosomatics* (2000) **41**: 5–14.

Coffey CE, Figiel GS, Djang WT, Saunders WB, Weiner RD, White matter hyperintensity on magnetic resonance imaging: clinical and neuroanatomic correlates in the depressed elderly, *J Neuropsychiatry Clin Neurosci* (1989) **1**: 135–44.

Coffey CE, Wilkinson WE, Weiner RD et al, Quantitative cerebral anatomy in depression. A controlled magnetic resonance imaging study, *Arch Gen Psychiatry* (1993) **50**: 7–16.

Coyle PK, Sterman AB, Focal neurologic symptoms in panic attacks, *Am J Psychiatry* (1986) **143**: 648–9.

Cummings JL, Frontal-subcortical circuits and human behavior, *Arch Neurol* (1993) **50**: 873–80.

Duffy JD, Kant R, Apathy secondary to neurologic disease. *Psychiatric Ann* (1997) **27**: 39–43.

Dupont RM, Jernigan TL, Butters N et al, Subcortical abnormalities detected in bipolar affective disorder using magnetic resonance imaging. Clinical and neuropsychological significance, *Arch Gen Psychiatry* (1990) **47**: 55–9.

Dupont RM, Jernigan TL, Heindel W et al, Magnetic resonance imaging and mood disorders. Localization of white matter and other subcortical abnormalities, *Arch Gen Psychiatry* (1995) **52**: 747–55.

Eastwood MR, Rifat SL, Nobbs H, Ruderman J, Mood disorder following cerebrovascular accident, *Br J Psychiatry* (1989) **154**: 195–200.

Erkinjuntti T, Gao F, Lee DH et al, Lack of difference in brain hyperintensities between patients with early Alzheimer's disease and control subjects, *Arch Neurol* (1994) **51**: 260–8.

Everson SA, Goldberg DE, Kaplan GA, Julkunen J, Salonen JT, Anger expression and incident hypertension, *Psychosom Med* (1998) **60**: 730–5.

Fedoroff JP, Starkstein SE, Parikh RM, Price TR, Robinson RG, Are depressive symptoms nonspecific in patients with acute stroke? *Am J Psychiatry* (1991) **148**: 1172–6.

Figiel GS, Krishnan KR, Doraiswamy PM et al, Subcortical hyperintensities on brain magnetic resonance imaging: a comparison between late age onset and early onset elderly depressed subjects, *Neurobiol Aging* (1991a) **12**: 245–7.

Figiel GS, Krishnan KR, Rao VP et al, Subcortical hyperintensities on brain magnetic resonance imaging: a comparison of normal and bipolar subjects, *J Neuropsychiatry Clin Neurosci* (1991b) **3**: 18–22.

Finset A, Andersson S, Coping strategies in patients with acquired brain injury: relationships between coping, apathy, depression and lesion location, *Brain Inj* (2000) **14**: 887–905.

Fujikawa T, Yokota N, Muraoka M, Yamawaki S, Response of patients with major depression and silent cerebral infarction to antidepressant drug therapy, with emphasis on central nervous system adverse reactions, *Stroke* (1996) **27**: 2040–2.

Gass CS, Lawhorn L, Psychological adjustment following stroke: an MMPI study, *Psycholog Ass* (1991) **3**: 628–33.

Goldstein K, *The Organism. A Holistic Approach to Biology Derived from Pathological Data in Man* (American Book: New York, 1939).

Greenwald BS, Kramer-Ginsberg E, Krishnan RR et al, MRI signal hyperintensities in geriatric depression, *Am J Psychiatry* (1996) **153**: 1212–5.

Gross CR, Shinar D, Mohr JP et al, Interobserver agreement in the diagnosis of stroke type, *Arch Neurol* (1986) **43**: 893–8.

Hamilton M, A rating scale for depression, *J Neurol, Neurosurg Psychiatry* (1960) **23**: 56–61.

Herrmann M, Bartels C, Schumacher M, Wallesch CW, Poststroke depression: is there a pathoanatomic correlate for depression in the postacute stage of stroke? *Stroke* (1995) **26**: 850–6.

Hickie I, Scott E, Mitchell P et al, Subcortical hyperintensities on magnetic resonance imaging: clinical correlates and prognostic significance in patients with severe depression, *Biol Psychiatry* (1995) **37**: 151–60.

Hickie I, Scott E, Wilhelm K, Brodaty H, Subcortical hyperintensities on magnetic resonance imaging in patients with severe depression – a longitudinal evaluation, *Biol Psychiatry* (1997) **42**: 367–74.

House A, Dennis M, Mogridge L et al, Mood disorders in the year after first stroke, *Br J Psychiatry* (1991) **158**: 83–92.

Kauhanen M, Korpelainen JT, Hiltunen P et al, Poststroke depression correlates with cognitive impairment and neurological deficits, *Stroke* (1999) **30**: 1875–80.

Kempster PA, Gerraty RP, Gates PC, Asymptomatic cerebral infarction in patients with chronic atrial fibrillation, *Stroke* (1988) **19**: 955–7.

Kiosses DN, Alexopoulos GS, Murphy C, Symptoms of striatofrontal dysfunction contribute to disability in geriatric depression, *Int J Geriatr Psychiatry* (2000) **15**: 992–9.

Krishnan KR, Ellinwood EJ, Goli V, Structural brain changes revealed by MRI [letter], *Am J Psychiatry* (1988) **145**: 1316.

Krishnan KR, Hays JC, Blazer DG, MRI-defined vascular depression, *Am J Psychiatry* (1997) **154**: 497–501.

Krishnan KR, Hays JC, George LK, Blazer DG, Six-month outcomes for MRI-related vascular depression, *Depress Anxiety* (1998) **8**: 142–6.

Krishnan KR, Doraiswamy PM, Clary CM, Clinical and treatment response characteristics of late-life depression associated with vascular disease: a pooled analysis of two multicenter trials with sertraline, *Prog Neuropsychopharmacol Biol Psychiatry* (2001) **25**: 347–61.

Kumar A, Bilker W, Jin Z, Udupa J, Atrophy and high intensity lesions:

complementary neurobiological mechanisms in late-life major depression, *Neuropsychopharmacology* (2000) **22**: 264–74.

Kumar A, Cummings J, Depression in neurodegenerative disorders and related conditions in Alzheimer's disease and related conditions. In: Gauthier S, Cummings J, eds, *Alzheimer's Disease and Related Disorders, Annual 2001* (Martin Dunitz: London, 2001) 123–41.

Kumar A, Mintz J, Bilker W, Gottlieb G, Autonomous neurobiological pathways to late-life major depressive disorder: clinical and pathophysiological implications, *Neuropsychopharmacology* (2001) (in press).

Lavretsky H, Kumar A, Non-major clinically significant depression. Old concepts, new insights? *Am J Geriatr Psychiatry* (2001) (in press).

Lesser IM, Miller BL, Boone KB et al, Brain injury and cognitive function in late-onset psychotic depression, *J Neuropsychiatry Clin Neurosci* (1991) **3**: 33–40.

Lesser IM, Boone KB, Mehringer CM et al, Cognition and white matter hyperintensities in older depressed patients, *Am J Psychiatry* (1996) **153**: 1280–7.

Levy ML, Cummings JL, Fairbanks LA et al, Apathy is not depression, *J Neuropsychiatry Clin Neurosci* (1998) **10**: 314–9.

Lipsey JR, Spencer WC, Rabins PV, Robinson RG, Phenomenological comparison of poststroke depression and functional depression, *Am J Psychiatry* (1986) **143**: 527–9.

Marin RS, Differential diagnosis and classification of apathy, *Am J Psychiatry* (1990) **147**: 22–30.

Marin RS, Apathy and related disorders of diminished motivation, *Am Psychiatric Press Rev Psychiatry* (1996) **15**: 205–42.

Marin RS, Differential diagnosis of apathy and related disorders of diminished motivation, *Psychiatric Ann* (1997) **27**: 30–3.

Marin RS, Fogel BS, Hawkins J, Duffy J, Krupp B, Apathy: a treatable syndrome, *J Neuropsychiatry Clin Neurosci* (1995) **7**: 23–30.

Mathew RJ, Wilson WH, Nicassio PM, Cerebral ischemic symptoms in anxiety disorders [letter], *Am J Psychiatry* (1987) **144**: 265.

Matsumoto Y, Uyama O, Shimizu S et al, Do anger and aggression affect carotid atherosclerosis? *Stroke* (1993) **24**: 983–6.

Mayberg HS, Parikh RM, Morris PL, Robinson RG, Spontaneous remission of post-stroke depression and temporal changes in cortical S2–serotonin receptors, *J Neuropsychiatry Clin Neurosci* (1991) **3**: 80–83.

Mayer-Gross W, Slater E, Roth M, *Clinical Psychiatry* (Cassell and Co.: London, 1960).

Mendez MF, Adams NL, Lewandowski KS, Neurobehavioral changes associated with caudate lesions, *Neurology* (1989) **39**: 349–54.

Morris PL, Robinson RG, Raphael B, Prevalence and course of depressive disorders in hospitalized stroke patients, *Int J Psychiatry Med* (1990) **20**: 349–64.

Morris PL, Robinson RG, Andrzejewski P, Samuels J, Price TR, Association of depression with 10–year poststroke mortality, *Am J Psychiatry* (1993) **150**: 124–9.

Morris PL, Robinson RG, Personality neuroticism and depression after stroke, *Int J Psychiatry Med* (1995) **25**: 93–102.

Musselman DL, Tomer A, Manatunga AK et al, Exaggerated platelet reactivity in major depression, *Am J Psychiatry* (1996) **153**: 1313–7.

Mylecharane EJ, Ventral tegmental area 5–HT receptors: mesolimbic dopamine release and behavioural studies, *Behav Brain Res* (1996) **73**: 1–5.

National Institute of Neurological Disorders and Stroke (special report), Classification of cerebrovascular diseases III, *Stroke* (1990) **21**: 637–76.

O'Brien J, Ames D, Chiu E et al, Severe deep white matter lesions and outcome in elderly patients with major depressive disorder: follow up study, *BMJ* (1998) **317**: 982–4.

O'Brien J, Perry R, Barber R, Gholkar A, Thomas A, The association between white matter lesions on magnetic resonance imaging and noncognitive symptoms. *Ann NY Sci* (2000) **903**: 482–9.

O'Brien JT, Ames D, Schweitzer I, White matter changes in depression and Alzheimer's disease: a review of magnetic resonance imaging studies, *Int J Geriatr Psychiatry* (1996) **11**: 681–94.

Okada K, Kobayashi S, Yamagata S, Takahashi K, Yamaguchi S, Poststroke apathy and regional cerebral blood flow, *Stroke* (1997) **28**: 2437–41.

Parikh RM, Robinson RG, Lipsey JR et al, The impact of poststroke depression on recovery in activities of daily living over a 2–year follow-up, *Arch Neurol* (1990) **47**: 785–9.

Post F, *The Significance of Affective Symptoms in Old Age, a Follow-up Study of One Hundred Patients* (Oxford University Press: London, 1962).

Primeau F, Post-stroke depression: a critical review of the literature. *Can J Psychiatry* (1988) **33**: 757–65.

Rabkin JG, Charles E, Kass F, Hypertension and DSM-III depression in psychiatric outpatients, *Am J Psychiatry* (1983) **140**: 1072–4.

Radloff LS, The CES-D Scale: a self-report depression scale for research in the general population, *App Psychol Meas* (1977) **1**: 385–401.

Ramasubbu R, Relationship between depression and cerebrovascular disease: conceptual issues, *J Affect Disord* (2000) **57**: 1–11.

Ramasubbu R, Flint A, Brown G, Awad G, Kennedy S, A neuroendocrine study of serotonin function in depressed stroke patients compared to non depressed stroke patients and healthy controls, *J Affect Disord* (1999) **52**: 121–33.

Rao R, Cerebrovascular disease and late life depression: an age old association revisited, *Int J Geriatr Psychiatry* (2000) **15**: 419–33.

Rieger D, Burke J Jr, Comorbidity of affective and anxiety disorders in the NIMH Epidemiologic Catchment Area Program. In: Maser JD, Cloninger CR, eds, *Comorbidity of Mood and Anxiety Disorders* (American Psychiatric Press, Inc.: Washington, DC, 1990) 113–22.

Robinson R, Starr L, Kubos K, Price T, A two-year longitudinal study of post-stroke mood disorders: findings during the initial evaluation, *Stroke* (1983) **14**: 736–41.

Robinson RG, Neuropsychiatric consequences of stroke, *Annu Rev Med* (1997) **48**: 217–29.

Robinson RG, Bolduc PL, Price TR, Two-year longitudinal study of post-stroke mood disorders: diagnosis and outcome at one and two years, *Stroke* (1987) **18**: 837–43.

Robinson RG, Price TR, Post-stroke depressive disorders: a follow-up study of 103 patients, *Stroke* (1982) **13**: 635–41.

Robinson RG, Starkstein SE, Current research in affective disorders following stroke, *J Neuropsychiatry Clin Neurosci* (1990) **2**: 1–14.

Robinson RG, Szetela B, Mood change following left hemispheric brain injury, *Ann Neurol* (1981) **9**: 447–53.

Ross ED, The aprosodias. Functional-anatomic organization of the affective components of language in the right hemisphere, *Arch Neurol* (1981) **38**: 561–9.

Sackeim HA, Brain structure in late-life depression. In: Morisha JM, ed, *Advances in Brain Imaging*. Review of Psychiatry, Volume 20 (American Psychiatric Publishing Inc.: Washington DC, London, 2001) 83–122.

Schmidt R, Fazekas F, Hayn M et al, Risk factors for microangiopathy-related cerebral damage in the Austrian stroke prevention study, *J Neurol Sci* (1997) **152**: 15–21.

Schultz SK, Castillo CS, Kosier JT, Robinson RG, Generalized anxiety and depression: assessment over 2 years after stroke, *Am J Geriatr Psychiatry* (1997) **5**: 229–37.

Sharpe M, Hawton K, House A et al, Mood disorders in long-term survivors of stroke: associations with brain lesion location and volume, *Psychol Med* (1990) **20**: 815–28.

Shinar D, Gross CR, Price TR et al, Screening for depression in stroke patients: the reliability and validity of the Center for Epidemiologic Studies Depression Scale, *Stroke* (1986) **17**: 241–5.

Simonsick EM, Wallace RB, Blazer DG, Berkman LF, Depressive symptomatology and hypertension-associated morbidity and mortality in older adults, *Psychosom Med* (1995) **57**: 427–35.

Simpson S, Baldwin RC, Jackson A, Burns AS, Is subcortical disease associated with a poor response to antidepressants? Neurological, neuropsychological and neuroradiological findings in late-life depression, *Psychol Med* (1998) **28**: 1015–26.

Simpson SW, Jackson A, Baldwin RC, Burns A, Subcortical hyperintensities in late-life depression: acute response to treatment and neuropsychological impairment, *Int Psychogeriatr* (1997) **9**: 257–75.

Starkstein SE, Robinson RG, Price TR, Comparison of cortical and subcortical lesions in the production of poststroke mood disorders, *Brain* (1987) **110**: 1045–59.

Starkstein SE, Robinson RG, Price TR, Comparison of patients with and without poststroke major depression matched for size and location of lesion, *Arch Gen Psychiatry* (1988) **45**: 247–52.

Starkstein SE, Robinson RG, Honig MA et al, Mood changes after right-hemisphere lesions, *Br J Psychiatry* (1989) **155**: 79–85.

Starkstein SE, Cohen BS, Fedoroff P et al, Relationship between anxiety disorders and depressive disorders in patients with cerebrovascular injury, *Arch Gen Psychiatry* (1990) **47**: 246–51.

Starkstein SE, Mayberg HS, Berthier ML et al, Mania after brain injury: neuroradiological and metabolic findings, *Ann Neurol* (1990b) **27**: 652–9.

Starkstein SE, Bryer JB, Berthier ML et al, Depression after stroke: the importance of cerebral hemisphere asymmetries, *J Neuropsychiatry Clin Neurosci* (1991) **3**: 276–85.

Starkstein SE, Fedoroff JP, Price TR, Leiguarda R, Robinson RG, Catastrophic reaction after cerebrovascular lesions: frequency, correlates, and validation of a scale, *J Neuropsychiatry Clin Neurosci* (1993a) **5**: 189–94.

Starkstein SE, Fedoroff JP, Price TR, Leiguarda R, Robinson RG, Apathy following cerebrovascular lesions, *Stroke* (1993b) **24**: 1625–30.

Starkstein SE, Sabe L, Vazquez S et al, Neuropsychological, psychiatric, and cerebral perfusion correlates of leukoaraiosis in Alzheimer's disease, *J Neurol Neurosurg Psychiatry* (1997) **63**: 66–73.

Steffens DC, Krishnan KR, Structural neuroimaging and mood disorders: recent findings, implications for classification, and future directions, *Biol Psychiatry* (1998) **43**: 705–12.

Stern R, Hooper S, Morey C, Development of visual analogue scales to measure mood in aphasia, *Clinical Neuropsychol* (1990) **4**: 300.

Stern RA, Bachman DL, Depressive symptoms following stroke, *Am J Psychiatry* (1991) **148**: 351–6.

Sultzer DL, Levin HS, Mahler ME, High WM, Cummings JL, A comparison of psychiatric symptoms in vascular dementia and Alzheimer's disease, *Am J Psychiatry* (1993) **150**: 1806–12.

Sunderland T, Hill JL, Lawlor BA, Molchan SE, NIMH Dementia Mood Assessment Scale (DMAS), *Psychopharmacol Bull* (1988) **24**: 747–53.

World Health Organization, *The International Classification of Mental and Behavioral Disorders. Clinical Description and Diagnostic Guidelines.* (WHO: Geneva, 1992).

Zubenko G, Sullivan P, Nelson J, et al, Brain imaging abnormalities in mental disorders of late life, *Arch Neurol* (1990) **47**: 1107–11.

10
Vascular depression: a new subtype of depressive disorder?

Warren D Taylor, David C Steffens and
K Ranga Rama Krishnan

Introduction

Depression is a clinical syndrome that likely has multiple aetiologies, including environmental and psychosocial origins, the result of medical illnesses or injuries, and genetic predisposition. Various researchers and clinicians have attempted to identify subtypes of depression that may have clinical significance, but these subtypes are often based on subtle differences in clinical presentation rather than on possible aetiologies of the symptoms.

As geriatric psychiatry developed into a distinct specialty, clinicians recognized that new-onset depression in the elderly differed from depression in younger individuals. Clinically, it may be associated with greater psychomotor retardation, less guilt (Alexopoulos et al, 1997b), and greater cognitive impairment. Late-onset depression is less associated with genetic factors than early-onset depression (Mendlewicz and Baron, 1981), while structural brain changes appear to be more important (Coffey et al, 1988; Lesser et al, 1991). These data prompted further research demonstrating that specific cortical and subcortical brain lesions contribute to the development of depression in the elderly.

This syndrome, which has been proposed as a distinct subtype of late-life depression, is termed 'vascular depression' (Krishnan and McDonald, 1995; Alexopoulos et al, 1997a,b; Krishnan et al, 1997). In this chapter, we will review the evidence supporting and contradicting this hypothesis, the clinical relevance of such a distinction, and proposed diagnostic criteria.

Associations between vascular disease and depression

The incidence of depression in the elderly is estimated to range from 1.3 to 3.1 per 100 person-years at risk (Palsson and Skoog, 1997), while in the subset of elderly with vascular illnesses such as hypertension or coronary artery disease, the incidence is even higher. For example, elderly people with hypertension reportedly have a three–fold increased risk of depression (Rabkin et al, 1983). The frequency is also higher with cardiac disease: studies find depression in 15–25% of the elderly with coronary artery disease

(Carney et al, 1987; Forrester et al, 1992; Gonzalez et al, 1996), and in 15–20% of survivors of myocardial infarction (Schleifer et al, 1989; Frasure-Smith et al, 1993). There is also some cross-sectional evidence demonstrating associations between depression and both diabetes (Littlefield et al, 1990; Lustman et al, 1992) and cigarette smoking (Kendler et al, 1993). Despite the numerous positive studies, these findings are not universal. A study comparing elderly depressed psychiatric inpatients with normal controls failed to show a significant difference between the two groups using a cumulative cerebrovascular risk factor score (Lyness et al, 1998).

Depression itself is a risk factor for increased morbidity and mortality related to vascular disease. Data from a large, longitudinal study of 4367 elderly hypertensive subjects demonstrated that for every 5–point increase in the Center for Epidemiology-Depression Scale, there is an 18% increased risk of myocardial infarction or stroke, and a 25% increase in overall mortality (Wassertheil-Smoller et al, 1996). Additionally, several studies have found depression that develops following a myocardial infarction to be associated with increased risk of future infarction and death, with adjusted odds ratios for the latter between 4 and 6 (Frasure-Smith et al, 1993, 1995; Barefoot and Schroll, 1996; Pratt et al, 1996).

If vascular disease is related to depression, is it related to antidepressant response or non-response? Most data suggest no relationship. A large, pooled study of the use of sertraline to treat late-life depression demonstrated that subjects with vascular disease exhibited comparable response rates to those without vascular disease (Krishnan et al, 2001). There was also no difference in rates of adverse events. Another study comparing paroxetine with nortriptyline in subjects with ischaemic heart disease found the two agents comparably effective, however the authors did note a significantly higher rate of adverse cardiac events in the nortriptyline group (18% vs 2%; $P < 0.03$) (Roose et al, 1998).

Stroke and depression

Depression is a frequent complication of stroke, developing in 20–30% of cases (Ebrahim et al, 1987; Wade et al, 1987; Tiller, 1992; Astrom et al, 1993). Initial research reported an association between depression and left hemispheric stroke (Robinson et al, 1984); some subsequent studies reached similar conclusions (Greenwald et al, 1998), but others failed to replicate it, while some demonstrated an association with right hemispheric lesions. These conflicting results are often limited by small sample size and lack quantification of lesion severity or extent.

But stroke with neurological symptoms may not be as common as 'silent stroke,' or ischaemia without neurological symptoms. Japanese studies demonstrate that 80–90% of elderly subjects with late-onset depression exhibit silent strokes greater than 5 mm in diameter (Fujikawa et al, 1993). As a comparison, an American study examining cerebrovascular risk factors independent of the presence or absence of depression demonstrated that infarct-like lesions were present in 23% of the participants without history of stroke. In those with such lesions, 79% of the lesions were over 3 mm in size (Bryan et al, 1994). These reports suggest that such small lesions may be seen more often in depressed than non-depressed elderly people.

Neuroimaging findings

Neuroimaging studies in the depressed elderly are generally divided into two types of studies: studies of lesions and studies of brain volume. Although it is well documented that the brain's volume decreases with normal ageing (Passe et al, 1997; Coffey et al, 1998; Kumar et al, 1999), the depressed elderly also exhibit selective regional atrophy, particularly of the frontal lobe (Krishnan et al, 1992; Coffey et al, 1993; Parashos et al, 1998). This finding is not universal (Pantel et al, 1997). It is thought that atrophy and vascular disease may represent two distinct pathways to a common clinical syndrome, and it has been demonstrated that a combination of atrophy and vascular disease significantly increases the risk of developing depression (Kumar et al, 2000, 2001).

Lesion studies have primarily focused on MRI hyperintensities – regions in the brain parenchyma that appear bright on T2–weighted imaging and are thought to represent vascular injury, although not all researchers agree on this point. Research consistently demonstrates that hyperintensities are more common in late-onset depressed subjects than controls (Krishnan et al, 1988; Coffey et al, 1990; Rabins et al, 1991; Greenwald et al, 1996; Kumar et al, 1997; Lenze et al, 1999). As they may represent injury to brain tissue, hyperintensities are thought to potentially play a critical role in the pathogenesis of depression in these individuals.

Beyond depression, hyperintensities are associated with increased age (Awad et al, 1986; Longstreth et al, 1996; Kumar et al, 1999) and are seen in normal ageing (Fazekas et al, 1988a; Guttmann et al, 1998). Although many studies associate hyperintensities in specific regions with increased age (Hickie et al, 1995; Kumar et al, 1997; Sato et al, 1999), at least one study has not associated subcortical or deep white matter hyperintensities with increased age (Kumar et al, 1997).

In addition to age, hyperintensities are also associated with medical comorbidity. Hyperintensities appear in Alzheimer's dementia (Bennett et al, 1992; Kumar et al, 1997) and multiple sclerosis (Fazekas et al, 1998). Increased hyperintensity severity also correlates strongly with cerebrovascular risk factors (Fazekas et al, 1988a; Ylikoski et al, 1995; Longstreth et al, 1996), including hypertension (Awad et al, 1986; Fazekas et al, 1988a; Longstreth et al, 1996), diabetes (Fazekas et al, 1988a), history of smoking

(Longstreth et al, 1996), low cerebral blood flow velocity (Fazekas et al, 1988a; Tzourio et al, 2001), carotid artery disease (Fazekas et al, 1988a) and prior episodes of cerebral ischaemia (Awad et al, 1986; Longstreth et al, 1996; Sato et al, 1999). However, hyperintensities may occur in subjects without such risk factors. A recent study using diffusion tensor imaging, a MRI variation exquisitely sensitive to ischaemic disease, demonstrated that hyperintensities had diffusion characteristics similar to chronic ischaemic lesions (Taylor et al, 2001).

Although hyperintensity severity is associated with depression, hyperintensity location may be an even more critical factor. Evidence is strongest for a contributory effect of subcortical hyperintensities, particularly basal ganglia hyperintensities. Basal ganglia hyperintensities are more common in late-onset depressed subjects than in controls (Rabins et al, 1991; Greenwald et al, 1996; Iidaka et al, 1996; Steffens et al, 1999; MacFall et al, 2001), although one large study of community-dwelling elderly concluded that non-basal ganglia lesions (i.e. white matter lesions) were more strongly associated with depression than basal ganglia lesions (Sato et al, 1999). The putamen may be particularly important, as one study has found that left putaminal hyperintensities predicted assignment into the depressive or control group (Greenwald et al, 1998).

Studies of periventricular hyperintensities – hyperintensities that ring the ventricles – are more mixed. Some research found increased frequency in depressed elderly subjects compared with controls (Coffey et al, 1993), and in late-onset compared with early-onset depressed subjects (Salloway et al, 1996). Others have not found these correlations (Rabins et al, 1991; Steffens et al, 1999; de Groot et al, 2000; Nebes et al, 2001).

Studies examining deep white matter hyperintensities (DWMH) are more promising. Late-onset depressed subjects have more significant disease than do controls (Rabins et al, 1991; Kumar et al, 2000; Nebes et al, 2001) or early-onset subjects (Figiel et al, 1991; Krishnan et al, 1993; Lesser et al, 1996; Salloway et al, 1996). Research has also demonstrated that increased deep white matter hyperintensities (DWMH) severity is associated with a greater risk of depression (de Groot et al, 2000; Kumar et al, 2000). Despite this strong evidence, one large study of over 3600 community elderly found that white matter hyperintensities were overall not associated with depressive symptoms (Steffens et al, 1999).

This supports the idea that the location of the hyperintensities may be even more important than their overall severity. The orbital frontal cortex (OFC) may be particularly important in the pathogenesis of depression. Depressed subjects have smaller OFC volumes than do control subjects (Lai et al, 2000), and post-mortem studies of depressed elderly patients demonstrate OFC and dorsolateral prefrontal cortex atrophy (Rajkowska et al, 1999). Increased depression severity is also associated with increased hyperintensity density in the medial OFC (MacFall et al, 2001).

Neuropsychological findings

Older individuals with depression may experience deficits in a variety of neuropsychological domains, including deficits in attention and concentration (Palsson et al, 2000), mental processing speed (Burt et al, 1995; Beats et al, 1996; Palsson et al, 2000), executive dysfunction (Stromgren, 1977; Channon and Green, 1999), amongst others. Individuals with vascular depression have been found to exhibit a specific pattern of frontal lobe dysfunction and psychomotor slowing (Krishnan et al, 1997; Simpson et al, 1997; Dahabra et al, 1998).

Involvement of the prefrontal cortex may be particularly important in late-life depression. Research indicates that prefrontal dysfunction, specifically psychomotor retardation and abnormal initiation/perseveration scores on the Mattis Dementia Rating Scale (MDRS) (Mattis, 1988), is associated with poor or delayed response to antidepressant therapy (Kalayam and Alexopoulos, 1999), and increased rates of relapse and recurrence of geriatric depression (Alexopoulos et al, 2000). Depressed elderly people also exhibit performance feedback deficits, wherein they cannot correct performance errors even after corrective feedback; these deficits are thought to be related to impairment in the orbital frontal cortex (Steffens et al, 2001b).

How do hyperintense lesions affect cognitive function? Most research associates increased hyperintensity severity with impaired attention and psychomotor speed (Ylikoski et al, 1993; Hickie et al, 1995; Simpson et al, 1998), executive dysfunction (Harrell et al, 1991; Hickie et al, 1995; Salloway et al, 1996; Simpson et al, 1998), and impairment in verbal and non-verbal memory (Austrom et al, 1990; Salloway et al, 1996; Kramer-Ginsberg et al, 1999), although negative findings do exist (Tupler et al, 1992). One large study of community dwelling elderly people found impaired cognitive function correlated with global severity of white matter hyperintensities (Longstreth et al, 1996). Damage to specific regions is probably the more important factor. Increased severity of grey matter hyperintensities is associated with the subsequent development of frank dementia (Steffens et al, 2000).

The combination of depression and neuropsychological impairment leads to increased disability. Increased hyperintensity severity is associated with greater impairment in the activities of daily living (ADLs) (Cahn et al, 1996). One study found this association to be strongest for greater white matter lesion severity (Steffens et al, 2002), while a large study of over 3300 elderly subjects found that ADL and IADL (instrumental ADL) impairment was associated with basal ganglia hyperintensities. The risk of impairment further increased if hyperintensities were present both in and outside of the basal ganglia. This study also found that difficulty in one or more IADLs was strongly associated with depression severity, indicating a complex relationship between impairment, mood, and neuroradiological abnormalities (Sato et al, 1999). This relationship is further complicated by findings associating prefrontal dysfunction, such as deficits in psychomotor retardation and the initiation/perseveration scale of the MDRS, with greater impairment in IADLs (Kiosses et al, 2000).

Clinical significance

Beyond the satisfaction of potentially demonstrating a firm biological basis for depression, do these findings matter? How do they relate to individual patients? To answer these questions, we need to examine how imaging findings relate to adverse treatment events and treatment response.

Adverse events

Cerebral lesions are associated with a higher occurrence of adverse central nervous system reactions to somatic antidepressant therapies (Fujikawa et al, 1996). Hyperintensities are specifically associated with a higher risk of delirium from both antidepressant drug therapy (Figiel et al, 1989) and electroconvulsive therapy (ECT) (Figiel et al, 1990; Steffens et al, 2001a). Moreover, caudate hyperintensities are associated with increased risk of antipsychotic-induced Parkinsonism (Figiel et al, 1991).

Treatment response

Increased hyperintensity severity is associated with poor treatment response to both pharmacotherapy and ECT (Hickie et al, 1995; Simpson et al, 1998; Steffens et al, 2001a). One author, having previously coined the term 'silent cerebral infarction' (SCI) in referring to hyperintensities (Fujikawa et al, 1993), retrospectively found that individuals with more severe SCI had more hospitalizations for depression (Yanai et al, 1998) that lasted significantly longer than those with moderate SCI (Fujikawa et al, 1996).

Diagnostic criteria

Based on these data, researchers have proposed that vascular depression may be a subtype of depression as it may be accompanied by specific clinical features, neuropsychological impairment, and neuroimaging findings. Initially termed 'arteriosclerotic depression' (Krishnan and McDonald, 1995), the subtype was later identified as 'vascular depression'. Analogous to vascular dementia, this term implies both a biological basis and a specific clinical syndrome.

But researchers had differing opinions on how to define the syndrome. Krishnan and colleagues initially defined the syndrome using magnetic resonance imaging to identify cerebral lesions (Krishnan and McDonald, 1995; Krishnan et al, 1997). Alexopoulos and colleagues took a different approach, defining the syndrome based on clinical cerebrovascular risk factors (Alexopoulos et al, 1997a,b). Ultimately, Steffens and Krishnan (1998) proposed criteria that combined these two concepts and added the further criteria of neuropsychological impairment and functional impairment (see Table 10.1).

Conclusions

There exists significant evidence to support the establishment of a 'vascular' subtype of major depressive disorder. Research criteria have in fact already been proposed, incorporating the neurological, neuropsychological, and clinical features of this syndrome.

Although this theory includes a biological basis for the syndrome, its full clinical significance is currently unclear and worthy of further research. Implications for treatment response, and potentially new therapeutics designed to specifically treat this subtype of depression, need to be investigated.

Table 10.1   Proposed criteria for vascular depression subtype.

Specify vascular subtype (can be applied to the current or most recent major depressive episode in major depressive disorder or bipolar disorder) if A and either B1, B2, or B3:

A. Major depression occurring in the context of clinical and/or neuroimaging evidence of cerebrovascular disease or neuropsychological impairment.

B1. Clinical manifestations may include history of stroke or transient ischaemic attacks, or focal neurological signs or symptoms (e.g. exaggeration of deep tendon reflexes, extensor plantar response, pseudobulbar palsy, gait disturbance, weakness of an extremity).

B2. Neuroimaging findings may include white or grey matter hyperintensities (Fazekas criteria >2 (Fazekas et al, 1988b); or lesion >5 mm in diameter and irregular in shape), confluent white matter lesions, or cortical or subcortical infarcts.

B3. Cognitive impairment manifested by disturbance of executive function (e.g. planning, organizing, sequencing, abstracting), memory, or speed of processing of information.

The diagnosis is supported by the following features:

1) Depression onset after 50 years of age or change in course of depression after the onset of vascular disease in patients with onset before 50 years of age.

2) Marked loss of interest or pleasure.

3) Psychomotor retardation.

4) Lack of family history of mood disorders.

5) Marked disability in instrumental or self-maintenance of activities of daily living.

Source: Reprinted with permission from the Society of Biological Psychiatry [*Biological Psychiatry* (1998) **43**:705–12] (Steffens and Krishnan, 1998).

Acknowledgement

Work on this chapter was supported by National Institute of Mental Health grants P50 MH60451, R01 MH54846, and K07 MH01367.

References

Alexopoulos GS, Meyers BS, Young RC, et al, Vascular depression hypothesis, *Arch Gen Psychiatry* (1997a) **54**(10):915–22.

Alexopoulos GS, Meyers BS, Young RC, et al, Clinically defined vascular depression, *Am J Psychiatry* (1997b) **154**(4):562–5.

Alexopoulos GS, Meyers BS, Young RC et a, Executive dysfunction and long-term outcomes of geriatric depression, *Arch Gen Psychiatry* (2000) **57**:285–90.

Astrom M, Adolfsson R, Asplund K, Major depression in stroke patients. A 3-year longitudinal study, *Stroke* (1993) **24**:976–82.

Austrom MG, Thompson RFJ, Hendrie HC et al, Foci of increased T2 signal intensity in MR images of healthy elderly subjects. A follow-up study, *J Am Geriatr Soc* (1990) **38**:1133–8.

Awad IA, Spetzler RF, Hodak JA et al, Incidental subcortical lesions identified on magnetic resonance imaging in the elderly. I. Correlation with age and cerebrovascular risk factors, *Stroke* (1986) **17**:1084–9.

Barefoot JC, Schroll M, Symptoms of depression, acute myocardial infarction, and total mortality in a community sample, *Circulation* (1996) **93**:1976–80.

Beats BC, Sahakian BJ, Levy R Cognitive performance in tests sensitive to frontal lobe dysfunction in the elderly depressed, *Psychol Med* (1996) **26**(3):591–603.

Bennett DA, Gilley DW, Wilson RS et al, Clinical correlates of high signal lesions on magnetic resonance imaging in Alzheimer's disease, *J Neurol* (1992) **239**:186–90.

Bryan RN, Manolio TA, Schertz LD et al, A method for using MR to evaluate the effects of cardiovascular disease on the brain: the cardiovascular health study, *AJNR Am J Neuroradiol* (1994) **15**:1625–33.

Burt DB, Zembar MJ, Niederene G, Depression and memory impairment: a meta-analysis of the association, its pattern, and specificity, *Psychol Bull* (1995) **117**:285–305.

Cahn DA, Malloy PF, Salloway S et al, Subcortical hyperintensities on MRI and activities of daily living in geriatric depression, *J Neuropsychiatry Clin Neurosci* (1996) **8**(4):404–11.

Carney RM, Rich WM, Tevelde A et al, Major depressive disorder in coronary artery disease, *Am J Cardiol* (1987) **60**:1273–5.

Channon S, Green PS, Executive function in depression: the role of performance strategies in aiding depressed and non-depressed participants, *J Neurol Neurosurg Psychiatry* (1999) **66**:162–71.

Coffey CE, Figiel GS, Djang WT et al, Leukoencephalopathy in elderly depressed patients referred for ECT, *Biol Psychiatry* (1988) **24**(2):143–61.

Coffey CE, Figiel GS, Djang WT et al, Subcortical hyperintensity on magnetic resonance imaging: a comparison of normal and depressed elderly subjects, *Am J Psychiatry* (1990) **147**(2):187–9.

Coffey CE, Wilkinson WE, Weiner RD et al, Quantitative cerebral anatomy in depression: a controlled magnetic resonance imaging study, *Arch Gen Psychiatry* (1993) **50**(1):7–16.

Coffey CE, Lucke JF, Saxton JA et al, Sex differences in brain imaging, *Arch Neurol* (1998) **55**:169–79.

Dahabra S, Ashton CH, Bahrainian M et al, Structural and functional abnormalities in elderly patients clinically recovered from early- and late-onset depression, *Biol Psychiatry* (1998) 34–46.

de Groot JC, de Leeuw F, Oudkerk M et al, Cerebral white matter lesions and depressive symptoms in elderly adults, *Arch Gen Psychiatry* (2000) **57**:1071–6.

Ebrahim S, Barer K, Nouri F, Affective illness after stroke, *Br J Psychiatry* (1987) **154**:170–82.

Fazekas F, Niederkor K, Schmidt R et al, White matter signal abnormalties in normal individuals: correlation with carotid ultrasonography, cerebral blood flow measurements, and cerebrovascular risk factors, *Stroke* (1988a) **19**:1285–8.

Fazekas F, Offenbacher H, Fuchs S et al, Criteria for an increased specificity of MRI interpretation in elderly subjects with suspected multiple sclerosis, *Neurology* (1988b) **38**:1822–5.

Fazekas F, Barkhof F, Filippi M, Unenhanced and enhanced magnetic resonance imaging in the diagnosis of multiple sclerosis, *J Neurol Neurosurg Psychiatry* (1998) **64**:S2–S5.

Figiel GS, Krishnan KRR, Breitner JC et al, Radiologic correlates of antidepressant-induced delirium: the possible significance of basal-ganglia lesions, *J Neuropsychiatry Clin Neurosci* (1989) **1**:188–90.

Figiel GS, Coffey CE, Djang WT et al, Brain magnetic resonance imaging findings in ECT-induced delirium, *J Neuropsychiatry Clin Neurosci* (1990) **2**:53–8.

Figiel GS, Krishnan KRR, Doraiswamy PM et al, Subcortical hyperintensities on brain magnetic resonance imaging: a comparison between late age onset and early onset elderly depressed subjects, *Neurobiol Aging* (1991a) **12**(3):245–7.

Figiel GS, Krishnan KRR, Doraiswamy PM et al, Caudate hyperintensities in elderly depressed patients with neuroleptic-induced parkinsonism, *J Geriatr Psychiatry Neurol* (1991b) **4**:86–9.

Forrester AW, Lipsey JR, Teitelbaum ML et al, Depression following myocardial infarction, *Int J Psychiatry Med* (1992) **22**:33–46.

Frasure-Smith N, Lesperance F, Talajic M, Depression following myocardial infarction. Impact on 6-month survival, *JAMA* (1993) **270**:1819–25.

Frasure-Smith N, Lesperance F, Talajic M, Depression and 18-month prognosis after myocardial infarction, *Circulation* (1995) **91**:999–1005.

Fujikawa T, Yamawaki S, Touhouda Y, Incidence of silent cerebral infarction in patients with major depression, *Stroke* (1993) **24**:1631–4.

Fujikawa T, Yokota N, Muraoka M et al, Response of patients with major depression and silent cerebral infarction to antidepressant drug therapy, with emphasis on central nervous system adverse reactions, *Stroke* (1996) **27**:2040–2.

Gonzalez MB, Snyderman TB, Colket JT et al, Depression in patients with coronary artery disease, *Depression* (1996) **4**:57–62.

Greenwald BS, Kramer-Ginsberg E, Krishnan KRR et al, MRI signal hyperintensities in geriatric depression, *Am J Psychiatry* (1996) **153**:1212–5.

Greenwald BS, Kramer-Ginsberg E, Krishnan KRR et al, Neuroanatomic localization of magnetic resonance imaging signal hyperintensities in geriatric depression, *Stroke* (1998) **29**(3):613–7.

Guttman CRG, Jolesz FA, Kikinis R et al, White matter changes with normal aging, *Neurology* (1998) **50**:972–8.

Harrell LE, Duvall E, Folks DG et al, The relationship of high-intensity signals on magnetic resonance images to cognitive and psychiatric state in Alzheimer's disease, *Arch Neurol* (1991) **48**:1136–40.

Hickie I, Scott E, Mitchell P et al, Subcortical hyperintensities on magnetic resonance imaging: clinical correlates and prognostic significance in patients with severe depression, *Biol Psychiatry* (1995) **37**(3):151–60.

Iidaka T, Nakajima T, Kawamoto K et al, Signal hyperintensities on brain magnetic resonance imaging in elderly depressed patients, *Eur Neurol* (1996) **36**(5):293–9.

Kalayam B, Alexopoulos GS, Prefrontal dysfunction and treatment response in geriatric depression, *Arch Gen Psychiatry* (1999) **56**:713–8.

Kendler KS, Neale MC, MacLean CJ et al, Smoking and major depression. A causal analysis, *Arch Gen Psychiatry* (1993) **50**:36–43.

Kiosses DN, Alexopoulos GS, Murphy C, Symptoms of striatofrontal dysfunction contribute to disability in geriatric depression, *Int J Geriatr Psychiatry* (2000) **15**:992–9.

Kramer-Ginsberg E, Greenwald BS, Krishnan KRR et al, Neuropsychological functioning and MRI signal hyperintensities in geriatric depression, *Am J Psychiatry* (1999) **156**:438–44.

Krishnan KRR, Goli V, Ellinwood EH et al, Leukoencephalopathy in patients diagnosed as major depressive, *Biol Psychiatry* (1988) :519–22.

Krishnan KRR, McDonald WM, Escalona PR et al, Magnetic resonance imaging of the caudate nucleus in depression. Preliminary observations, *Arch Gen Psychiatry* (1992) **49**:553–7.

Krishnan KRR, McDonald WM, Doraiswamy PM et al, Neuroanatomical substrates of depression in the elderly, *Eur Arch Psychiatry Clin Neurosci* (1993) **241**:41–6.

Krishnan KRR, McDonald WM, Arteriosclerotic depression, *Med Hypotheses* (1995) **44**:111–5.

Krishnan KRR, Hays JC, Blazer DG, MRI-defined vascular depression, *Am J Psychiatry* (1997) **154**(4):497–501.

Krishnan KRR, Doraiswamy PM, Clary CM, Clinical and treatment response characteristics of late-life depression associated with vascular disease: a pooled analysis of two multicenter trials with sertraline, *Prog Neuropsychopharmacol Biol Psychiatry* (2001) **25**:347–51.

Kumar A, Miller D, Ewbank D et al, Quantitative anatomic measures and comorbid medical illness in late-life major depression, *Am J Geriatr Psychiatry* (1997) **5**:15–25.

Kumar A, Bilker W, Jin Z et al, Age of onset of depression and quantitative neuroanatomic measures: absence of specific correlates, *Psychiatry Res* (1999) **91**:101–10.

Kumar A, Bilker W, Zhisong J et al, Atrophy and high intensity lesions: Complementary neurobiological mechanisms in late-life depression, *Neuropsychopharmacology* (2000)**22**:264–74.

Kumar A, Mintz J, Bilker W et al, Autonomous neurobiological pathways to late-life major depressive disorder: clinical and pathophysiological implications, *Neuropsychopharmacology* (2002) **26**:229–36.

Lai TJ, Payne ME, Byrum CE et al, Reduction of orbital frontal cortex volume in geriatric depression, *Biol Psychiatry* (2000) **48**(10):971–5.

Lenze E, DeWitte C, McKeel D et al, White matter hyperintensities and gray matter lesions in physically healthy depressed subjects, *Am J Psychiatry* (1999) **156**:1602–7.

Lesser IM, Miller BL, Boone KB et al, Brain injury and cognitive function in late-onset psychotic depression, *J Neuropsychiatry Clin Neurosci* (1991) **3**:33–40.

Lesser IM, Boone KB, Mehringer CM et al, Cognition and white matter hyperintensities in older depressed patients, *Am J Psychiatry* (1996) **153**:1280–7.

Littlefield CH, Rodin GM, Murray MA et al, Influence of functional impairment and social support on depressive symptoms in persons with diabetes, *Health Psychol* (1990) **9**:737–49.

Longstreth WTJ, Manolio TA, Arnold A et al, Clinical correlates of white matter findings on cranial magnetic resonance imaging of 3301 elderly people: the cardiovascular health study, *Stroke* (1996) **27**:1274–82.

Lustman PJ, Griffith LS, Gavard JA et al, Depression in adults with diabetes, *Diabetes Care* (1992) **15**:1631–9.

Lyness JM, Caine ED, Cox C et al, Cerebrovascular risk factors and later-life major depression. Testing a small-vessel brain disease model, *Am J Geriatr Psychiatry* (1998) **6**:5–13.

MacFall JR, Payne ME, Provenzale JE et al, Medial orbital frontal lesions in late-onset depression, *Biol Psychiatry* (2001) **49**:803–6.

Mattis S, Dementia Rating Scale (DRS). Odessa, Florida, Psychological Assessment Resources (1988).

Mendlewicz J, Baron M, Morbidity risks in subtypes of unipolar depressive illness: differences between early and late onset forms, *Br J Psychiatry* (1981) **139**:463–6.

Nebes Rd, Vora IJ, Meltzer CC et al, 'Relationship of deep white matter hyperintensities and apolipoprotein E genotype to depressive symptoms in older adults without clinical depression, *Am J Psychiatry* (2001) **158**:878–84.

Palsson S, Johansson B, Berg S et al, A population study on the influence of depression on neuropsychological functioning in 85-year-olds, *Acta Psychiatr Scand* (2000) **101**:185–93.

Palsson S, Skoog I, The epidemiology of affective disorders in the elderly: a review, *Int Clin Psychopharmacol* (1997) **12** (Supp 7):S3–13.

Pantel J, Schroder J, Essig M et al, Quantitative magnetic resonance imaging in geriatric depression and primary degenerative dementia, *J Affect Disord* (1997) **42**:69–83.

Parashos IA, Tupler LA, Blitchington T et al, Magnetic-resonance morphometry in patients with major depression, *Psychiatry Res* (1998) **84**:7–15.

Passe TJ, Rajagopalan P, Tupler LA et al, Age and sex effects on brain morphology, *Prog Neuropsychopharmacol Biol Psychiatry* (1997) **21**:1231–7.

Pratt LA, Ford DE, Crum RM et al, Coronary heart disease / myocardial infarction: depression, psychotropic medication, and risk of myocardial infarction: prospective data from the Baltimore ECA follow-up, *Circulation* (1996) **94**:3123–9.

Rabins PV, Pearlson GD, Aylward E et al, Cortical magnetic resonance imaging changes in elderly inpatients with major depression, *Am J Psychiatry* (1991) **148**:617–20.

Rabkin JG, Charles E, Kass F, Hypertension and DSM-III depression in psychiatric outpatients, *Am J Psychiatry* (1983) **140**:1072–4.

Rajkowska G, Miguel-Hidalgo JJ, Wei J et al, Morphometric evidence for neuronal and glial prefrontal cell pathology in major depression, *Biol Psychiatry* (1999) **45**(9):1085–98.

Robinson RG, Kubos KL, Starr LB et al, Mood disorders in stroke patients. Importance of lesion location, *Brain* (1984) **107**:81–93.

Roose SP, Laghrissi-Thode F, Kennedy JS et al, Comparison of paroxetine and nortriptyline in depressed patients with ischemic heart disease, *JAMA* (1998) **279**:287–91.

Salloway S, Malloy P, Kohn R et al, MRI and neuropsychological differences in early- and late-life-onset geriatric depression, *Neurology* (1996) **46**(6):1567–74.

Sato R, Bryan RN, Fried LP, Neuroanatomic and functional correlates of depressed mood: the cardiovascular health study, *Am J Epidemiol* (1999) **150**:919–29.

Schleifer SJ, Macari-Hinson MM, Coyle DA et al, The nature and course of depression following myocardial infarction, *Arch Intern Med* (1989) **149**:1785–9.

Simpson S, Baldwin RC, Jackson A et al, Is subcortical disease associated with a poor response to antidepressants? Neurological, neuropsychological and neuroradiological findings in late-life depression, *Psychol Med* (1998) **28**:1015–26.

Simpson SW, Jackson A, Baldwin RC et al, Subcortical hyperintensities in late-life depression: acute response to treatment and neuropsychological impairment, *Int Psychogeriatr* (1997) **9**:257–75.

Steffens DC, Krishnan KRR, Structural neuroimaging and mood disorders: recent findings, implications for classification, and future directions, *Biol Psychiatry* (1998) **43**:705–12.

Steffens DC, Helms MJ, Krishnan KRR et al, Cerebrovascular disease and depression symptoms in the cardiovascular health study, *Stroke* (1999) **30**(10):2159–66.

Steffens DC, MacFall JR, Payne ME et al, Grey-matter lesions and dementia *Lancet* (2000) **356**:1686–7.

Steffens DC, Conway CR, Dombeck CB et al, Severity of subcortical gray matter hyperintensity predicts ECT response in geriatric depression. *J ECT* (2001a) **17**:45–9.

Steffens DC, Wagner HR, Levy RM et al, Performance feedback deficit in geriatric depression, *Biol Psychiatry* (2001b) **50**:358–63.

Steffens DC, Bosworth HB, Provenzale JM et al, Subcortical white matter lesions and functional impairment in geriatric depression, *Depress Anxiety* (2002) **15**:23–8.

Stromgren LS, The influence of depression on memory, *Acta Psychiatr Scand* (1977) **56**:109–28.

Taylor WD, Payne ME, Krishnan KRR et al, Evidence of white matter tract disruption in MRI hyperintensities, *Biol Psychiatry* (2001) **50**:179–83.

Tiller JW, Post-stroke depression, *Psychopharmacology* (1992) **106** (Suppl): S130–33.

Tupler LA, Coffey CE, Logue PE et al, Neuropsychological importance of subcortical white matter hyperintensity, *Arch Neurol* (1992) **49**:1248–52.

Tzourio C, Levy C, Dufouil C et al, Low cerebral blood flow velocity and risk of white matter hyperintensities, *Ann Neurol* (2001) **49**:411–4.

Wade DT, Legh-Smith J, Hewer RA, Depressed mood after stroke. A community study of its frequency, *Br J Psychiatry* (1987) **151**:200–5.

Wassertheil-Smoller S, Applegate WB, Berge K et al, Change in depression as a precursor of cardiovascular events, *Arch Intern Med* (1996) **156**:553–61.

11
Cerebrovascular risk factors and depression: data, deductions, and directions

Jeffrey M Lyness and Eric D Caine

Introduction

During the past century, psychopathologists have depended on the precise description of clinical phenomena and specific syndromes to establish psychiatric diagnoses and develop empirically tested therapeutic interventions (Caine and Lyness, 2000). Colleagues in other fields of medicine, however, moved away from syndrome classifications to those based on a clearer theoretical understanding of disease mechanisms, and an appreciation of those risk-enhancing pathobiological and social processes that lead to the eventual emergence of clinically evident symptoms and signs. As a result of these endeavors, they have been able to prevent disease expression (e.g. reduce the incidence of myocardial infarctions). Also, they have discerned once more, as infectious disease specialists have long known, that common risk factors underpin apparently disparate disorders (e.g. cigarette smoking leading to cardiac diseases and stroke).

Cerebrovascular risk factors (CVRFs) are individual characteristics or systemic diseases that enhance the probability of developing cerebrovascular diseases. Considerable evidence implicates the following as risk factors for the subsequent development of stroke: older age, male sex, hypertension or elevated systolic blood pressure, coronary artery disease, atrial fibrillation, left ventricular hypertrophy, diabetes mellitus, and cigarette smoking (Dyken et al, 1985; American Heart Association, 1990). The role of hypercholesterolaemia in stroke is less clear, although it is certainly an important independent risk factor for other atherosclerotic conditions such as coronary artery disease (American Heart Association, 1990). We will consider in this chapter the evidence that such CVRFs also are risk factors for the development of small vessel brain disease, which in turn may lead to the development of clinically significant mood disorders.

The study of CVRFs as risk factors for depression is of interest for at least two reasons. Examination of these relationships offers important supportive evidence for specific theoretical models of the pathogenesis of depression in later life. Also, such study provides a useful context in which to consider conceptual and methodological issues involving risk factor research for psychiatric conditions, issues that are relevant to a host of studies regarding mood (and other) disorders.

Accordingly, this chapter will begin by reviewing the theoretical models of depression pertaining to the CVRF–depression dynamic. It will then consider the broader conceptual and methodological contexts in which one may examine CVRFs as risk factors for depression or other psychiatric conditions. Next it will review the available empirical data about CVRFs and depression. It will conclude with a summary, including consideration of directions for further research.

Even as this review is conducted we recognize an inherent limitation of this approach. Assume for the moment that CVRFs are pathobiologically tied to the development of depression. Clearly they are also tied to other disease manifestations. As psychiatrists, we view the 'system' through the lens of disturbances in mood, seeking to discern a specific causal association and its mechanism(s). *We acknowledge as we pursue this goal that we have a fundamental observer bias, an artifact of our training, clinical practice, and research interests.* As human biologists, we recognize that it would always be preferable to proceed from a hypothesized aetiology toward the manifestations of disease, rather than in the opposite direction. We likely would find, of course, that there is not a single or specific clinical presentation, and again confront the challenge that depression, like other psychopathological conditions, can arise from multiple aetiologies.

Theoretical models relevant to the CVRF–depression dynamic

The 'structural' cerebrovascular disease model of depression

In this model, often referred to as 'vascular depression', otherwise clinically occult small vessel brain disease may 'predispose, precipitate, or perpetuate' (Alexopoulos et al, 1997) some depressive episodes, especially those of first onset later in life. Evidence in favour of this model, as described previously (Alexopoulos et al, 1997; Krishnan et al, 1997), will be summarized briefly. There is considerable data to indicate that strokes, that is clinically apparent cerebrovascular disease, can cause or contribute physiologically to depression. It appears that depression in later life, especially that with an older age of onset, is more often associated with acquired factors such as medical illnesses than with genetic influences or stressors earlier in life. The association of a variety of cognitive deficits with elderly depression suggests the presence of fairly widespread brain dysfunction. Structural neuroimaging studies have shown that later-life depression is associated with central and cortical atrophy, consistent with widespread brain parenchymal loss due to cerebrovascular disease. More specifically, magnetic resonance imaging (MRI) scans show more diffuse hyperintensities on T2-weighted images in people who are depressed than in age-matched controls, hyperintensities that may reflect small vessel disease given both CVRF correlative studies and post-mortem findings in other populations. Other findings using techniques assessing brain function, including functional neuroimaging and electrophysiological methods, have also demonstrated diffuse dysfunction consistent with cerebrovascular disease.

More recently, Alexopoulos and colleagues have proposed an extension of the cerebrovascular model in which some late-onset depression reflects the effects of cerebrovascular disease on striato-frontal circuitry (Alexopoulos et al, 2000; Alexopoulos, 2001). This model is based on findings of a distinctive clinical profile, including greater psychomotor retardation, difficulty with executive functioning, disability, and poorer outcome. This proposal is highly useful and provocative, one that lends itself to testing by a variety of methods including more detailed neuropsychological assessments, functional neuroimaging, electrophysiology (Kindermann et al, 2000), and other tests of brain functioning, as well as by the risk factor approaches described below.

Cytokine-mediated model of atherosclerosis and depression

Recognizing that other routes might help us understand the potential relationships between cerebro- and cardiovascular diseases and depression, our group has proposed a model (Lyness and Caine, 2000) which we will summarize briefly here. In this model, atherosclerotic disease burden leads to elevated levels of inflammatory cytokines, specifically interleukin-1-b (IL-1b). Chronically elevated IL-1b levels stimulate central monoamine turnover, which over time leads to decreased activity of these systems due to autotoxicity. Decreased monoamine system function then manifests as depressive symptoms or syndromes. As described previously (Lyness and Caine, 2000), there is evidence to support each of the individual steps in this model, but to date no direct evidence supporting the overall theory. Our own pilot data failed to note a correlation between serum IL-1b level and depression in cardiac patients undergoing cardiac rehabilitation (Lyness et al, 2001). However, more definitive work needs to be done, including the use of a comparison group without evident atherosclerotic disease. As well, while the central effects of cytokines on monoamine systems may be less clear, the role of other cytokines such as IL-6 may be important in other diseases' relationships to depression (Musselman et al, 2001) and remains to be explored in cardiovascular disorders.

Depression contributing to cardiovascular disease

To this point, this chapter has focused on models in which CVRFs, either individually (cardiovascular disorders) or cumulatively, contribute to the pathogenesis of depression. One must recognize, however, that depression may itself contribute to the pathogeneses of CVRFs. Again, the bulk of the evidence for this is about cardiovascular disorders. There is small but growing support for potential mechanisms underlying this model, including the role of negative emotions in cardiac disease, potentially through autonomically-mediated increase in myocardial workload and thus ischaemia (Gullette et al, 1997), or in ventricular irritability (Frasure-Smith et al, 1995a; Musselman et al, 1998); diminished beat-to-beat heart rate variability (Miyawaki and Salzman, 1991); or worsened atherogenesis due to the effects of depression, through relatively direct effects on platelet function (Musselman et al, 1998) or hypercortisolaemia-mediated effects on other CVRFs such as blood pressure or lipid levels.

With these models as a backdrop, we now turn to consider the usefulness of a risk-factor approach to determining pathogenesis.

Risk factors: conceptual and definitional issues

It has long been recognized that the study of risk factors, which by implication are tied to pathogenesis of an illness (Evans, 1978), can yield insight into disease mechanisms. However, terminology has often been used imprecisely. As reviewed by Kraemer and colleagues (1997, 2001), the following definitions will prove useful:

- *Risk* is the probability of an outcome.
- A *correlate* is a variable associated with an outcome.
- A *risk factor* is a correlate that precedes the outcome.

It is important to note, then, that a specific temporal sequence is required; thus, for example, CVRFs cannot be true risk factors for stroke, or for depression, unless they are present prior to the development of stroke or depression.

Having said that, let us re-examine the statement that risk factors are by implication tied to pathogenesis of an illness. In fact, too often it is assumed that 'risk factor' is synonymous with 'causal factor'. A *causal risk factor* is defined as a risk factor that, when changed, changes the outcome (Kraemer et al, 2001). Yet not all causal risk factors are equally proximate to the disease mechanism. In addition, most conditions have multiple risk factors and even multiple causal risk factors. Kraemer and colleagues (2001), building on prior work, have proposed that there are five ways in which risk factors can work together. Considering the case in which both A and B are risk factors for outcome O:

(1) B may be a *proxy risk factor* for A if A and B are correlated, if there is no temporal precedence of either A or B (or if A precedes B), and if A predominates (that is, if B's correlation with O weakens or disappears when A is included). Proxy risk factors ultimately may prove incidental to the disease mechanisms, but they may aid the search for causal risk factors.
(2) A and B are *overlapping risk factors* if A and B are correlated, if neither has temporal precedence, and if they are codominant (that is, each

individual correlation with O remains the same when considering the other). Overlapping risk factors may each relate to the same construct, and consideration of each may improve the assessment of this construct and its relationship to the outcome.

(3) A and B are *independent risk factors* if they are not correlated with each other, neither has temporal precedence, and they are codominant.

(4) B is a *mediator* of A's relationship to O if B explains *how* A relates to the outcome. Thus there is a relationship chain, in which A is correlated with and precedes B, and B is dominant in its relationship to O (or codominant, in the case of partial mediation). A mediator role is consistent with (although by itself does not prove) a causal chain.

(5) B is a *moderator* of A if B affects A's relationship to O, but A and B are not correlated. A statistical interaction between A and B in their association with O is an example of a moderator effect.

These conceptualizations and definitions provide the backdrop for consideration of CVRFs' relationships to depression.

CVRFs and depression

Much of the previously described work regarding models of the CVRF–depression dynamic assumes, implicitly or explicitly, that there is some type of association between the two. What is the direct evidence for this?

As reviewed previously (Hayward, 1995; Lyness et al, 1998), studies examining whether there is an association between CVRFs and depression in psychiatric patient populations have found mixed results. Yet most of this work involved cross-sectional assessments; while admittedly the CVRFs assessed may have been present for some time, perhaps predating the depression, as noted above cross-sectional studies can only directly address correlations, not true risk factors. For example, our own group did not find a cross-sectional association between CVRFs and depression in older subjects recruited from primary care settings (Lyness et al, 1999). However, using this same subject group we found that cumulative CVRF severity predicted depressive symptoms and disorders at 1-year follow-up (Lyness et al, 2000). Further complicating the interpretation of findings, though, this association was not significant after covarying overall medical burden, suggesting that CVRFs are a proxy risk factor for global medical burden, either due to the lack of specificity to the CVRF–depression association or to the methodological difficulty in disentangling CVRFs (and their end-organ effects) from global medical burden (Lyness et al, 2000).

We also note that the above-described modifications to the cerebrovascular model of depression proposed by Alexopoulos and colleagues, that is, the role of striato-frontal dysfunction, introduce a mediator to the CVRF–depression dynamic. That is, CVRFs would not have an independent association with depression; rather, this association would be mediated by striato-frontal deficits presumed to originate in localized cerebrovascular disease. Longitudinal risk factor analyses testing this mediator model remain to be published.

Similarly, the analyses required to best test the cytokine-mediated model described above also would require longitudinal data. Indeed, given the model, one would ideally have predictor variables (atherosclerosis, IL-1b level) at a point in time years prior to the assessment of depression. As noted above, only limited pilot data exist at this time, and these are cross-sectional data that therefore cannot fully test the model.

The strongest risk factor data regarding CVRFs and depression relate to depression's contributions to cardiovascular disease. These data include both cross-sectional and longitudinal data demonstrating that depression is an independent risk factor for the subsequent development of cardiovascular disease (cardiovascular death or myocardial infarction), even after controlling for CVRFs (Ford et al, 1998; Glassman and Shapiro, 1998; Musselman et al, 1998; Penninx et al, 1998). In patients' status post-myocardial infarction, depression has also been shown to be an independent predictor of cardiac outcome over periods of time ranging from 6 to 18 months (Frasure-Smith et al, 1993, 1995b). Indeed, it is precisely these risk factor studies that have led to the informed speculations about possible mechanisms by which depression may contribute to the pathogeneses of cardiovascular disease. However, such a causal relationship is not the only possible explanation for depression's association with cardiovascular outcome. Since atherosclerotic cardiac disease takes years to decades to manifest clinically, the apparent temporal precedence of depression to 'newly developed' cardiac disorders may be illusory. It may be that depression is merely an early clinical manifestation of cardiovascular disorders, that is, of its own risk factor. Alternatively, depression may be a proxy risk factor for a predominant, causal relationship between other CVRFs (e.g. hypertension) and cardiac disease, albeit this argument is not supported by the finding that depression retained its association with cardiac outcome after covarying other measurable CVRFs (Ford et al, 1998; Glassman and Shapiro, 1998; Musselman et al, 1998; Penninx et al, 1998).

Summary

A summary of our risk factor discussion is shown in Figure 11.1. CVRFs may, via a series of steps involving small vessel brain disease, cytokines, or other mechanisms, contribute to depression as well as to other disorders. At the same time, a variety of other factors (biological, psychological, and social) may also contribute to depression, as well as to other disorders. And depression may contribute to cardiac disease (which itself is one of the CVRFs, and is contributed to by other CVRFs) and to other disorders.

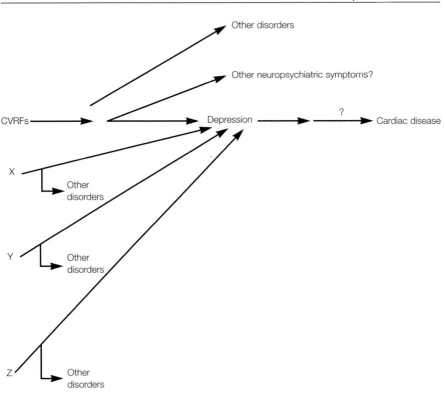

Figure 11.1

Risk factors.

While the broad spectrum of other risk factors for depression – 'X, Y, and Z' in Figure 11.1 – is beyond the scope of this chapter, we again note that the breadth of such risk factors is indicative of the heterogeneity of depression as a syndromically defined entity. That is, depression is not one disorder, but a final common psychopathological pathway for a number of processes across the biopsychosocial spectrum. Presumably, common neurobiological processes are disrupted, as well as common psychological functions, suggesting that *what we consider to be 'depression' is the fundamental reflection of its mediating substrates rather than a specific or unique manifestation of its 'causes', that is, those 'aetiologies' that are involved.*

Current treatment strategies, while often effective, essentially target this final common pathway regardless of aetiology. The hope is that identification of specific aetiologies or pathogenic mechanisms will lead to more specific and effective treatments for those subsets of depression, including the potential for primary or secondary prevention.

However, the investigation of aetiologies – that is, studies that begin from the left side of Figure 11.1 – will have to confront the lack of specificity of such aetiologies. Thus the 'other disorders' caused by CVRFs likely include a variety of cognitive disturbances, ranging from mild cognitive impairment to frank dementia, and perhaps also other neuropsychiatric symptoms or syndromes. The same processes can also lead to 'pure' neurological conditions, such as lacunar infarcts. Whether CVRFs produce dementia, depression, or other psychiatric symptoms in a given individual may depend on the mechanistic route (e.g. the cytokine-mediated model), an 'accident' of the brain regions affected (e.g. whether the small vessel disease predominantly involves striato-frontal circuitry), or more complex interplay of the affected regions with underlying individual vulnerabilities. Recognition of these issues must inform future work at the interface of CVRFs and depression, and in turn may serve as a model for other avenues of mechanistic research in psychiatric conditions.

Acknowledgement

This work was supported by a grant from the National Institute of Mental Health, R01 MH61429 (Dr Lyness).

References

Alexopoulos GS, The depression-executive dysfunction syndrome of late life, A specific target for D3 agonists? *Am J Geriatr Psychiatry* (2001) **9**: 22–9.

Alexopoulos GS, Meyers BS, Young RC et al, 'Vascular depression' hypothesis, *Arch Gen Psychiatry* (1997) **54**: 915–22.

Alexopoulos GS, Meyers BS, Young RC et al, Executive dysfunction and long-term outcomes of geriatric depression, *Arch Gen Psychiatry* (2000) **57**: 285–90.

American Heart Association *Stroke Risk Factor Prediction Chart* (American Heart Association: Dallas, 1990).

Caine ED, Lyness JM, Delirium, dementia, and amnestic and other cognitive disorders. In: Kaplan HI, Sadock BJ, eds, *Comprehensive Textbook of Psychiatry*, 7th edn (Lippincott and Wilkins: Baltimore, 2000) 854–923.

Dyken ML, Wolf PA, Barnett HJM et al, Risk factors for stroke. In: *A Statement for Physicians by the Subcommittee on Risk Factors and Stroke of the Stroke* Council (Reprint No. 71–022–A) (American Heart Association: Dallas, 1985).

Evans AS, Causation and disease. A chronological journey, *Am J Epidemiol* (1978) **108**: 249–58.

Ford DE, Mead LA, Chang PP, Coopertrick L et al, Depression is a risk factor for coronary artery disease in men. The Precursors study, *Arch Int Med* (1998) **158**: 1422–6.

Frasure-Smith N, Lesperance F, Talajic M, Depression following myocardial infarction. Impact on 6–month survival, *JAMA* (1993) **270**: 1819–25.

Frasure-Smith N, Lesperance F, Talajic M, The impact of negative emotions on prognosis following myocardial infarction. Is it more than depression? *Health Psychol* (1995a) **14**: 388–98.

Frasure-Smith N, Lesperance F, Talajic M, Depression and 18–month prognosis after myocardial infarction, *Circulation* (1995b) **91**: 999–1005.

Glassman AH, Shapiro PA, Depression and the course of coronary artery disease, *Am J Psychiatry* (1998) **155**: 4–11.

Gullette ECD, Blumenthal JA, Babyak M et al, Effects of mental stress on myocardial ischemia during daily life, *JAMA* (1997) **277**: 1521–6.

Hayward C, Psychiatric illness and cardiovascular disease risk, *Epidemiol Rev* (1995) **17**: 129–38.

Kindermann SS, Kalayam B, Brown GG, Burdick KE, Alexopoulos GS, Executive functions and P300 latency in elderly depressed patients and control subjects, *Am J Geriatr Psychiatry* (2000) **8**: 57–65.

Kraemer HC, Kazdin AE, Offord DR et al, Coming to terms with the terms of risk, *Arch Gen Psychiatry* (1997) **54**: 337–43.

Kraemer HC, Stice E, Kazdin A, Offord D, Kupfer D, How do risk factors work together? Mediators, moderators, and independent, overlapping, and proxy risk factors, *Am J Psychiatry* (2001) **158**: 848–56.

Krishnan KRR, Hays JC, Blazer DG, MRI-defined vascular depression, *Am J Psychiatry* (1997) **154**: 497–501.

Lyness JM, Caine ED, Vascular disease and depression. Models of the interplay between psychopathology and medical comorbidity. In: Williamson GM, Shaffer DR, Parmelee PA, eds, *Physical Illness and Depression in Older Adults: a Handbook of Theory, Research, and Practice* (Kluwer Academic/Plenum: New York, 2000) 31–49.

Lyness JM, Caine ED, Cox C et al, Cerebrovascular risk factors and later-life major depression. Testing a small-vessel brain disease model, *Am J Geriatr Psychiatry* (1998) **6**: 5–13.

Lyness JM, Caine ED, King DA et al, Cerebrovascular risk factors and depression in older primary care patients. Testing a vascular brain disease model of depression, *Am J Geriatr Psychiatry* (1999) **7**: 252–8.

Lyness JM, King DA, Conwell Y, Cox C, Caine ED, Cerebrovascular risk factors and 1–year depression outcome in older primary care patients, *Am J Psychiatry* (2000) **157**: 1499–501.

Lyness JM, Moynihan JA, Williford DJ, Cox C, Caine ED, Depression, medical illness, and interleukin-1b in older cardiac patients, *Int J Psychiatry Med* (2001) **31**: 321–6.

Miyawaki E, Salzman C, Autonomic nervous system tests in psychiatry. Implications and potential uses of heart rate variability, *Integrated Psychiatry* (1991) **7**: 21–8.

Musselman DL, Evans DL, Nemeroff CB, The relationship of depression to cardiovascular disease. Epidemiology, biology, and treatment, *Arch Gen*

Psychiatry (1998) **55**: 580–92.

Musselman DL, Miller AH, Porter MR et al, Higher than normal plasma interleukin-6 concentrations in cancer patients with depression. Preliminary findings, *Am J Psychiatry* (2001) **158**: 1252–7.

Penninx BWJH, Guralnik JM, Mendes de Leon CF et al, Cardiovascular events and mortality in newly and chronically depressed persons >70 years of age, *Am J Cardiol* (1998) **81**: 988–94.

12
Basal ganglia and mood disorders

David C Steffens and K Ranga Rama Krishnan

Introduction

From an anatomical standpoint, there is no precise definition of the basal ganglia. For most clinicians and researchers the term basal ganglia includes the caudate nucleus and the lentiform nucleus, the latter with its two subdivisions, the putamen and the globus pallidus. By convention, many also include the claustrum, the subthalamic nucleus, and the substantia nigra in the basal ganglia (Adams and Victor, 1993). As this chapter focuses on neuroimaging findings in clinical populations, the term basal ganglia will largely refer to the caudate and putamen nuclei and, to a lesser extent, to the globus pallidus.

There is a growing literature linking the basal ganglia with expression of mood disorders, both unipolar depression and bipolar disorder. Much of the evidence for this association is provided by structural and functional neuroimaging studies. Additional information has emerged from neuropathological studies. As the basal ganglia are rich in dopaminergic neurons, their apparent role in mood disorders may implicate dopamine as an important neurotransmitter in the development and expression of mood disorders. This chapter will focus on neuroimaging and other research that has examined the basal ganglia in patients with mood disorders.

Neuroimaging studies in unipolar depression

Structural imaging

Structural imaging studies using computed tomography (CT) and magnetic resonance imaging (MRI) have been undertaken in patients with unipolar depression. These studies have concentrated largely on two areas, volumetric measurements and assessment of burden of hyperintensities. Early work utilizing CT brain scans focused on areas of hyperintense signal, usually in the form of punctate lesions or larger clusters of lesions. Generally, investigators examined the severity of hyperintensities in the basal ganglia, particularly in the caudate nucleus, comparing a group of depressed patients with a group of age-matched non-depressed control subjects.

For example, Beats et al (1991) examined 25 elderly patients (mean age 73 years, range 61–88 years) with major depression and 25 healthy age- and sex-matched controls using CT. The radiodensity of the left and right heads of the caudate was significantly higher in the depressed patients. Densitometric measurements of the grey and white matter did not show significant correlations with age, number or frequency of depressive episodes, age of onset, or duration of illness.

Starkstein et al (1988) examined patients with CT scan-verified unilateral lesions in the basal ganglia or thalamus for the presence of post-stroke mood disorders. Patients with left-sided basal ganglia lesions (mainly in the head of the caudate nucleus) showed a significantly higher frequency and severity of depression, as compared with patients with right-sided basal ganglia or thalamic (left- or right-sided) lesions. Results suggest that damage to biogenic amine pathways and/or frontocaudate projections may play an important role in the modulation of mood.

Morris et al (1996) examined a consecutive series of 41 first-ever stroke patients with single small lesions on CT scan for the presence and severity of post-stroke depressive disorder. Lesions involving left prefrontal or basal ganglia structures were compared with other left hemisphere lesions and all right hemisphere lesions. Patients with lesions involving left hemisphere prefrontal or basal ganglia structures had a higher frequency of depressive disorder (9/12; 75%) than other left hemisphere lesions (1/12; 8%) or those with right hemisphere lesions (5/17; 29%), $P = 0.002$. These findings suggest that damage to neural pathways within left hemisphere prefrontal or basal ganglia structures is associated with depressed mood following stroke.

With the advent of MRI, investigators began to examine both volumes of specific structures and the burden of hyperintensities. Advances in MRI technology have allowed for higher spatial resolution and therefore greater visualization of small neuronal structures. Volumetric or area measurement using MRI has been used to assess a variety of brain structures in depression, including the constituent parts of the basal ganglia, especially the caudate and putamen.

Krishnan et al (1992) used MRI and an unbiased stereological technique to estimate the volumes of the caudate nuclei in 50 patients who met DSM-III criteria for major depression and 50 age- and gender-matched nondepressed controls free of psychiatric illness. Depressed patients had smaller caudate nucleus volumes (5.2 +/- 1.6 cm^3) compared with controls (6.2 +/- 1.7 cm^3). Right and left caudate nucleus volumes were smaller in depressed patients compared with controls. Age was negatively correlated with caudate nucleus volumes in depressed patients as well as in controls. Caudate nucleus volumes in depressed patients were inversely correlated with the bicaudate and bifrontal indices. These were among the first reported results of diminished caudate nucleus volumes in depression and suggested a role for the caudate nucleus in the pathogenesis of major depression.

Husain et al (1991) used high-resolution magnetic resonance images and a systematic sampling stereological method to assess putamen nuclei volumes in 41 patients with major depression (DSM-III) and 44 healthy volunteer controls of similar age. Depressed patients had significantly smaller putamen nuclei compared with controls. Age was negatively correlated with putamen size in both groups. These results were among the first reports of diminished putamen volumes in depression.

Krishnan et al (1993) used MRI to evaluate basal ganglia volume and hyperintensity burden in depressed elderly patients and non-depressed matched controls. Elderly depressed patients had smaller caudate nuclei, smaller putaminal complexes, and increased frequency of subcortical hyperintensities compared with controls. These findings were more pronounced in patients with late-onset depression.

Parashos et al (1998) used MRI to study 72 patients with major depression compared with 38 control subjects and found statistically significant reductions in the volumes of the caudate and putamen in depressed patients. Age of first depressive episode was related to putamen volume after accounting for chronological age, and a correlation of 0.26 ($P < 0.04$) was observed between caudate volume and global mental status. Results are in accord with previous reports of basal ganglia abnormalities in depressed patients and support the role of subcortical structures in mediating affective disorder.

Greenwald et al (1997) used qualitative criteria-based scales to compare brain morphology on MRI of 30 elderly depressives and 36 normal controls. Significant differences between depressed and control groups were not demonstrated on ratings of lateral and third ventricle enlargement, or cortical, medial temporal, and caudate atrophy. However, later-onset depressives had significantly more left medial temporal and left caudate atrophy than early-onset counterparts of similar age. The investigators were interested in examining the association between MRI abnormalities and risk factors for cerebrovascular disease (e.g., hypertension, diabetes, and atrial fibrillation), given the hypothesis that certain structural brain changes may be due to cerebrovascular disease. However, the authors found that cerebrovascular risk factors did not predict MRI abnormalities. Cerebrovascular disease risk factors did not predict MRI abnormalities.

However, some volumetric studies have failed to demonstrate this relationship. Lenze & Sheline (1999) failed to find significant caudate or putamen volume differences between 24 depressed and 24 matched non-depressed women. The age range was 24–86 years, with a mean of 53 for each group. These results may differ from other studies because the authors excluded subjects with cerebrovascular risk factors from the study. Dupont et al (1995) failed to find a significant difference in caudate volume between 30 depressives and 26 controls, although the trend in this relatively small sample was for depressives to have smaller volumes.

There are several studies assessing basal ganglia hyperintensities seen on MRI. Normally, these are visualized on T2-weighted images, although newer techniques using FLAIR procedures have also been used to examine hyperintensities. Both qualitative and quantitative methods are used to assess hyperintensities. The qualitative methods include those of Fazekas and Boyko (McDonald et al, 1999), in which hyperintense lesion severity is graded on an ordinal scale. In addition, semi-automated methods have been developed that allow for quantitative measure of hyperintensities, usually expressed as a volume.

Figiel et al (1991a) found a higher occurrence of caudate hyperintensities (60% vs 11%) in late-onset elderly depressed subjects compared with early-onset elderly depressed subjects. These results suggest that late-onset depression may be mediated by caudate and white matter structural changes in some patients.

Greenwald et al (1996) compared hyperintensity ratings on MRI brain scans of 48 elderly depressed patients with those of 39 normal elderly subjects. Older depressed patients manifested significantly more severe hyperintensity ratings in the subcortical grey matter than age-matched comparison subjects. These findings support those of neuroimaging studies implicating the basal ganglia in depression and geriatric depression.

Lauterbach et al (1997) studied subjects with focal subcortical lesions (SCLs) and investigated the frequency of pallidal lesions in secondary major depression presenting after but not before lesion onset. Forty-five subjects were selected for focal SCLs from 10 000 hospital MRI films. Lauterbach et al compared pallidal lesions among SCL subjects who did not have lifetime histories of mood disorders and depressed SCL subjects. Pallidal lesions were present in eight of nine (89%) subjects with secondary major depression, and in 13 of 22 (59%) controls. Left posterior pallidal lesions occurred in four of the nine (44%) depressed subjects and two of the 22 (9%) controls. Demographic and other factors did not differ between subjects with secondary major depression and controls. These data suggest the possibility that abnormal pallidal function may contribute to depressive pathophysiology, and the left-sided finding is consistent with previous findings in depression.

Investigators have examined clinical consequences of volumetric differences. For example, Pillay et al (1998) examined 38 unipolar depressed patients and 20 matched comparison subjects using MRI. Patients were of mild-to-moderate severity of depression and were treated with 10 weeks of fluoxetine 20 mg. There were no group mean differences in caudate and lenticular nucleus volumes between patients and comparison subjects. Baseline Hamilton Depression Rating Scale scores correlated negatively with left caudate nucleus volume in depressed patients. The authors found that female treatment responders tended to have larger caudate volumes than male responders, and also larger right caudate nucleus volumes.

Investigators have examined specific symptoms to determine whether they are associated with localized brain structures. Kim et al (1999) examined 19 deluded depressed patients and 26 non-psychotic depressed patients, all older than 55 years of age. They found that psychotic depressives had smaller absolute volume of prefrontal cortex (PFC) than non-psychotic depressives, but there were no group differences observed in basal ganglia volume.

Steffens et al (1998) examined signal hypointensity in the putamen nuclei (a measure of iron deposition) in 68 elderly depressed patients and a group of 28 age-matched non-depressed control subjects. Among the depressed patients, older age of depression onset and greater severity of depression were associated with increased putamen nuclei iron deposition. When depressed patients were compared with control subjects, the patient group demonstrated greater putamen nuclei iron, but the finding was significant only for the left hemisphere. These findings support previous neuroimaging studies linking both changes in the basal ganglia and greater left-sided brain pathology to late-life depression.

Elderly patients are particularly sensitive to the neurological side effects of psychotropic medications. This increased sensitivity may be related to brain structural changes associated with ageing. Figiel et al (1991b) reported on the occurrence of caudate hyperintensities, using brain MRI, in seven elderly depressed subjects who developed neuroleptic-induced Parkinsonism. Caudate hyperintensities were not observed in any of the seven healthy elderly controls examined. These results suggest that caudate hyperintensities may render some elderly depressed patients susceptible to neuroleptic-induced Parkinsonism.

Several investigators have examined lesion location in post-stroke depression to help identify brain regions and structures that may be involved in the development of functional mood disorders. For example, Beblo et al (1999) examined 20 patients with post-stroke depression and found that nine out of 10 subjects with left hemisphere strokes exhibited a major depression and seven out of 10 subjects with right hemisphere infarcts had a minor depression. For both major and minor depression the maximal overlap of lesions was found in subcortical areas, including parts of the caudate nucleus, posterior parts of the putamen, and the deep white matter. The authors suggest that post-stroke depression is related to the dysfunction of (cortico-)striato-pallido-thalamic-cortical projections that modulate cortico-thalamo-cortical loop systems.

The Cardiovascular Health Study, an NIH-supported multi-site study of risk factors for cardiovascular and cerebrovascular disease, included a neuroimaging component and an abbreviated depression measure, a modified version of the Centers for Epidemiologic Studies Depression (CES-D) scale. Using the Cardiovascular Health Study data base, Steffens et al (1999) examined the association of depression score and hyperintensities in the subcortical white and grey matter in 3660 subjects after controlling for a variety of demographic and medical variables as well as functional status and Modified Mini-Mental State Examination score. They found that the number of small (<3 mm) basal ganglia lesions was significantly associated with reported depressive symptoms, but white matter grade (the Cardiovascular Health Study's measure of subcortical white matter severity) was not. In subsequent logistic regression models, number of basal ganglia lesions remained a significant predictor after controlling for non-MRI variables and severity of white matter lesions. These findings extend previous reports linking the basal ganglia and depression that were based on relatively small clinical populations to a much larger community-based population of individuals not referred for depression.

MRI hyperintensities and depression outcomes

Simpson et al (1998) followed 75 consecutive elderly (aged 65–85) patients with DSM-III-R major depression in a naturalistic treatment study consisting of three outcome groups: 1) those treated with medication monotherapy; 2) monotherapy-refractory patients treated with lithium augmentation; and 3) monotherapy-refractory patients treated with electro-convulsive therapy (ECT). Subcortical hyperintensities were significantly increased in the more resistant patients. These included confluent deep white matter, multiple (> 5) basal ganglia lesions and pontine reticular formation lesions. Extrapyramidal, frontal, and pyramidal neurological signs characterized the resistant groups.

Krishnan et al (1998) followed 57 depressed elderly subjects to estimate the relative probabilities of 6-month recovery from an index episode of major depression for individuals with and without MRI-confirmed vascular brain changes, defined as moderate to severe hyperintensities in subcortical white or grey matter. Overall, the recovery rate in this sample was 57.9%. Subjects with MRI-related vascular depression demonstrated outcomes similar to subjects with non-vascular depression (crude risk ratio = 0.67, confidence interval = 0.32–1.43). There was a trend that demonstrated that MRI-related vascular depression placed elderly subjects and subjects with first onset of depression after age 40 at increased risk of non-recovery. Thus, overall, the study demonstrated no significant difference in course between patients with and without vascular depression. It also suggests that patients with vascular depression may have a different course depending on their age and age of onset of the disease.

Severity of MRI hyperintensities in the basal ganglia also appears to affect treatment response. Steffens et al (2000) examined depressed elderly patients receiving treatment with ECT who had undergone a brain MRI scan. Patients with greater severity of subcortical grey matter hyperintensities were found to be less responsive to an acute course of ECT.

O'Brien and colleagues (1998) followed 54 elderly patients with major depression for up to 4 years, and found that the presence of severe deep white matter lesions on MRI at baseline was predictive of a very low likelihood of long-term survival free from depression or incident dementia.

Cognitive outcomes of depression have also been examined, with an eye toward the significance of the basal ganglia. Using survival analysis with dementia as the outcome of interest, Steffens et al (2000) followed 182 elderly non-demented patients for up to 5 years. Twenty-six patients developed dementia. In addition to higher age and lower baseline Mini-Mental State Examination score, greater grey matter lesion volume was significantly associated with later dementia.

Functional imaging

Investigators have used various functional imaging technologies to examine patients with affective disorders. These include positron emission tomography (PET), single photon emission computerized tomography (SPECT), magnetic resonance spectroscopy (MRS) and functional MRI.

Baxter et al (1985) examined cerebral glucose metabolic rates in patients with unipolar depression ($N = 11$), bipolar depression ($N = 5$), mania ($N = 5$), bipolar mixed states ($N = 3$), and in normal controls ($N = 9$) using PET and fluorodeoxyglucose F18. Bipolar depressed and mixed patients had supratentorial whole brain glucose metabolic rates that were significantly lower than those of the other comparison groups. The whole brain metabolic rates for patients with bipolar depression increased going from depression or a mixed state to a euthymic or manic state. Patients with unipolar depression showed a significantly lower ratio of the metabolic rate of the caudate nucleus divided by that of the hemisphere as a whole when compared with normal controls and patients with bipolar depression.

Laasonen-Balk et al (1999) examined the binding of [123I]beta-CIT (2beta-carbomethoxy-3beta-(4-iodophenyl-tropane) to the dopamine transporter sites in the basal ganglia in 15 drug-naïve depressed patients and 18 healthy controls using SPECT. They found a significantly higher [123I]beta-CIT uptake in both sides of the basal ganglia in patients with major depression than in the controls. This finding was somewhat unexpected, since it is generally believed that monoaminergic neurotransmission is lower in depression, and therefore it could be assumed that a reduction in dopamine transmission would lead to secondary down-regulation of DAT density. The authors suggest that it is possible that up-regulation of the DAT may be the primary alteration, as this leads to lower intrasynaptic dopamine concentration and to lower dopamine neural transmission.

Hamakawa et al (1998) recorded proton magnetic resonance spectra from a subcortical region containing the basal ganglia in 40 patients with affective disorders (18 with bipolar disorder and 22 with major depression) and in 20 normal controls. The absolute concentration of the choline-containing compounds (Cho) in the patients with bipolar disorder was significantly higher than that in the normal controls. The patients with bipolar disorder had significantly higher levels of the Cho/creatine + phosphocreatine (Cr-PCr) and Cho/N-acetly-1-aspartate (NAA) peak ratio compared with the normal controls, in both the depressive and euthymic states but with a tendency to higher levels in the depressive state. The Cho/NAA peak ratio was also significantly higher in the patients with major depression compared with the normal controls. These results suggest that the membrane phospholipid metabolism in the basal ganglia is altered in affective disorders.

Moore et al (1997) sought to determine whether the concentration of beta-nucleoside triphosphate is lower in the basal ganglia of depressed subjects using in vivo 31P MRS. There were 35 unmedicated depressed subjects and

18 comparison subjects. Beta-nucleoside triphosphate was 16% lower in the depressed subjects than in the comparison subjects. This finding is consistent with an abnormality of high-energy phosphate metabolism in the basal ganglia of subjects with major depression.

Functional imaging can also be used to investigate whether functional brain changes associated with the affect disturbance seen in major depression are similar to those that accompany transient sadness in normal subjects. To address this question, Beauregard et al (1998) used an emotional activation paradigm that involved assessment of brain activity associated with passive viewing of an emotionally laden film clip aimed at inducing a transient state of sadness contrasted with that associated with passive viewing of an emotionally neutral film clip in patients suffering from unipolar depression and in normal control subjects. Transient sadness produced significant activation in the medial and inferior prefrontal cortices, the middle temporal cortex, the cerebellum, and the caudate in both depressed and normal subjects. These results strongly support the view that activation paradigms represent an extremely useful and powerful way of delineating the functional anatomy of the various symptoms that characterize major depression.

Martinot et al (2001) used [18F]-fluorodopa PET imaging to study six depressed patients with affective flattening and psychomotor retardation, six depressed patients with high impulsivity and anxiety, and 10 healthy control subjects. The two depressed patient groups were matched for severity of depression. [18F]-DOPA uptake values in the left caudate were significantly lower in patients with psychomotor retardation than in patients with impulsivity and in control subjects.

Similarly, Hickie et al (1999) utilized a split-dose SPECT scanning technique in association with a two-stage test of psychomotor speed to examine psychomotor slowing in 25 patients with primary depressive disorder. Patients were injected with technetium-99m hexamethylpropylene amine oxime (99mTc-HMPAO) while performing each component of a two-stage psychomotor task. The first stage, 'simple reaction time' (RT), and the second stage, 'choice reaction time' (CRT), were each followed by 30-minute SPECT scans. Regions of interest (ROIs) corresponding to the left and right neo-striatum (caudate-putamen) were drawn, and regional cerebral blood flow (rCBF) values were calculated. Importantly, the change in rCBF measure in the left neo-striatum was inversely correlated with RT ($R = -0.48$, $P < 0.05$). That is, the patients with the greatest psychomotor slowing initially showed the least increase in rCBF during the CRT condition. This effect was independent of age.

Functional imaging and depression treatment studies

There is evidence from treatment studies employing functional imaging to support a role for the basal ganglia in recovery from depression after acute treatment. Martin et al (2001) examined 28 middle-aged depressives treated with either interpersonal therapy or venlafaxine. Sequential SPECT scans were obtained before treatment and after 6 weeks of treatment. In both treatment groups a statistical parametric mapping analysis showed significant activation of the basal ganglia for both treatment groups. Similarly, Brody et al (2001) studied 24 depressed subjects and 16 normal controls with PET before and after 12 weeks of treatment with either paroxetine or interpersonal psychotherapy. At baseline, depressed subjects had higher normalized metabolism than controls in the prefrontal cortex, caudate, and thalamus, and lower metabolism in the temporal lobes. With treatment, there were metabolic changes in the direction of normalization in these regions.

Renshaw et al (1997) investigated proton magnetic resonance spectra of the basal ganglia in 41 medication-free outpatients with major depression prior to starting an 8-week standardized trial of open-label fluoxetine, and 22 matched comparison subjects. Upon completing the trial, depressed subjects were classified as treatment responders ($N = 18$) or non-responders ($N = 23$), based on changes in scores on the Hamilton Depression Rating Scale. Depressed subjects had a lower area ratio of the choline resonance to the creatine resonance (Cho/Cr) than comparison subjects. This statistically significant difference between the depressed subjects and comparison subjects was more pronounced in the treatment responders than in non-responders. There were no differences in the relative volumes of grey matter or white matter in the voxel used for proton spectroscopy in depressed subjects relative to comparison subjects. These results are consistent with an alteration in the metabolism of cytosolic choline compounds in the basal ganglia of depressed subjects and, in particular, those who are responsive to fluoxetine.

Larisch et al (1997) characterized cerebral dopamine-D2 receptors in 13 patients with major depression (treated with a selective serotonin reuptake inhibitor) using the dopamine-D2 receptor antagonist iodobenzamide and SPECT. Dopamine receptor binding was assessed twice, before and during serotonin reuptake inhibition. An increase in dopamine-D2 receptor binding during serotonin reuptake inhibition was found in the striatum and anterior cingulate gyrus in treatment responders, but not in non-responders. The increase in dopamine-D2 receptor binding correlated significantly with clinical recovery from depression as assessed with the Hamilton depression scale. The data strengthen the concept that the striatum and the anterior cingulate gyrus are involved in mood regulation, and that dopamine-D2 receptors may constitute a central role in this domain.

Henry et al (2001) used [18F]-fluorodeoxyglucose PET imaging to examine six patients with major depression before and after an acute course of ECT. In a region of interest analysis of absolute metabolic rate, they found a decrease in metabolism after ECT in all 61 regions examined. When normalized to global metabolic rate, metabolism was decreased in most areas, but increased metabolism was found in eight regions, including the basal ganglia, upper brainstem, and occipital lobe. These relative increases in metabolism in regions with known dopaminergic innervation (e.g. caudate and upper brainstem) are interesting and have not been previously reported.

Awata et al (1998) examined patterns of regional cerebral blood flow (rCBF) abnormalities in 18 elderly depressed patients using SPECT and 99mTc-hexamethylpropyleneamine oxime (99mTc-HMPAO). Compared with 13 age-matched controls, relative rCBF was significantly decreased bilaterally in the anterior cingulate gyrus, the prefrontal cortex, the temporal cortex, the parietal cortex, the hippocampus, and the caudate nucleus. In 10 patients with a prolonged depressive episode or prolonged residual symptoms (the refractory subgroup), robust and extensive decreases in rCBF were found compared with controls, and the rCBF decreased significantly in the anterior cingulate gyrus and the prefrontal cortex compared with that in the non-refractory subgroup. In the non-refractory subgroup, rCBF decreased significantly in the caudate nucleus and tended to decrease in the anterior cingulate gyrus compared with controls. These findings indicate that dysfunction of the limbic system, the cerebral association cortex, and the caudate nucleus may be implicated in late-life depression.

Neuroimaging studies in bipolar disorder

Structural studies

Aylward et al (1994) hypothesized that patients with bipolar disorder would demonstrate smaller basal ganglia volumes and a greater number of hyperintensities on MRI than comparison subjects who were matched for age, race, sex, and education. They measured volumes of the caudate, putamen, and globus pallidus in 30 patients with bipolar disorder and 30 matched normal comparison subjects and assessed the presence, number, and location of hyperintensities. Male patients with bipolar disorder demonstrated larger caudate volumes than male comparison subjects. Older, but not younger, patients with bipolar disorder demonstrated more hyperintensities than comparison subjects, primarily in frontal lobe white matter. These results are not consistent with those of previous studies showing reduced basal ganglia volume in subjects with affective disorders, but they are consistent with previous findings of increased white matter hyperintensities, especially in older patients with bipolar disorder. Considered together with results from other studies, the findings suggest that the nature of basal ganglia/subcortical white matter involvement may vary according to the type of depression (unipolar vs bipolar) and the age and sex of the patient.

Strakowski et al (1999) also found striatal enlargement in a group of 24 bipolar patients compared with non-psychiatric controls. In addition, they reported an enlargement of the globus pallidus, a finding not seen by Aylward et al (1994). However, Strakowski et al found no significant differences in any structure between patients who were categorized into first-episode (N = 12) and those into multiple-episode (N = 12) subgroups.

Brain structural volumes were not significantly associated with duration of illness, prior medication exposure, number of previous hospital admissions, or duration of substance abuse.

Despite these positive studies, some investigators have failed to find any significant differences in the volumes of the caudate or putamen when comparing bipolar patients and normal controls. Swayze et al (1992) compared volumetric measurements of 48 bipolar patients and 47 normal controls. They found no differences in caudate or putamen volumes. Likewise, Sax et al (1999) failed to find differences in volumes of basal ganglia structures between 17 manic hospitalized patients and 12 group-matched comparison subjects.

Structural imaging research in bipolar disorder also extends to the examination of basal ganglia hyperintensities. McDonald et al (1999) evaluated 70 bipolar inpatients (mean age = 49.9 +/- 19.7 years) and 70 age- and gender-matched control subjects (mean age = 53.2 +/- 18.1 years) and rated MR scans to assess for the presence of hyperintensities. Compared with control subjects, the bipolar patients demonstrated hyperintense lesions in the subependymal region, subcortical grey nuclei, and the deep white matter.

Functional studies

Buchsbaum et al (1986) examined 20 affective disorder patients (16 with bipolar disorder and four with unipolar depression) and 24 normal controls using PET with [18F]2-deoxyglucose (FDG) as a tracer. Subjects received a series of brief electrical stimuli to their right arms during FDG uptake. Patients with bipolar affective illness had significantly lower frontal to occipital glucose metabolic rate ratios (relative hypofrontality) and significantly lower metabolic rates in their basal ganglia in comparison to whole slice metabolism than normal controls. Patients with unipolar illness showed significantly higher frontal to occipital ratios, and also showed relatively reduced metabolism in the basal ganglia. All results in unipolar patients should be considered exploratory due to the small number of patients. Clinical depression ratings correlated negatively with whole slice metabolic rate.

MRS has been used to examine choline membrane transport in bipolar disorder. Lithium has been shown to affect this transport system, with particular inhibitory effects on the phosphotidylinositol (PI) second messenger system, and lesser effects on the phosphatidylcholine (PC) system. Stoll et al (1996) hypothesized that some treatment refractory manic patients may circumvent lithium-induced suppression of the PI system by activating the PC system, the suggestion being that the combination of both lithium and choline would inhibit both the PI and PC systems and provide a more effective treatment. To test this, they added choline to lithium in four refractory patients with rapid-cycling bipolar disorder. The four patients experienced clinical improvement, and MRS choline resonance in the basal ganglia was shown to increase.

Sharma et al (1992) examined four patients with bipolar disorder treated with lithium and nine normal control subjects. They found elevations in the ratios of NAA/Cr-PCr, Cho/Cr-PCr, and inositol/Cr-PCr in the basal ganglia in the patient group when compared with the control group.

However, these results linking lithium to specific choline elevations are not supported by other work. For example, Kato et al (1996) examined 19 subjects with bipolar disorder treated with lithium and other psychotropic drugs. They found increases in Cho/Cr-PCr levels in the basal ganglia of bipolar patients compared with normal controls, regardless of lithium treatment. Also, as noted in the depression section above, Hamakawa et al (1998) demonstrated that the basal ganglia Cho/NAA ratio was elevated not only in depressed and euthymic bipolar patients, but in patients with unipolar depression. This study suggests that altered membrane phospholipid metabolism is not specific to bipolar disorder.

PET has been used to examine dopamine binding and density in three studies with bipolar patients. Wong et al (1985) examined bipolar patients and healthy controls and found no difference in the caudate/cerebellum dopamine D_2-binding ratio between the two groups. Suhara et al (1992) found no difference in dopamine D_1-receptor binding potentials in the caudate between bipolar patients and healthy controls. However, Pearlson et al (1995) observed that psychotic bipolar patients, compared with normal volunteers, had increased density of dopamine D_2-receptors in the caudate.

Neuropathological studies

Several neuropathological studies indicate that the basal ganglia are smaller in patients with depressive episodes, whether they have unipolar or bipolar disorder (for a review see Baumann and Bogerts, 2001).

Bowden et al (1997) measured the concentrations of dopamine, and the dopamine metabolites homovanillic acid (HVA) and dihydroxyphenylacetic acid (DOPAC), in five brain regions from suicide victims with a firm retrospective diagnosis of depression, and matched controls. The suicides were divided into those free of antidepressant drugs and those in whom prescription of antidepressant drugs was clearly documented. DOPAC concentrations were significantly lower in the caudate, putamen, and nucleus accumbens of antidepressant-free suicides compared with controls. In antidepressant-treated suicides, lower concentrations of DOPAC were observed in the basal ganglia, reaching statistical significance in the caudate. Lower DOPAC concentrations were largely restricted to those suicides who died by non-violent methods. There were no significant differences in dopamine and HVA concentrations in either suicide group compared to controls, although there was a trend for HVA concentrations to be lower in suicides. This study provides evidence for reduced dopamine turnover, as judged from reduced DOPAC levels, in depressed suicides.

In a post-mortem study, Allard and Norlen (1997) examined the binding of the ligand [3H]WIN 35,428 to dopamine uptake sites in the caudate nucleus of 13 depressed suicide victims and 19 controls. There were no differences in Bmax or Kd between the suicide group and controls. Subdividing the suicide group according to the presence of major depression, antidepressant medication, and suicide method, respectively, did not yield any differences. Thus, this study did not support previous findings of striatal dopaminergic biochemical and receptor changes in depression. At least, those findings were not reflected by alterations in density or affinity of dopamine uptake sites in depressed suicide victims.

Summary: Why the basal ganglia?

At first blush, it may not seem intuitive that the basal ganglia should have a role in mood disorders. The prevailing biological theories usually invoke the serotonergic and noradrenergic systems. Most somatic treatments are thought to affect either or both of these neurotransmitters. Thus, the basal ganglia, rich in dopaminergic neurons, challenges traditional notions of the biological underpinnings of depression. We have summarized the evidence implicating the basal ganglia in mood disorders (Table 12.1).

Many experts in neuroanatomy and mood disorders favour the concept of a disconnection syndrome, particularly for unipolar depression. The basal ganglia, especially the caudate and putamen, are connected to the prefrontal cortex and to the thalamus. Thus, a cortico-striatal-thalamo-cortical mood

Table 12.1   Summary of evidence linking mood disorders and basal ganglia.

1. Basal ganglia lesions seen on computed tomography and magnetic resonance imaging are related to occurrence of unipolar depression, especially in the elderly

2. Post-stroke depression occurs more frequently in left frontal areas or left basal ganglia compared with other left hemispheric areas or right hemispheric areas

3. Volumes of caudate and putamen, seen on magnetic resonance imaging, are smaller among depressed patients than matched controls

4. Individuals with late-age-onset mania may have more severe basal ganglia hyperintensities on magnetic resonance imaging

5. Presence and severity of basal ganglia lesions are associated with poor short-term response to antidepressant treatment

6. Functional imaging studies show a decrease in brain glucose metabolism in depression

7. There are no consistent volumetric findings for the basal ganglia in bipolar disorder

Figure. 12.1 Five proposed basal ganglia-thalamocortical circuits. Each circuit consists of a loop of connections from cortex to striatum to pallidum/substantia nigra (SN) to thalamus and back to the cortex (adapted from Alexander et al, 1986)

	MOTOR	OCULOMOTOR	DORSOLATERAL PREFRONTAL	LATERAL ORBITO-FRONTAL	ANTERIOR CINGULATE
CORTEX →	SUPPLEMENTARY MOTOR AREA	FRONTAL EYE FIELDS	DORSOLATERAL PREFRONTAL CORTEX	LATERAL ORBITO-FRONTAL CORTEX	ANTERIOR CINGULATE AREA
STRIATUM	PUTAMEN	CAUDATE BODY	DORSOLATERAL CAUDATE HEAD	VENTROMEDIAL CAUDATE HEAD	VENTRAL STRIATUM
PALLIDUM	VENTRO-LATERAL GLOBUS PALLIDUS	CAUDAL DORSOMEDIAL GLOBUS PALLIDUS	LATERAL DORSOMEDIAL GLOBUS PALLIDUS	MEDIAL DORSOMEDIAL GLOBUS PALLIDUS	ROSTRO-LATERAL GLOBUS PALLIDUS, VENTRAL PALLIDUM
SUBSTANTIA NIGRA (SN) →	CAUDOLATERAL SN – PARS RETICULATA	VENTRO-LATERAL SN – PARS RETICULATA	ROSTRO-LATERAL SN – PARS RETICULATA	ROSTRO-MEDIAL SN – PARS RETICULATA	ROSTRODORSAL SN – PARS RETICULATA
THALAMUS	VENTRALIS LATERALIS, PARS ORALIS AND PARS MEDIALIS	LATERAL VENTRALIS ANTERIOR PARS MAGNO-CELLULARIS, MEDIALIS DORSALIS PARS PARALA-MELLARIS	VENTRALIS ANTERIOR PARS PARVO-CELLULARIS, MEDIALIS DORSALIS PARS PARVO-CELLULARIS	MEDIAL VENTRALIS ANTERIOR PARS MAGNO-CELLULARIS, MEDIALIS DORSALIS PARS MAGNA-CELLULARIS	POSTERO-MEDIAL MEDIALIS DORSALIS

circuit has been proposed. Basal ganglia pathology would therefore disrupt the circuit. Drevets (2000) and Krishnan et al (1993) have articulated this circuit well for depression. Others have proposed a similar neuroanatomical model for bipolar disorder (Strakowski et al, 2000).

The basal ganglia consist of input nuclei and output nuclei. The input nuclei are the caudate, putamen, and nucleus accumbens. Fibres from the input nuclei project to the globus pallidus (output nuclei) and substantia nigra (not usually considered a functional part of the basal ganglia). Afferents packaged as parallel modular units from sensorimotor association areas and the limbic cortex project to specific zones within the caudate and putamen (Graybiel, 1990). A similar organization has been described through both nigrothalamic and thalamocortical loops, but with these components there may be some degree of integration (Parent, 1990). These parallel modular units can be anatomically, and likely functionally, grouped into at least five basic basal ganglia-thalamocortical circuits (Alexander et al, 1986) (Fig. 12.1). Three of these five have relevance for mood disorders: the dorsolateral prefrontal circuit (with additional input from the parietal cortex), the lateral orbitofrontal circuit (with additional input from the superior and inferior temporal gyri), and the anterior cingulate circuit (with additional input from the hippocampus and amygdala). The key feature of these circuits is their termination in prefrontal association areas. The exact role of each of these circuits in affective disorders is unclear; discovering their role is an important focus of ongoing basic science studies. As structural and functional imaging becomes more sophisticated, we may also be able to employ these modalities to understand the circuitry of the basal ganglia, possibly providing valuable clinical information for diagnosis and prognosis in mood disorders.

Acknowledgement

Work on this chapter was supported by National Institute of Mental Health grants P50 MH60451, R01 MH54846, and K07 MH01367.

References

Adams RD, Victor M (eds), *Principles of Neurology*, 5th edn, (New York, NY: McGraw-Hill, Inc., 1993) 57–9.

Alexander GE, Delong MR, Strick PL, Parallel organization of functionally segregated circuits linking basal ganglia and cortex, *Ann Rev Neurosci* (1986) **9**:357–81.

Allard P, Norlen M, Unchanged density of caudate nucleus dopamine uptake sites in depressed suicide victims, *J Neural Transm* (1997) **104**:1353–60.

Awata S, Ito H, Konno M et al, Regional cerebral blood flow abnormalities in late-life depression: relation to refractoriness and chronification, *Psychiatry Clin Neurosci* (1998) **52**:97–105.

Aylward EH, Roberts-Twillie JV, Barta PE, et al, Basal ganglia volumes and white matter hyperintensities in patients with bipolar disorder, *Am J Psychiatry* (1994) **151**:687–93.

Baumann B, Bogerts B, Neuroanatomical studies on bipolar disorder, *Br J Psychiatry* (2001) **41** (Suppl): 142–7.

Baxter LR Jr, Phelps ME, Mazziotta JC et al, Cerebral metabolic rates for glucose in mood disorders. Studies with positron emission tomography and fluorodeoxyglucose F 18, *Arch Gen Psychiatry* (1985) **42**:441–7.

Beats B, Levy R, Forstl H, Ventricular enlargement and caudate hyperdensity in elderly depressives, *Biol Psychiatry* (1991) **30**:452–8.

Beauregard M, Leroux JM, Bergman S et al, The functional neuroanatomy of major depression: an fMRI study using an emotional activation paradigm, *Neuroreport* (1998) **9**:3253–8

Beblo T, Wallesch CW, Herrmann M, The crucial role of frontostriatal circuits for depressive disorders in the postacute stage after stroke, *Neuropsychiatry Neuropsychol Behav Neurol* (1999) **12**:236–46.

Bowden C, Cheetham SC, Lowther S et al, Reduced dopamine turnover in the basal ganglia of depressed suicides, *Brain Res* (1997) **769**:135–40.

Brody AL, Saxena S, Stoessel P et al, Regional brain metabolic changes in patients with major depression treated with either paroxetine or interpersonal therapy: preliminary findings, *Arch Gen Psychiatry* (2001) **58**:631–40.

Buchsbaum MS, Wu J, DeLisi LE et al, Frontal cortex and basal ganglia metabolic rates assessed by positron emission tomography with [18F]2-deoxyglucose in affective illness, *J Affect Disord* (1986) **10**:137–52.

Drevets WC, Neuroimaging studies of mood disorders, *Biol Psychiatry* (2000) **48**:813–29.

Dupont RM, Jernigan TL, Heindel W et al, Magnetic resonance imaging and mood disorders. Localization of white matter and other subcortical abnormalities, *Arch Gen Psychiatry* (1995) **52**:747–55.

Figiel GS, Krishnan KR, Doraiswamy PM, Nemeroff CB, Caudate hyperintensities in elderly depressed patients with neuroleptic-induced parkinsonism, *J Geriatr Psychiatry Neurol* (1991a) **4**:86–9.

Figiel GS, Krishnan KR, Doraiswamy PM et al, Subcortical hyperintensities on brain magnetic resonance imaging: a comparison between late age onset and early onset elderly depressed subjects, *Neurobiol Aging* (1991b) **12**:245–7.

Graybiel AM, Neurotransmitters and neuromodulators in the basal ganglia, *Trends Neurosci* (1990) **13**:244–53.

Greenwald BS, Kramer-Ginsberg E, Bogerts B et al, Qualitative magnetic resonance imaging findings in geriatric depression. Possible link between later-onset depression and Alzheimer's disease? *Psychol Med* (1997) **27**:421–31.

Greenwald BS, Kramer-Ginsberg E, Krishnan RR et al, MRI signal hyperintensities in geriatric depression, *Am J Psychiatry* (1996) **153**:1212–5.

Hamakawa H, Kato T, Murashita J, Kato N, Quantitative proton magnetic resonance spectroscopy of the basal ganglia in patients with affective disorders, *Eur Arch Psychiatry Clin Neurosci* (1998) **248**:53–8.

Henry ME, Schmidt ME, Matochik JA, Stoddard EP, Potter WZ, The effects of ECT on brain glucose: a pilot FDG PET study, *J ECT* (2001) **17**:33–40.

Hickie I, Ward P, Scott E et al, Neostriatal rCBF correlates of psychomotor slowing in patients with major depression, *Psychiatry Res* (1999) **92**:75–81.

Husain MM, McDonald WM, Doraiswamy PM et al, A magnetic resonance imaging study of putamen nuclei in major depression, *Psychiatry Res* (1991) **40**:95–9.

Kato T, Hamakawa H, Shioiri T et al, Choline-containing compounds detected by proton magnetic resonance spectroscopy in the basal ganglia in bipolar disorder, *J Psychiatry Neurosci* (1996) **21**:248–54.

Kim DK, Kim BL, Sohn SE et al, Candidate neuroanatomic substrates of psychosis in old-aged depression, *Prog Neuropsychopharmacol Biol Psychiatry* (1999) **23**:793–807.

Krishnan KR, McDonald WM, Escalona PR et al, Magnetic resonance imaging of the caudate nuclei in depression. Preliminary observations, *Arch Gen Psychiatry* (1992) **49**:553–7.

Krishnan KR, McDonald WM, Doraiswamy PM et al, Neuroanatomical substrates of depression in the elderly, *Eur Arch Psychiatry Clin Neurosci* (1993) **243**:41–6.

Krishnan KR, Hays JC, George LK, Blazer DG, Six-month outcomes for MRI-related vascular depression. *Depress Anxiety* (1998) **8**:142–6.

Laasonen-Balk T, Kuikka J, Viinamäki H et al, Striatal dopamine transporter density in major depression, *Psychopharmacology (Berl)* (1999) **144**:282–5.

Larisch R, Klimke A, Vosberg H et al, In vivo evidence for the involvement of dopamine-D2 receptors in striatum and anterior cingulate gyrus in major depression, *Neuroimage* (1997) **5**: 251–60.

Lauterbach EC, Jackson JG, Wilson AN, Dever GE, Kirsh AD, Major depression after left posterior globus pallidus lesions, *Neuropsychiatry Neuropsychol Behav Neurol* (1997) **10**:9–16.

Martin SD, Martin E, Rai SS, Richardson MA, Royall R, Brain blood flow changes in depressed patients treated with interpersonal psychotherapy or venlafaxine hydrochloride: preliminary findings, *Arch Gen Psychiatry* (2001) **58**:641–8.

Martinot M, Bragulat V, Artiges E et al, Decreased presynaptic dopamine function in the left caudate of depressed

patients with affective flattening and psychomotor retardation, *Am J Psychiatry* (2001) **158**:314–6.

McDonald WM, Tupler LA, Marsteller FA et al, Hyperintense lesions on magnetic resonance images in bipolar disorder, *Biol Psychiatry* (1999) **45**:965–71.

Moore CM, Christensen JD, Lafer B, Fava M, Renshaw PF, Lower levels of nucleoside triphosphate in the basal ganglia of depressed subjects: a phosphorous-31 magnetic resonance spectroscopy study, *Am J Psychiatry* (1997) **154**:116–8.

Morris PL, Robinson RG, Raphael B, Hopwood MJ, Lesion location and post-stroke depression, *J Neuropsychiatry Clin Neurosci* (1996) **8**:399–403.

O'Brien JT, Ames D, Chiu E, Schweitzer I, Desmond P, Tress B, Severe deep white matter lesions and outcome in elderly patients with major depressive disorder: follow-up study, *BMJ* (1998) **317**: 982–4.

Parashos IA, Tupler LA, Blitchington T, Krishnan KR, Magnetic-resonance morphometry in patients with major depression, *Psychiatry Res* (1998) **84**:7–15.

Parent A, Extrinsic connections of the basal ganglia, *Trends Neurosci* (1990) **13**:254–8.

Pearlson GD, Wong DF, Tune LE et al, In vivo D_2 dopamine receptor density in psychotic and nonpsychotic patients with bipolar disorder, *Arch Gen Psychiatry* (1995) **52**:471–7.

Pillay SS, Renshaw PF, Bonello CM et al, A quantitative magnetic resonance imaging study of caudate and lenticular nucleus gray matter volume in primary unipolar major depression: relationship to treatment response and clinical severity, *Psychiatry Res* (1998) **84**:61–74.

Renshaw PF, Lafer B, Babb SM et al, Basal ganglia choline levels in depression and response to fluoxetine treatment: an in vivo proton magnetic resonance spectroscopy study, *Biol Psychiatry* (1997) **41**:837–43.

Sax KW, Strakowski SM, Zimmerman ME et al, Frontosubcortical neuroanatomy and the Continuous Performance Test in mania, *Am J Psychiatry* (1999) **156**:139–41.

Sharma R, Venkatasubramaniam PN, Barany M, Davis JM, Proton magnetic spectroscopy of the brain in schizophrenic and affective patients, *Schizophr Res* (1992) **8**:43–9.

Simpson S, Baldwin RC, Jackson A, Burns AS, Is subcortical disease associated with a poor response to antidepressants? Neurological, neuropsychological and neuroradiological findings in late-life depression, *Psychol Med* (1998) **28**:1015–26.

Starkstein SE, Robinson RG, Berthier ML, Parikh RM, Price TR, Differential mood changes following basal ganglia vs thalamic lesions, *Arch Neurol* (1988) **45**:725–30.

Steffens DC, Tupler LA, Ranga K, Krishnan R, Magnetic resonance imaging signal hypointensity and iron content of putamen nuclei in elderly depressed patients, *Psychiatry Res* (1998) **83**:95–103.

Steffens DC, Helms MJ, Krishnan KR, Burke GL, Cerebrovascular disease and depression symptoms in the cardiovascular health study, *Stroke* (1999) **30**:2159–66.

Steffens DC, MacFall JR, Payne ME, Welsh-Bohmer KA, Krishnan KRR, Grey-matter lesions and dementia, *Lancet* (2000) **356**:1686–7.

Stoll AL, Sachs GS, Cohen BM et al, Choline in the treatment of rapid-cycling bipolar disorder: clinical and neurochemical findings in lithium-treated patients, *Biol Psychiatry* (1996) **40**:382–8.

Strakowski SM, DelBello MP, Sax KW, Zimmerman ME, Shear PK et al, Brain magnetic resonance imaging of structural abnormalities in bipolar disorder, *Arch Gen Psychiatry* (1999) **56**:256–60.

Strakowski SM, DelBello MP, Adler C, Cecil KM, Sax KW, Neuroimaging in bipolar disorder, *Bipolar Disorders* (2000) **2**:148–64.

Suhara T, Nakayama K, Inoue O et al, D_1 dopamine receptor binding in mood disorders measured by positron emission tomography, *Psychopharmacology* (1992) **106**:14–8.

Swayze VW, Andreasen NC, Alliger RJ, Yuh WTC, Ehrhardt JC, Subcortical and temporal structures in affective disorder and schizophrenia: a magnetic resonance imaging study, *Biol Psychiatry* (1992) **31**:221–40.

Wong DF, Wagner HN Jr, Pearlson G et al, Dopamine receptor binding of C-11-3-N-methylspiperone in the caudate in schizophrenia and bipolar disorder: a preliminary report, *Psychopharmacol Bull* (1985) **21**:595–8.

13

The interface between cerebrovascular disease, depression and dementia

Robert Stewart

Cerebrovascular disease, depression and dementia are common conditions in older populations. Associations between any of these factors are therefore important because an intervention affecting one at a population level may have a large impact on risk for another. For example, treatment or prevention of cerebrovascular disease in a community might substantially reduce incidence rates of depression and dementia. Alternatively, treatment of depression might substantially reduce cerebrovascular disease and dementia. Clearly an understanding of the nature and direction of cause and effect is vital in order to make these predictions. However, methodological obstacles are substantial and research in this area has a long way to go.

Mixed pathology and mixed clinical disease are common in older populations. A substantial overlap between cerebrovascular disease, depression and dementia would be expected through chance alone. Interactions between comorbid conditions complicate the picture still further. In discussing an 'interface' between two (let alone three) processes, simple solutions or models are an attractive option. However, these may amount to wishful thinking. After considering important methodological issues, individual associations will be reviewed before considering potential pathways linking the three disorders.

Methodological issues

Limitations of diagnostic criteria

'Dementia', 'depression' and 'stroke' are frequently defined as present/absent categories. However all three are, to a greater or lesser extent, imposed on physiological/pathological systems which exist as dimensions. Normality and abnormality are not so easily distinguished as 'diagnoses' suggest:

1. Dementia, viewed cross-sectionally, merges seamlessly with milder levels of cognitive impairment, and is principally distinguished in a research setting by a subjective decision concerning the extent to which 'function' has been impaired. Investigated prospectively, no absolute distinction can be drawn between individuals whose declining cognitive function is consistent with early dementia, those with more slow and subtle decline which may or may not result in dementia, and those whose function is essentially stable.

2. No absolute boundaries exist between categories such as major depression, moderate depression, mild depression, dysthymia and normality.
3. Cerebrovascular disease can be considered as a spectrum from normality, through 'brain at risk' and subclinical ischaemia/infarction, to clinically significant single/multiple major infarctions.

A reasonable alternative approach might therefore be to measure the dimension rather than the category. However, dimensions themselves may be multiple, overlapping and/or interacting. Single cortical infarctions, multiple infarctions, subcortical lacunar infarctions and white matter ischaemia may be heterogeneous conditions which do not fit well into a single axis of 'cerebrovascular disease severity'. However, common underlying mechanisms are likely to exist and it may be equally problematic to consider them as entirely separate dimensions. Dementia has traditionally been classified into separate syndromes including Alzheimer's disease and vascular dementia. However, increasing evidence suggests that vascular risk factors for dementia fail to observe this simplistic model and are associated with both clinical syndromes. Depression as a continuous variable is most often quantified in terms of numbers of depressive symptoms on a screening instrument. However, the extent to which this represents a single parameter is uncertain. Recent data have suggested that at least two 'axes' of depression (diminished motivation and affective distress) can be defined for older populations which have different aetiological features (Prince et al, 1999).

Long prodromal periods

As discussed above, understanding the nature and direction of cause and effect is important in order to draw implications from an observed association. However, disorders manifesting in later life may have developed over long periods. The period between the development of early pathological changes and the emergence of a clinical dementia syndrome may be over 10 years for Alzheimer's disease. Cerebrovascular disease may exist in a mild, subclinical form for a similar length of time before detection. For depression which has apparently arisen in later life, an unknown factor is the extent to which it has been preceded by dysthymic traits, mild depressive episodes, or even by episodes of severe depression which have subsequently been forgotten. The direction of cause and effect cannot therefore be assumed around the time of an observed association. This is true even for prospective studies, unless the duration of follow-up is longer than the latent period for the outcome under investigation.

Time/stage-specific effects

Associations between slowly evolving and overlapping conditions cannot be assumed to remain constant or consistent. Depression may be associated with mild, and possibly preclinical stages of dementia. However, associations may diminish with further progression. Subclinical cerebrovascular disease may precipitate clinical symptoms of dementia in the presence of mild Alzheimer's disease but have little influence on further cognitive decline. These stage-specific effects have important implications for interpreting research findings. In particular, associations with depression and cerebrovascular disease may be strongest for mild stages of cognitive decline before diagnostic criteria for dementia can be reliably applied.

Bilateral directions of causation

It is also possible that, for an association between two conditions, the direction of cause and effect may change over time. High blood pressure may exacerbate dementia in its early stages through associated cerebrovascular disease. Neurodegenerative processes may then result in lower blood pressure as the condition progresses. Mild levels of depression in early adult life, through effects on lifestyle, may increase the risk of cerebrovascular disease. Clinical or subclinical stroke may then in turn precipitate the onset of a more severe depressive syndrome in later life.

Individual associations

Vascular disease and dementia

The traditional distinction between vascular dementia and Alzheimer's disease involves a circular argument where cerebrovascular disease is assumed to cause a specific type of dementia and that type of dementia is then defined according to its presumed cause. However, it is becoming increasingly evident that cerebrovascular disease as a risk factor for dementia is poorly represented by this simplistic system:

1. Prospective epidemiological studies have found that principal risk factors for cerebrovascular disease, such as hypertension, diabetes, and raised cholesterol, are not only risk factors for 'vascular' dementia but also for clinically defined Alzheimer's disease (Skoog et al, 1996; Notkola et al, 1998; Ott et al, 1999; Kivipelto et al, 2001).
2. Large post-mortem studies have found that Alzheimer and vascular pathology are frequently mixed in samples with dementia, especially in older age groups (Holmes et al, 1999; Neuropathology Group of the Medical Research Council Cognitive Function and Ageing Study, 2001). Cerebrovascular disease is rarely found to be associated with dementia in the absence of comorbid Alzheimer pathology (Hulette et al, 1997).
3. Prospective studies following up patients with clinical stroke have found that previous dementia is common (Pohjasvaara et al, 1999). Also, in a substantial proportion of cases, subsequent dementia occurs in the

absence of further infarction (Tatemichi et al, 1994), and follows a course similar to Alzheimer's disease (Kokmen et al, 1996).

Comorbid Alzheimer's disease therefore appears to be an important factor in dementia associated with cerebrovascular disease. Potential interactions at a pathological level include inflammatory responses to cerebral infarction, disturbances in blood–brain barrier function, excitotoxicity, oxidative stress and abnormal protein glycation (Stewart, 1998). However, these interactions remain largely theoretical, and evidence to date suggests instead that the two processes principally interact in their clinical manifestations. Two large studies have found that cognitive impairment is associated with earlier stages of Alzheimer pathology if cerebrovascular disease is also present (Snowdon et al, 1997; Esiri et al, 1999). Neither study found associations between cerebrovascular disease and the severity of Alzheimer pathology. Cerebrovascular disease does not therefore appear to influence Alzheimer processes directly. However, in the presence of mild Alzheimer's disease, cerebrovascular disease may bring forward the age of onset for clinical symptoms of dementia.

Evidence from prospective studies with long follow-up periods suggests strongly that vascular disorders such as hypertension and type 2 diabetes mellitus are risk factors for dementia. In this respect they appear to influence relatively early cognitive decline, but there is little evidence so far to support a substantial effect on the subsequent course of dementia once this has developed (Lee et al, 2000). Dementia may also influence cerebrovascular disease. Early cognitive decline may lead to suboptimal control of pre-existing hypertension or diabetes, resulting in increased risk of stroke. Vascular abnormalities associated with Alzheimer's disease, such as microangiopathy and cerebral amyloid angiopathy, are also the subject of increasing research interest (de la Torre and Mussivand, 1993; Olichney et al, 2000).

In summary, a large body of evidence suggests that cerebrovascular disease is an important cause of dementia. The resulting clinical syndrome, however, does not fit well with traditional sub-categories of dementia, and accumulating research suggests that comorbid Alzheimer's disease may be present in most cases. The clinical impact of vascular abnormalities associated with Alzheimer's disease remains to be established.

Vascular disease and depression

Research into the association between cerebrovascular disease and depression is reviewed in other chapters. The two findings which are most consistent to date are: a) that risk of depression is high following clinical stroke, and b) that depression in older people is associated with white matter hyperintensities on magnetic resonance imaging, suggesting mild cerebrovascular disease.

The association between stroke and onset of depression has been found in prospective studies (Pohjasvaara et al, 1998; Gainotti et al, 1999), and suggests a clear direction of causality. However, poor general physical health is known to be a strong risk factor for depression in later life (Prince et al, 1998), and the association between stroke and depression may not necessarily be mediated through vascular damage. A recent meta-analysis found little consistent evidence to support an association between depression and specific lesion location in stroke (Carson et al, 2000). One cross-sectional survey found a strong association between stroke and depression which was not explained by levels of disability and handicap (Stewart et al, 2001a). However, other psychological sequelae arising from the impact of a clinical stroke may be important (Dam, 2001). In summary, there is strong evidence that stroke is a risk factor for onset of depression but less evidence to support a vascular/neurological basis for this.

Depression has been found to be associated with more mild manifestations of cerebrovascular disease such as transient ischaemic episodes (Rao et al, 2001) and, consistently, with the presence and/or extent of white matter hyperintensities on magnetic resonance imaging (de Groot et al, 2000). However, studies to date have been cross-sectional in design. If subclinical cerebrovascular disease caused depression, prevalence rates of depression would be expected to be increased in groups with vascular risk factors such as hypertension and diabetes. Epidemiological evidence for this is weak and no associations were found between any measures of risk for cerebrovascular disease and mild to moderate levels of depression in a recent community survey of a vulnerable population (Stewart et al, 2001a). Furthermore, several prospective studies have found a positive association between depressive symptoms and risk of later cerebrovascular disease (Everson et al, 1998; Jonas & Mussolino, 2000; Ohira et al, 2001). It is therefore possible that depression earlier in life may be a risk factor both for later depressive episodes and for later cerebrovascular disease. Against this, some studies have found white matter hyperintensities to be more specifically associated with 'late-onset' depression (de Groot et al, 2000). However, recall of previous psychiatric morbidity has been found to be poor for major depression (Andrews et al, 1999), let alone for more mild syndromes or dysthymic traits. Age of 'onset' therefore may be difficult to establish reliably and the direction of causality between cerebrovascular disease and depression remains to be clearly established.

Depression and dementia

Several prospective studies have found that mild to moderate depression in older people is associated with an increased risk of later dementia (Devenand et al, 1996; Berger et al, 1999; Geerlings et al, 2000). Mechanisms underlying this association have yet to be fully clarified. Depression may be a reaction to perceived difficulties with memory. Adjustment for baseline memory complaints was found to make little difference to the association between depressive symptoms and risk of dementia in one study (Berger et al, 1999). On the other hand, in a cross-sectional survey a stronger association between depression and the apolipoprotein E e4 allele (a marker of risk for dementia) was found if subjective memory impairment was also present (Stewart et al, 2001b).

Depression may be a symptom of dementia. The prospective studies cited above suggest that this occurs at an early stage before cognitive decline has become severe enough to cause functional impairment and attract a diagnosis of 'dementia'. However, another longitudinal study with multiple follow-up points found that depression *followed* rather than predicted the onset of dementia (Chen et al, 1999). One prospective study found that depression was only associated with cognitive decline in participants whose baseline cognitive function was already impaired (Bassuk et al, 1998). However, in two other samples, depression was associated with increased risk of Alzheimer's disease and cognitive decline in participants *without* cognitive impairment, albeit only in those with higher educational attainment (Geerlings et al, 2000). The nature of depressive symptoms appears to change as Alzheimer's disease becomes more apparent, moving from loss of motivation to agitation and motor slowing (Ritchie et al, 1999).

The uncertain boundary between dementia and mild cognitive impairment may underlie inconsistent findings. Change in cognitive function may be a more appropriate outcome measure. Transient improvement in cognitive function following recovery from depression may obscure associations with underlying decline. This may explain why two large studies have found no association between depression in older people and subsequent cognitive decline (Dufouil et al, 1996; Henderson et al, 1997). One study with a 9–12-year follow-up period found that lower crystallized intelligence scores (associated with depression at baseline) explained the association between depression and later cognitive impairment (Cervilla et al, 2000). Low 'pre-morbid' cognitive function may therefore be a risk factor both for depression and subsequent cognitive decline and dementia.

Depression, dementia and cerebrovascular disease

Depression may be an early symptom of dementia. Exactly how early this manifests is less certain. Some studies have suggested that it precedes detectable cognitive impairment, others the opposite. Cerebrovascular disease is associated with both disorders and might therefore be a common underlying factor. If this was so, adjustment for cerebrovascular disease would be expected to weaken the association between depression and later dementia. One prospective study found that depression and later dementia were more strongly associated in people with higher levels of risk for cerebrovascular disease (Bassuk et al, 1998). The association between depression and dementia may not therefore be *explained* by cerebrovascular disease. However, the results do suggest that depression may be a more accurate 'marker' of early dementia if other risk factors for the latter are also present.

The 'vascular depression' hypothesis proposes a distinguishable syndrome of late-onset depression caused by cerebrovascular disease. Key editorials highlight adverse outcomes potentially associated with this syndrome including a less favourable response to antidepressant treatment and a raised risk of cognitive decline and dementia (Alexopoulos et al, 1997; Hickie and Scott, 1998). Research findings reviewed in this chapter are predominantly derived from epidemiological studies. People with late-onset 'major' depression are likely to form a minority of 'screen-positive' cases and community samples have not, in general, been large enough to investigate this group specifically. Research findings for mild to moderate depression cannot be assumed to be generalizable to groups with more florid clinical syndromes. However, depression, dementia and cerebrovascular disease are common in older populations and a substantial degree of overlap would be expected purely by chance. People with combinations of these disorders, particularly if severe, will be more likely to be referred for secondary care services and will be over-represented in outpatient or inpatient samples (and therefore be more obvious to clinical researchers). If an 'interface' is to be investigated between cerebrovascular disease, depression and dementia, an important consideration is the extent to which the three conditions co-occur more often than would be expected. This has yet to be established conclusively. Further investigation of potential interactions between these disorders is also required:

a) Patients with late-onset depression and cerebrovascular disease may be likely to experience cognitive decline. However, cerebrovascular disease is a well-recognized risk factor for dementia. Is, therefore, the risk of dementia associated with cerebrovascular disease any higher in patients with depression than would be found in non-depressed samples? The prospective study by Bassuk et al (1998) supports this. However, the statistical significance of interaction terms between depression and vascular risk was not formally investigated and the findings require confirmation.

b) Depression and/or symptoms of apathy have been found to be more common in patients with 'vascular' dementia compared to groups with Alzheimer's disease (Hargrave et al, 2000). As discussed above, clinical stroke is known to be a powerful risk factor for depression. Is this therefore any stronger in samples with dementia compared to those without cognitive impairment?

The problem for community surveys is that the large sample sizes required to detect an association between any two conditions have to be multiplied still further to detect effect modification by a third. A case control design reduces the numbers required and would permit more severe syndromes of depression, for example, to be investigated. However, sample sizes would still be considerable and it is often difficult to identify appropriate control groups for cases recruited from secondary or tertiary referral centres.

Mechanisms of association

An understanding of mechanisms underlying associations between the three disorders is crucial for considering potential interventions. A popular proposal is that subclinical cerebrovascular disease disrupts fronto-subcortical function, which in turn causes a syndrome of late-onset depression and, with accumulated vascular damage, cognitive decline and dementia. However, there are drawbacks with this explanation. First, the relationship between subclinical cerebrovascular disease and onset of depression has yet to be investigated prospectively. Second, prospective evidence to date is more supportive of the opposite direction of association, albeit in younger samples. Third, a recent post-mortem study found no evidence of increased generalized or frontal microvascular disease associated with late-onset depression, although cases did have more severe atherosclerosis in the aorta and cerebral arteries (Thomas et al, 2001).

The following pathways might underlie an interface between the three conditions:

a) As discussed above, subclinical cerebrovascular disease may cause depression and also cause or precipitate dementia.
b) Subclinical cerebrovascular disease may cause or precipitate dementia with depression occurring non-specifically as an early symptom.
c) Depression may exacerbate pre-existing cerebrovascular disease (e.g. through deteriorating control of underlying conditions such as hypertension and diabetes) and increase the risk of further cerebral damage and dementia.

These pathways consist essentially of precipitating events. Research in many fields of medicine has been limited by assumptions that, for disorders with an apparently recent onset, risk factors must also consist of recent co-occurrences. For 'late-onset' depression, research has focused on identifying precipitants and has paid less attention to predisposing factors. As suggested in Figure 13.1, cross-sectional associations between the three disorders might also arise from 'interfaces' much earlier in life. A prospective study found that, of people who had been hospitalized for a major depressive episode, 30% failed to recall this 25 years later and 50% were unable to recall the episode in sufficient detail for retrospective diagnostic criteria (Andrews et al, 1999). It is therefore not unreasonable to suppose that an important proportion of patients with apparently 'late-onset' depression (particularly in the context of mild cognitive impairment) have in fact suffered from clinically significant episodes earlier in life. Mild 'subclinical' episodes may be still more frequent and the role of personality traits as vulnerability factors for depression in older people has received scant investigation. Causal pathways underlying any association between cerebrovascular disease, depression and dementia may therefore operate over longer time periods than have generally been proposed:

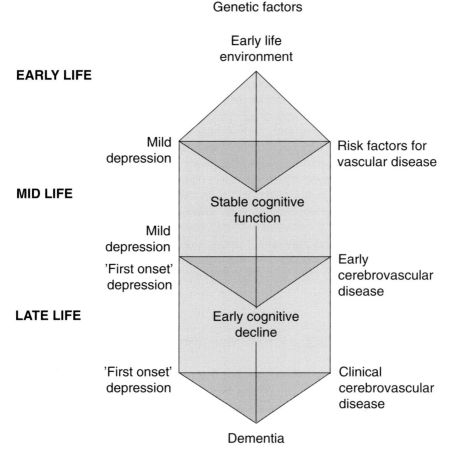

Figure 13.1

The interface between cerebrovascular disease, depression and dementia: a model of interactions across the life-course.

a) Mild depression in mid-life may increase the risk of later cerebrovascular disease which, in turn, causes dementia. More severe depression may then occur as an early symptom of dementia, or may be precipitated by deteriorating physical health.

b) Personality traits may underlie both risk of cerebrovascular disease and risk of 'late-onset' depression. Cerebrovascular disease or early dementia may also act as later precipitants for depression.

c) As suggested by Cervilla et al (2000), lower mid-life cognitive function may be associated with an increased risk of both depression and dementia. Lower cognitive function has also been found to be a risk factor for cerebrovascular disease (Ferucci et al, 1996; Gale et al, 1996).

d) Other vulnerability factors may be shared. For example, insulin resistance may underlie both cerebrovascular disease and Alzheimer's disease (Lovestone, 1999; Stewart and Liolitsa, 1999). Depression may occur later in life as an early symptom of the latter. Social factors in early life may also underlie later morbidity. Lower educational attainment has been found to be a risk factor for dementia although mechanisms underlying this association are controversial. Cardiovascular disease and affective disorder are associated with lower socio-economic status. Associations between early-life social environment and depression in later life have received less attention.

e) Genetic factors might, in part, explain later associations between the three disorders but their role has yet to be clearly established. Apolipoprotein E genotype has received most attention in this respect. However, the association between the $\epsilon 4$ allele and dementia has not been found to be mediated by cardiovascular factors (Slooter et al, 1999; Prince et al, 2000). Associations between $\epsilon 4$ and depression are inconsistent, and positive associations may reflect depression occurring as an early symptom of Alzheimer's disease. A recent family study found evidence of an inherited component for late-onset depression but no substantial shared inheritance with dementia (Heun et al, 2001).

Possible directions for future research

If causal pathways between cerebrovascular disease, depression and dementia are to be understood, the time period may have to be expanded over which risk factors are measured. At the very least, it should be established whether depression which is currently classified as 'late-onset' truly arises *de novo* without previous psychiatric morbidity. A difficulty is that, for cross-sectional surveys, recall may be unreliable and subject to bias. For prospective studies, considerable follow-up periods are required to investigate associations adequately between mid- and late-life, let alone early-life, factors. The most feasible way forward is to make use of existing cohorts where information of interest has already been gathered and where reasonable cohesion has been maintained. It is unlikely that single cohorts will provide all the answers and more specific objectives may have to be considered:

a) To investigate earlier, unrecalled psychiatric morbidity in samples with apparently 'late-onset' depression.

b) To investigate prospectively the association between mid-life depression and white matter hyperintensities in late-life.

c) To investigate the association between stable cognitive function, risk of depression and risk profile for cerebrovascular disease in mid-life. To investigate potential common sources of vulnerability for these factors, arising in early-life.

d) To investigate the association between early-life environmental factors and risk for cerebrovascular disease, depression and dementia in late-life.

e) To investigate the extent to which cerebrovascular disease, depression and dementia have a shared genetic basis.

As well as investigations of vulnerability factors earlier in life, further research is also indicated to clarify processes more proximal to the interface between the three disorders. For example, are white matter hyperintensities a risk factor for onset of depression? Why do some people with early dementia suffer from depression while others do not, and what is the role of cerebrovascular disease in this process? Current systems of diagnostic classification are unhelpful and new ways of thinking may be required. Depression frequently occurs at a stage where mild cognitive impairment merges into dementia and therefore where categorical 'diagnoses' have dubious validity. Since cognitive decline and its effects on global function are the principal dimensions being assessed, it may be better to measure these objectively as separate dimensions rather than combining them into a single category. For example, at what point does depression manifest along trajectories of declining cognition and increasing disability, and how is this influenced (if at all) by comorbid cerebrovascular disease? Cerebrovascular disease cannot be investigated as a risk factor if it is included in the diagnostic criteria for a given condition. Furthermore, now that successively milder levels of cerebrovascular disease can be quantified *in vivo* through neuroimaging, a 'present/absent' system of categorizing vascular comorbidity will become steadily more problematic.

Investigations in this area must face up to important challenges of overlapping and slowly developing conditions with long prodromal periods, changing directions of cause and effect, and complex interactions between precipitants and predisposing factors which may potentially operate over periods as long as a lifetime. These could be viewed as insuperable obstacles, or as exciting new challenges for a research field of growing importance.

References

Alexopoulos GS, Meyers BS, Young RC et al, 'Vascular depression' hypothesis, *Arch Gen Psychiatry* (1997) **54**:915–22.

Andrews G, Anstey K, Brodaty H, Issakidis C, Luscombe G, Recall of depressive episode 25 years previously, *Psychol Med* (1999) **29**:787–91.

Bassuk SS, Berkman LF, Wypij D, Depressive symptomatology and incident cognitive decline in an elderly community sample, *Arch Gen Psychiatry* (1998) **55**:1073–81.

Berger A-K, Fratiglioni L, Forsell Y, Winblad B, Bäckman L, The occurrence of depressive symptoms in the preclinical phase of AD, *Neurology* (1999) **53**:1998–2002.

Carson AJ, MacHale S, Allen K et al, Depression after stroke and lesion location: a systematic review, *Lancet* (2000) **356**:122–6.

Cervilla JA, Prince M, Joels S, Mann A, Does depression predict cognitive outcome 9 to 12 years later? Evidence from a prospective study of elderly hypertensives, *Psychol Med* (2000) **30**:1017–23.

Chen P, Ganguli M, Mulsant BH, DeKosky ST, The temporal relationship between depressive symptoms and dementia, *Arch Gen Psychiatry* (1999) **56**:261–6.

Dam H, Depression in stroke patients 7 years following stroke, *Acta Psych Scand* (2001) **103**:287–93.

de Groot JC, de Leeuw F-E, Oudkerk M et al, Cerebral white matter lesions and depressive symptoms in elderly adults, *Arch Gen Psychiatry* (2000) **57**:1071–6.

de la Torre JC, Mussivand T, Can disturbed brain microcirculation cause Alzheimer's disease? *Neurol Res* (1993) **15**:146–53.

Devenand DP, Sano M, Tang MX et al, Depressed mood and the incidence of Alzheimer's disease in the elderly living in the community, *Arch Gen Psychiatry* (1996) **53**:175–82.

Dufouil C, Fuhrer R, Dartigues J-F, Alpérovitch A, Longitudinal analysis of the association between depressive symptomatology and cognitive deterioration, *Am J Epidemiol* (1996) **144**:634–41.

Esiri MM, Nagy Z, Smith MZ, Barnetson L, Smith AD, Cerebrovascular disease and threshold for dementia in the early stages of Alzheimer's disease, *Lancet* (1999) **354**:919–20.

Everson SA, Roberts RE, Goldberg DE, Kaplan GA, Depressive symptoms and increased risk of stroke mortality over a 29-year period, *Arch Intern Med* (1998) **158**:1133–8.

Ferucci L, Guralnik JM, Salive ME et al, Cognitive impairment and risk of stroke in the older population, *J Am Geriatr Soc* (1996) **44**:237–41.

Gainotti G, Azzoni A, Marra C, Frequency, phenomenology and anatomical-clinical correlates of major post-stroke depression, *Br J Psychiatry* (1999) **175**:163–7.

Gale CR, Martyn CN, Cooper C, Cognitive impairment and mortality in a cohort of elderly people, *BMJ* (1996) **312**:608–11.

Geerlings MI, Schoevers RA, Beekman ATF et al, Depression and risk of cognitive decline and Alzheimer's disease, *Br J Psychiatry* (2000) **176**:568–75.

Hargrave R, Geck LC, Reed B, Mungas D, Affective behavioural disturbances in Alzheimer's disease and ischaemic vascular dementia, *J Neurol Neurosurg Psychiatry* (2000) **68**:41–6.

Henderson AS, Korten AE, Jacomb PA et al, The course of depression in the elderly: a longitudinal community-based study in Australia, *Psychol Med* (1997) **27**:119–29.

Heun R, Papassotiropoulos A, Jessen F, Maier W, Breitner JCS, A family study of Alzheimer disease and early- and late-onset depression in elderly patients, *Arch Gen Psychiatry* (2001) **58**:190–6.

Hickie I, Scott E, Late-onset depressive disorders: a preventable variant of cerebrovascular disease? *Psychol Med* (1998) **28**:1007–13.

Holmes C, Cairns N, Lantos P, Mann A, Validity of current clinical criteria for Alzheimer's disease, vascular dementia and dementia with Lewy bodies, *Br J Psychiatry* (1999) **174**:45–50.

Hulette C, Nochlin D, McKeel D et al, Clinical-neuropathological findings in multi-infarct dementia: a report of six autopsied cases, *Neurology* (1997) **48**:668–72.

Jonas BS, Mussolino ME, Symptoms of depression as a prospective risk factor for stroke, *Psychosom Med* (2000) **62**:472–3.

Kivipelto M, Helkala E-L, Laakso MP et al, Midlife vascular risk factors and Alzheimer's disease in later life: longitudinal, population based study, *BMJ* (2001) **322**:1447–51.

Kokmen E, Whistman JP, O'Fallon WM, Chu CP, Beard CM, Dementia after ischemic stroke: a population-based study in Rochester, Minnesota (1960-1984), *Neurology* (1996) **19**:154–9.

Lee J-H, Olichney JM, Hansen LA, Hofsetter CR, Thal LJ, Small concomitant vascular lesions do not influence rates of cognitive decline in patients with Alzheimer disease, *Arch Neurol* (2000) **57**:1474–79.

Lovestone S, Diabetes and dementia: is the brain another site of end-organ damage? *Neurology* (1999) **53**:1907–9.

Neuropathology Group of the Medical Research Council Cognitive Function and Ageing Study, Pathological correlates of late-onset dementia in a multicentre, community-based population in England and Wales, *Lancet* (2001) **357**:169–75.

Notkola I-L, Sulkava R, Pekkanen J et al, Serum total cholesterol, apolipoprotein E 4 allele, and Alzheimer's disease, *Neuroepidemiol* (1998) **17**:14–20.

Ohira T, Iso H, Satoh S et al, Prospective study of depressive symptoms and risk of stroke among Japanese, *Stroke* (2001) **32**:903–8.

Olichney JM, Hansen LA, Lee JH et al, Relationship between severe amyloid angiopathy, apolipoprotein E genotype, and vascular lesions in Alzheimer's disease, *Ann NY Acad Sci* (2000) **903**:138–48.

Ott A, Stolk RP, van Harskamp F et al, Diabetes mellitus and the risk of dementia, *Neurology* (1999) **53**:1937–42.

Pohjasvaara T, Leppavuori A, Siira I et al, Frequency and clinical determinants of poststroke depression, *Stroke* (1998) **29**:2311–7.

Pohjasvaara T, Mäntylä R, Aronen HJ et al, Clinical and radiological determinants of prestroke cognitive decline in a stroke cohort, *J Neurol Neurosurg Psychiatry* (1999) **67**:742–8.

Prince M, Lovestone S, Cervilla J et al, The association between APOE and dementia is mediated neither by vascular disease nor its risk factors in an aged cohort of survivors with hypertension, *Neurology* (2000) **54**:397–402.

Prince MJ, Beekman ATF, Deeg DJH et al, Depression symptoms in late-life assessed using the EURO-D scale, *Br J Psychiatry* (1999) **174**:339–45.

Prince MJ, Harwood RH, Thomas A, Mann AH, A prospective population-based cohort study of the effects of disablement and social milieu on the onset and maintenance of late-life depression. The Gospel Oak Project VII, *Psychol Med* (1998) **28**:337–50.

Rao R, Jackson S, Howard R, Depression in older people with mild stroke, carotid stenosis and peripheral vascular disease: a comparison with healthy controls, *Int J Geriatr Psychiatry* (2001) **16**:175–83.

Ritchie K, Gilham C, Ledesert B, Touchon J, Kotzki P-O, Depressive illness, depressive symptomatology and regional cerebral blood flow in elderly people with sub-clinical cognitive impairment, *Age Ageing* (1999) **28**:385–91.

Skoog I, Lernfelt B, Landahl S et al, 15-year longitudinal study of blood pressure and dementia, *Lancet* (1996) **347**:1141–5.

Slooter AJC, Cruts M, Ott A et al, The effect of APOE on dementia is not through atherosclerosis: The Rotterdam Study, *Neurology* (1999) **53**:1593–5.

Snowdon DA, Greiner LH, Mortimer JA et al, Brain infarction and the clinical expression of Alzheimer disease, *JAMA* (1997) **277**:813–7.

Stewart R, Cardiovascular factors in Alzheimer's disease, *J Neurol Neurosurg Psychiatry* (1998) **65**:143–7.

Stewart R, Liolitsa D, Type 2 diabetes mellitus, cognitive impairment and dementia, *Diabetic Med* (1999) **16**:93–112.

Stewart R, Prince M, Richards M, Brayne C, Mann A, Stroke, vascular risk factors and depression. A cross sectional study in a UK Caribbean-born population, *Br J Psychiatry* (2001a) **178**:23–8.

Stewart R, Russ C, Richards M et al, Depression, APOE genotype and subjective memory impairment: a cross-sectional study in an African Caribbean population, *Psychol Med* (2001b) **31**:431–40.

Tatemichi TK, Paik M, Bagiella E et al, Risk of dementia after stroke in a hospitalised cohort: results of a longitudinal study, *Neurology* (1994) **44**:1885–91.

Thomas AJ, Ferrier IN, Kalaria RN et al, A neuropathological study of vascular factors in late-life depression, *J Neurol Neurosurg Psychiatry* (2001) **70**:83–7.

14(i)
Post-stroke depression

Risto Vataja, Tarja Pohjasvaara, Antero Leppävuori
and Timo Erkinjuntti

Introduction

Depression as a consequence of stroke is a field of intense research, with 40–50 new papers on the topic coming out each year in scientific journals registered in the MEDLINE database. The reasons for this interest are obvious. Stroke is one of the leading causes of death in Western societies and causes often devastating consequences to the surviving individuals in the form of loss of ability to work, loss of independence in activities of daily living and nursing home placement. Post-stroke depression (PSD) has been shown to be an important and independent correlate of poor functional outcome (Herrmann et al, 1998; Pohjasvaara et al, 2000) and mortality (Morris et al, 1993; House et al, 2001). Effective prevention and therapy of PSD could thus be expected to diminish the human suffering and economic burden associated with stroke (Hachinski, 1999). Also, PSD provides a valuable model for understanding the neurobiology of mood regulation in normal individuals and in patients suffering from endogenous depression. Mood changes and disorders associating to localized brain damage help identify critical cerebral structures and connections as well as neurochemical changes that may be involved in functional depression.

The diversity of definitions and instruments in diagnosing depression as well as heterogeneity in study populations and designs probably explain why some of the core questions of PSD still remain far from settled. Is depression more frequent or more severe in stroke patients than in individuals suffering from other serious medical illnesses? Is PSD a product of disturbed neural function or merely a reaction to the psychosocial stress accompanying severe disease? Are PSD and endogenous depression identical with regard to phenomenology and treatment? In this chapter, we present the current knowledge and views on these issues.

Prevalence of post-stroke depression: is depression more common following stroke than in other chronic diseases?

Folstein et al reported in 1977 that in their study comparing 20 stroke patients with 10 orthopaedic patients whose activities of daily living were equally compromised, depression was found in 45% of the stroke patients, whereas only 10% of the orthopaedic patients were depressed. This is to our knowledge the only study with such a direct comparative setting. In a recent population-based study in the USA focusing on a general elderly population aged 65–100 years (Steffens et al, 2000), the point prevalence of major depression was estimated to be 4.4% in non-demented female and 2.7% in male individuals. However, in elderly general practice outpatients the prevalence of depression has been reported to be significantly higher, between 17 and 30% (Evans and Katona, 1993; Callahan et al, 1994). Depression has been reported to be common in patients with various medical conditions. For example, 16–23% of patients with coronary heart disease (Musselmann et al, 1998), 20% of cancer patients (Bottomley, 1998) and 23% of patients with rheumatoid arthritis (Abdel-Nasser et al, 1998) have been reported to suffer from significant depression. The reported prevalence of depression in neurological disorders is somewhat higher. Major depression was present in 27% of the patients referred to general neurology outpatient clinics for any reason (Carson et al, 2000b). The prevalence of depression in Parkinson's disease (Cummings and Masterman, 1999), in multiple sclerosis (Ron and Logsdail, 1989) and in outpatients with traumatic brain injury (Kreutzer et al, 2001) is around 40%.

Numerous studies have addressed the prevalence of depression in stroke patients. The percentages of depressed patients vary from study to study, depending on the time elapsed from the onset of stroke symptoms, study setting (acute inpatient, rehabilitation hospital, outpatient) and diagnostic criteria used. Some of the essential studies reporting prevalence rates of post-stroke depression are presented in Table 14.1. In the most recent studies, the estimated prevalence of depressive disorders has been around 40% (Pohjasvaara et al, 1998).

Comparing the data from different patient populations is difficult. However, depression is clearly more prevalent in post-stroke patients than in the general elderly population. It seems to be more common in patients with stroke than in patients with cancer, rheumatoid arthritis or coronary heart disease. In patients with Parkinson's disease, multiple sclerosis or traumatic brain injury, the reported prevalence of depression equals that of PSD. This indirect evidence suggests that brain injury associated with CNS disorders of different mechanisms may be an additional risk factor for depression, in addition to the psychosocial stress caused by severe disease.

The diagnosis and phenomenology of post-stroke depression

The clinician treating a patient with behavioural disturbance or change of mood after stroke faces a challenging task. In the acute phase, the patient may be worried and anxious, having to cope with frightening and invalidat-

Table 14.1 Studies of prevalence and significance of lesion location in Post-stroke depression.

	N	Setting	Prevalence of depression (%)	Association between lesion location and	Depression criteria	Time from stroke to assessment
Robinson et al (1984)	36	Inpatient	44	Left side more common	DSM-III Major and minor depression	Acute
Sinyor et al (1986)	35	Rehabilitation	40	Right side more common	DSM-III	2 weeks
Starkstein et al (1987)	45	Inpatient, rehabilitation	31	Left side more common	DSM-III Major and minor depression	Mean, 20 days
Dam et al (1989)	92	Inpatient, outpatient	30	No association	Research diagnostic criteria (RDC)	Mean, 35 days
MacHale et al (1998)	145	Inpatient	20	Right hemisphere more common	DSM-IV Major and minor depression	6 months
House et al (1990)	73	Community	11 (1 month) –5 (12 months)	No association	DSM-III Major depression	1, 6 and 12 months after stroke
Andersen et al (1995)	285	Inpatient, outpatient	30	No association	Hamilton Depression Rating Scale > 12 points	1 month
Schwartz et al (1993)	91	Rehabilitation	40	Right side more affected in depression	DSM-III Major and minor depression	3–9 months
Gainotti et al (1999)	153	Inpatient, rehabilitation	27 (<4 months) 40 (>4 months)	No association	DSM-III-R Major depression	2 weeks – 6 months
Sharpe et al (1990)	60	Community	18	No association	Any DSM-III-R depression	3 to 5 years
Åström et al (1993)	80	Inpatient	25 (acute stage), 31 (3 months), 16 (12 months), 29 (3 years)	Left anterior lesion more common in acute stage, not later	DSM-III Major depression	Acute phase–3 years
Herrmann et al. (1995)	47	Inpatient	36	Left basal ganglia lesions were correlated to depression	Any DSM-III-R depression	< 2 months
Kim and Choi-Kwon (2000)	148	Outpatient	18	No differences between hemispheres, but anterior more common than posterior	DSM-IV Major depression	2–4 months

ing symptoms like dysphasia or hemiparesis, often leading to loss of independent functioning in activities of daily living. Many depressive symptoms in
these circumstances may be regarded as part of the somatic symptoms
(e.g. slowness, loss of appetite, somatic complaints) or 'normal grief reaction', which may cause depression to go undetected. Also, typical stroke
symptoms of dysphasia, dementia, aprosodia (loss of melodic line of language) or anosognosia (lack of subjective awareness of disorder) may
confound the diagnosis of PSD (Ramasubbu and Kennedy, 1994). Of other
neuropsychiatric symptoms often mimicking or masking depression, apathy
and fatigue have recently received more attention. Apathy, defined as the
absence or lack of feeling, interest, emotion or concern, was reported in 18
(22.5%) of 80 consecutive stroke patients, nine of whom were also
depressed (Starkstein et al, 1993). Fatigue (feeling of early exhaustion developing during mental activity, with weariness, lack of energy and aversion to
effort) was present in 51% of stroke patients, compared with 16% of age-
matched controls (van der Werf et al, 2001). Of the patients with fatigue,
20% had elevated depression symptom scores. Thus, these post-stroke
symptoms may co-exist with depression but are often present also in the
non-depressed patients.

This large variability of symptoms and symptom clusters that is often present in post-stroke patients may explain why depression is recognized and
treated in only a minority of patients. In an unselected post-stroke patient
population (Kotila et al, 1998) 17% of the depressed stroke patients, and in
hospital-based cohorts (Morris and Robinson, 1990; Pohjasvaara et al,
1998), around 40% of the patients were using antidepressants suggesting
that a large majority of patients did not receive adequate treatment for their
depression.

The current diagnostic classifications of ICD-10 (WHO, 1992) and DSM-IV
(American Psychiatric Association, 1994) offer few diagnostic guidelines for
clinicians and are somewhat unsatisfactory for scientific purposes, forcing
different study groups to use modified criteria and thus adding confusion to
this study field. The ICD-10 criteria are commonly in use in clinical practice
in Europe. The diagnostic criteria of mental and behavioural disorders due to
organic brain damage as applied to patients with stroke are shown in Table
14.2. These criteria are very vague, allowing any depressive syndromes from
mild to severe depressive episodes or recurrent depressive disorders to dys-
thymia-like or unspecified depressive disorders to be diagnosed as organic
depressive disorder (F06.32). Further, it is presumed that the phenomenology of post-stroke depression is similar to 'endogenous' depression and that
the symptom lists of different endogenous depressive episodes and disorders are valid also for post-stroke patients.

The DSM-IV criteria for mood disorder due to a general medical condition
(298.83), on the other hand, require that there is evidence, after the clinician's 'careful and comprehensive assessment of multiple factors', that
mood disorder is due to stroke. As in ICD-10, patients with delirium and

Table 14.2   ICD-10 diagnostic criteria for organic depressive disorder as applied to PSD (F06.32).

G1.	Objective evidence of stroke (from clinical examination or laboratory tests, e.g. CT scan)
G2.	Presumed relationship between the stroke occurrence and subsequent depression (either immediate or delayed)
G3.	Recovery from, or significant improvement of, depression after improvement of stroke symptoms
G4.	Insufficient evidence for an alternative cause of the depression, e.g. a significant family history or a clinically similar disorder
	The condition must meet the diagnostic criteria of one of the depressive disorders (F32–F39) (Mild, moderate or severe depressive episode; recurrent depressive disorders; cyclo- and dysthymia; other depressive disorders)
	The condition is not associated with dementia or delirium

dementia must be excluded – an important notion here since approximately every fifth elderly stroke patient is also demented according to the DSM-IV criteria for dementia (Pohjasvaara et al, 1997). The DSM-IV specifies two subtypes of depression due to stroke. First, patients 'with depressive features' are defined as post-stroke patients whose predominant mood is depressed, but in whom full criteria for a major depressive episode are not met. This means that any patient whose depressed mood is judged to be a consequence of stroke may be diagnosed as PSD even though no other symptoms of the depression syndrome usually required for diagnosis is present. Second subtype 'with major depressive-like episode' specifies post-stroke patients whose depressive syndrome fulfils the DSM-IV criteria for major depressive episode. Again, it is presumed that the phenomenology of post-stroke depression is analogous to that of endogenous depression. Is this presumption justified?

Lipsey et al (1986) compared different depressive symptom clusters (based on the PSE semistructured interview) in 43 patients with major endogenous depression with 43 age- comparable (mean, 58 years) patients with post-stroke depression and found that the only symptom clusters differing between the two groups were slowness (more in the post-stroke group) and loss of interest and concentration (more in the functional depression group). Among the 16 symptom clusters of no difference were affective flattening, self-neglect, irritability, lack of energy, general anxiety and agitation. While the authors conclude that the symptomatology of these two depressive syndromes are alike, it must be noted that the patients with endogenous depression were recruited from an inpatient psychogeriatric unit. Silent, non-symptomatic brain infarcts are present in up to 51% of such elderly patient groups with major depression (Fujikawa et al, 1993), suggesting that many of the 'endogenous' depression group patients may actually have suffered from post-stroke or vascular depression. Further, contradicting data has been published by Gainotti et al (1999), who reported that patients with post-stroke depression have less depressed mood, anhedonia and suicidal thoughts, but more hyperemotionalism, catastrophic reactions and diurnal variations of the symptoms, than patients suffering from endogenous depression.

Different scales have been used to screen for depression in stroke patients. Agrell and Dehlin (1989) have compared six depression rating scales in geriatric stroke patients (the Geriatric Depression Scale, the Zung Scale, the Center for Epidemiologic Studies Depression Scale, the Hamilton Depression Rating Scale, the Comprehensive Psychopathology Rating Scale – Depression, and the Cornell Scale) using clinical examination or psychiatric interview as the independent variable to which scales were related. They found that with regard to internal consistency, sensitivity and predictive value the Geriatric Depression Scale and the Zung Scale were the best self-rating scales, and Comprehensive Psychopathology Rating Scale – Depression was the best examiner-rating scale. Schramke et al (1998), however, using better validated SCID-R as a reference, reported that the Center for Epidemiologic Studies Depression Scale and the Hamilton Depression Rating Scale actually indicated distress and were not specific for depression in post-stroke patients – which might hold true for many other current scales as well. Furthermore, there is evidence that when such scales are used in screening for PSD, the somatic items (i.e. sleep disorders, loss of appetite etc) are less specific and thus less reliable than non-somatic items (Stein et al, 1996). Clearly, there is need for caution when using existing depression rating scales as screening instruments in post-stroke patient populations.

In conclusion, the concept of post-stroke depression should be re-evaluated by studying different depressive and associated behavioural symptoms in post-stroke patients. The emerging syndrome may be different from that of endogenous depression. For example, if post-stroke depression is in part a result of dysfunction of the frontal-subcortical circuits (see 'mechanisms of post-stroke depression' below) it is to be expected that these patients would often present with other symptoms arising from disturbances within the same or adjacent frontal-subcortical loops. Clinically, symptoms like dysexecutive functions, apathy, anxiety, and disinhibition indeed often accompany depression post-stroke. If these features prove to be characteristic in future studies of post-stroke depression they should possibly be included in the diagnostic criteria of this syndrome.

A clinician should actively look for depression in his stroke patients, since almost half of them will suffer from it. In most of these cases, the depressed mood is clearly present and the diagnosis is not difficult. On the other hand, in patients with apathy, fatigue, loss of interest and lack of insight the task is more difficult. Depressive symptoms that are not mentioned in the diagnostic criteria should also be taken into consideration in these patients. For example, irritability, agitation, unexplained difficulties in the rehabilitation process and emotional lability are often present in patients with PSD.

Depression scales, e.g. Geriatric Depression Scale, may well be used as a part of diagnostic evaluation and follow-up but should not be relied on as a screening instrument.

The relationship between lesion location and post-stroke depression

The association between location of brain damage and subsequent changes in behaviour has been demonstrated in classic neuropsychology, i.e. in aphasic or amnestic disorders. The current knowledge in neurobiology emphasizes the model of wide-distributed neural networks, rather than strictly localized brain areas, as the anatomical basis of distinct brain functions. However, there may exist some critical 'relay areas' or areas of anatomical proximity of different neural networks that, when damaged, may give rise to disturbances in complex behaviour or affect. One mediating factor may be the changes in neural transmitter functions caused by the brain damage.

In association with depression after brain damage, such a hypothesis seemed to be supported by the early work by Robinson and colleagues (Robinson et al, 1975; Robinson, 1979). They showed in an experimental stroke model in rats that spontaneous activity increased in animals with induced right-sided brain lesions, but not in rats with left-sided lesions. The right-sided lesions were also associated with a decrease in the norepinephrine concentrations in the cerebral cortex. Thus, a lateralized behavioural change and an asymmetrical cathecolamine depletion could be produced in test animals. Robinson and colleagues then went on to study the association of depression and the distance of anterior lesion border from the anterior pole of the brain on CT images, first in patients with brain injury (Robinson and Szetela, 1981), and later in patients with stroke (Robinson et al, 1983; 1984; Starkstein et al, 1987). They reported that depression was significantly more common in patients with anterior and with left-sided lesions, and especially in patients with left anterior lesions, than in patients with lesions elsewhere. Also, the severity of depression seemed to be correlated to the distance of the lesion from the frontal pole of the brain.

More than 50 studies addressing the correlations between stroke lesion location and depression have been published after the seminal work by the Robinson group, and some of the most prominent studies are presented in Table 14.1. All studies shown here have applied CT methodology in localizing the stroke, and most of them have recruited only patients with a single stroke lesion. The results of the many studies in this field are conflicting: some report no association between the lesion location and depression; some find associations with right-sided lesion location and depression. Robinson (1998a) has suggested that the relationship between post-stroke depression and lesion location is dynamic, so that the association exists in the acute phase after stroke but not in later stages, i.e. 3 months after stroke. This dynamic change would explain the apparent discrepancies between studies carried out at different time periods after stroke. Some studies support this view (Åström et al, 1993; Shimoda and Robinson, 1999). However, the most powerful argument against the 'localization' hypothesis so far has been presented in a systematic review of the existing studies in this field by Carson et al (2000a). Their fixed-effects and random-effects meta-analysis of the pooled data from 48 studies found no evidence for the lesions of the left hemisphere or of the left anterior brain being critical in post-stroke depression. Among the suggested reasons for variable results between individual studies are different patient samples (i.e. differing social-class and racial characteristics of the patient populations) and admission criteria between studies. Carson et al also criticize poor description of the source of the patients as well as lack of detailed information about the patients who were excluded or refused to participate in many studies, and they suggest that multiple publication is a source of bias in this field. After warning that heterogeneity of the included studies limits the power of the meta-analysis, they concluded that 'the available data indicate that a patient's risk of depression is not related to where the cerebral lesion is located'. After reaching similar results in their review, Singh et al (1999) suggested methodological criteria for high-quality localisation studies (Table 14.3). This table illustrates how many clinical and radiological aspects should be accounted for in future studies.

Table 14.3   Methodological criteria for PSD localization studies as suggested by Singh et al (1999).

Subjects with single strokes only
Specified setting
Subjects with no history of neurological illness
Subjects with no previous psychiatric history
Subjects not using psychotropic medication
Subjects with no family history of psychiatric illness
Right-handed subjects only
Assessment of cognitive impairment
Assessment of physical and functional disability
Assessment of social support
Diagnostic criteria for depression
Standardized scales for depression
Standardized timing of psychiatric assessment
Standardized timing of CT scanning
CT-visible lesions only
CT assessed blind to outcome
Specified lesion volume method
Specified lesion localization method
Cerebral atrophy measurement

We have approached the question of radiological correlates of PSD in our study of 275 consecutive 55- – 85-year-old patients studied 3 months after ischaemic stroke (Vataja et al, 2001). The patients underwent 1.0 T MRI and a comprehensive psychiatric examination applying a semi-structured computer-based SCAN interview and various depression scales. Modified DSM-III-R and DSM-IV criteria were used to identify patients with any depressive disorder (major or minor depression). The severity of the stroke symptoms was assessed by different stroke scales; disability and handicap were assessed by different scales; and the cognitive status of the patients was evaluated by clinical neurological and neuropsychological examination. The MRI scans were rated by a neuroradiologist blind to the clinical data for lesion location, lesion volume estimation, white matter changes and cortical, central and mesial-temporal brain atrophy. The site and size of *all infarcts* (regardless of the assumed association with the stroke symptoms, i.e. symptomatic and non-symptomatic brain infarcts) detected in the MRI were evaluated in different brain lobes, vascular territories and specific locations of neuropsychiatric interest (i.e. putamen, pallidum, caudate, internal capsule, corona radiata, amygdala, etc). The volumes were estimated using the radii of largest diameter of the lesions. We also formed a sum variable for prefrontal-subcortical circuits (Alexander and Crutcher, 1986; Cummings, 1993, see below) including connections between frontal cortex, caudate, pallidum and thalamus.

In the univariate analysis, many central areas of the prefrontal-subcortical circuit, i.e. pallidum, genu of the internal capsule and caudate, were more often affected in the depressed patients, and left-sided lesions seemed to be more common in the depressed patients in many of these structures (Table 14.4). As

Table 14.4   The mean number (SD) of brain infarcts in patients with and without PSD in the Helsinki Stroke Aging Memory Study Cohort (Mann-Whitney non-parametric test).

Site	Without depression N=166	With depression N=109	P
Occipital lobe (right side)	0.18 (0.41)	0.09 (0.32)	0.04
Caudate (any side)	0.31 (0.60)	0.48 (0.69)	0.02
Caudate (left side)	0.15 (0.41)	0.27 (0.49)	0.01
Pallidum (any side)	0.32 (0.61)	0.54 (0.73)	0.005
Pallidum (right side)	0.17 (0.39)	0.27 (0.45)	0.03
Pallidum (left side)	0.15 (0.36)	0.27 (0.44)	0.02
Genu of internal capsule (left side)	0.03 (0.17)	0.11 (0.31)	0.007
Anterior capsule (left side)	0.06 (0.24)	0.16 (0.36)	0.009
Posterior corona radiata (any side)	0.32 (0.50)	0.49 (0.63)	0.03
Posterior corona radiata (left side)	0.15 (0.35)	0.26 (0.46)	0.03
Amygdala (any side)	0.006 (0.08)	0.05 (0.21)	0.03
Prefrontal–subcortical circuit (any side)	1.16 (1.39)	1.56 (1.61)	0.02
Prefrontal–subcortical circuit (left side)	0.57 (0.85)	0.86 (1.0)	0.01

a whole, the fronto-subcortical circuits were also more often affected in the depressed patients, with a left-sided predominance. We did not find any differences in the severity of brain atrophy or white matter changes using criteria proposed by Fazekas et al (1987) between the depressed and non-depressed patients. An adding multiple logistic regression analysis of the radiological variables suggested an increased risk of PSD with lesions affecting the left genu of internal capsule (OR 3.2) or the pallidum of any side (OR 1.6).

We did not find a correlation between the severity or extent of white matter changes or brain atrophy and PSD. This does not mean, however, that these more chronic ischaemic changes would not contribute to late-onset depression or PSD. Previously, left frontal deep white matter (and left putaminal) hyperintensities have been connected to late-onset depression (Greenwald et al, 1999). It is possible that a subtle effect of the white matter changes on function within neural circuits and on depression was masked by the more robust consequences of brain infarcts in our patients.

We believe that there are important methodological reasons why our results do not agree with the results of Carson and Singh. First, compared to computed tomography (CT), MRI is superior in detecting the site, type and extent of infarcts, especially in the deep grey matter structures, and small infarcts can also be more reliably estimated with MRI than with CT. Most elderly patients with their first symptomatic stroke already have previous clinically 'silent' lesions, usually small lacunes, that may well contribute to the depression following the clinical stroke; the sensitivity of MRI allows these lesions to be detected.

Second, most previous CT-based studies have used simple descriptions of lesion locations, e.g. distance from frontal pole. By using such robust methods, the critical neuroanatomical structures are easily missed. In our study the depressed patients did not have more infarcts affecting the basal ganglia area as a whole than the non-depressed patients. Significant differences were however detected in smaller substructures, i.e. caudate and pallidum, between the depressed and non-depressed patient groups. Clearly, MRI technology and more detailed radiological-anatomical variables relevant to neuropsychiatry should be used in future studies of lesion localization and PSD.

The mechanisms of post-stroke depression

The results of our study described in the previous paragraph suggest that the lesions affecting frontal-subcortical circuits within basal ganglia are connected to PSD. Such associations have also been reported in previous post-stroke studies, originally by Starkstein et al (1988). They found in their CT-based study of 25 patients with brain infarcts or intracerebral haematomas restricted to either thalamus or basal ganglia, that patients with left-sided basal ganglia lesions showed a higher frequency and severity of depression, as compared with patients with right-sided basal ganglia or thalamic lesions. Analogous findings in regards to significance of affected frontal-subcortical circuitry and PSD have been reported by Morris et al (1996) and Kim and Choi Kwon (2000).

Further, numerous functional (Drevets, 2000) and structural (Soares and Mann, 1997) neuroimaging studies of endogenous, 'non-organic' depression have also found correlations between neurophysiological and structural abnormalities of the prefrontal cortex, amygdala, striatum and thalamus.

Five different frontal-subcortical circuits have been recognized, three of which are associated with emotional and cognitive processes in man (Alexander and Crutcher, 1986; Cummings, 1993) (see Chapter 12). These three circuits have been named according to their site of origin on the frontal cortex as *dorsolateral prefrontal circuit* (originating from the convexity of the frontal lobe, Brodmann's areas 9 and 10), *lateral orbitofrontal circuit* (originating from the lower lateral parts of the prefrontal cortex, Brodmann's area 10) and *anterior cingulate circuit* (originating from the medially located cingular cortex, Brodmann's area 24). After their anatomically diverse areas of origin these circuits run closely adjacent to each other, although segregated, within the subcortical structures (Figure 14.1, Burrus et al, 2000) of caudate,

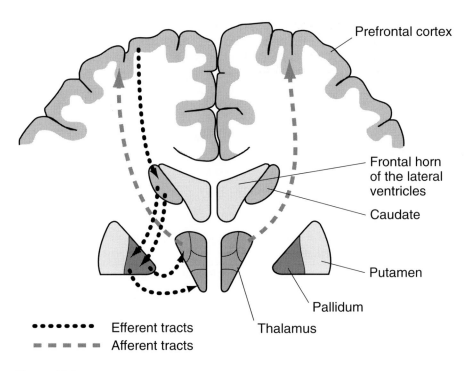

Figure 14.1

The schematic anatomical relationships of the frontal–subcortical circuits.

globus pallidus, substantia nigra, thalamic nuclei and interconnecting white matter structures, e.g. capsula interna and corona radiata, before returning to the frontal cortex, thus forming a closed circuit. These circuits also have rich connections with the structures of the limbic circuitry, e.g. amygdala and hippocampus.

Damage to the dorsolateral prefrontal circuit has been associated with cognitive changes, especially dysexecutive function; the orbitofrontal-subcortical circuit with irritability and agitation; and the anterior cingular circuit with apathy (Table 14.5). As the circuits run closely adjacent to each other after leaving the cortex, they are likely to get damaged together by large subcortical brain infarcts. The resulting clinical manifestations can thus be expected to be a variable mixture of the cognitive and psychiatric symptoms. Depression has not been specifically connected to any single circuit, and can probably be a result of functional or structural damage to one or more of these circuits. The association of PSD with other syndromes like apathy (Starkstein et al, 1993) and dysexecutive functions (Kauhanen et al, 1999; Leeds et al, 2001) is also understandable in the context of the frontal-subcortical circuitry model.

The role of specific neurotransmitters in PSD is unclear, although studies of receptor binding in animal models and human patients (Robinson, 1998b), as well as fenfluramine challenge studies (Ramasubbu et al, 1998), suggest that disturbances in the monoamine (dopamine, 5-HT and/or nor-epinephrine) metabolism may be involved. Also, the emerging model of depression as a result of neuroplastic changes in the limbic circuitry (Duman et al, 1997; Manji et al, 2001) might also apply to the pathophysiology of PSD. One could speculate that stroke causes deleterious plastic changes not only as a major psychological stress, but also by direct damage to the circuits involved.

Although the biological aspects of PSD are intriguing, it is clear that it is just as multidimensional a disorder as any other psychiatric condition. Among reported risk factors for PSD are premorbid neurotic peronality and

Table 14.5   Behavioural and psychological symptoms after damage to specific frontal-subcortical circuits.

Dorsolateral prefrontal circuit	Lateral orbitofrontal circuit	Anterior cingulate circuit
Impairment in goal formulation	Loss of tact	Apathy
Impairment in planning	Irritability	Lack of spontaneous speech
Impairment in set shifting	Apathy	Lack of emotion
Impairment in abstracting	Loss of initiative	Akinetic mutism
Impairment in verbal fluency	Elevated mood	(Depression)
Depression	Disinhibition	
	(Depression)	

previous family or personal history of depression (Morris et al, 1992); major life events other than stroke (Bush, 1999); living alone before stroke, female gender and social stress before stroke (Andersen et al, 1995); and stroke severity and disability after stroke (Pohjasvaara et al, 1998). The psychosocial factors of this disorder are not to be forgotten in clinical work or in research.

Treatment of post-stroke depression

If the pathophysiology of PSD is not identical to that of so-called endogenous depression, do the same therapeutic principles apply to both conditions? There are at present six controlled studies addressing this question (Table 14.6) in addition to open-label studies. The data from these studies show that PSD does respond to antidepressants with different modes of action with a rate comparable to that of endogenous depression. It is possible that antidepressive medication also improves cognitive functions and ability to perform activities of daily living, but the data is still not conclusive and negative results in these non-psychiatric outcomes have been published.

What is the drug of choice in these patients? Robinson et al (2000) have suggested that nortriptyline, a heterocyclic compound, is superior to fluoxetine (and placebo) in patients with PSD with regard to antidepressive effect. This is the only post-stroke study so far in which antidepressants have been compared with each other. However, in elderly patients with cerebrovascular disease the significance of possible adverse effects is highlighted, and the anticholinergic effects (i.e. glaucoma, urinary retention and cognitive deterioration) and potential cardiotoxic effects of nortriptyline clearly limit its usefulness post-stroke. The selective seratonin reputake inhibitors (SSRIs) probably have fewer side effects and contraindications in post-stroke patients (Cole et al, 2001) and are more feasible to use. Novel agents, e.g. venlafaxine, seem to be safe and effective in our clinical experience, supported by some open-label research data (Dahmen et al, 1999).

Electroconvulsive therapy (ECT) is probably also safe and effective in PSD (Currier et al, 1992). Although there are case reports (Weintraub and Lippmann, 2000) of safe ECT even in the post-acute phase (7–14 days after stroke), it is probably safer to wait for a few weeks before introducing ECT to avoid ischaemic complications (Miller and Isenberg, 1998).

Although no controlled trials of different psychotherapeutic approaches in patients with PSD exists, the value of supportive psychotherapy and psychoeducation and family support is hard to deny in clinical practice. Of the more structured therapy modalities, cognitive psychotherapy is probably worthy of consideration in patients with at most mildly disturbed communicative and cognitive abilities (Lincoln et al, 1997; Kneebone and Dunmore, 2000).

Table 14.6 Controlled pharmacological trials in Post-stroke depression.

Study group	Patient population	N	Criteria	Drug, dose	Effect
Reding et al (1986)	Stroke rehabilitation programme	27 patients	Zung scale score, clinical depression	Trazodone 200 mg/day	Improvement in Barthel ADL better in active medication group
Lipsey et al (1984)	Rehabilitation hospital, outpatients	34 patients	DSM-III	Nortriptyline 100 mg/day	Improvement in Hamilton, Zung, PSE in active medication group
Wiart et al (2000)	Rehabilitation unit patients	31 patients	ICD-10 major depression and MADRS>19	Fluoxetine 20 mg/day	Improvement in MADRS, not in function or cognition or motor
Andersen et al (1994)	Unselected inpatients and outpatients	66 patients	Hamilton depression score cutpoint	Citalopram 10–40 mg/day	Improvement in Hamilton depression score
Grade et al (1998)	Community-based rehabilitation unit patients	21 patients	Hamilton depression scale, Zung self-rating depression scale cutpoints	Methylphenidate 30 mg/day	Improvement in HAM-D and Zung
Robinson et al (2000)	Mostly rehabilitation unit patients	104 patients *with and without* depression	DSM-IV criteria for major or minor depression and HAM-D>11	Nortriptyline 100 mg/day vs. Fluoxetine 40 mg/day vs placebo	Nortriptyline superior to fluoxetine and placebo in treating depression; fluoxetine no different from placebo. No effect on cognitive or social functioning in any group

References

Abdel-Nasser AM, Abd El-Azim S, Taal E, El-Badawy SA, Rasker JJ, Valkenburg HA, Depression and depressive symptoms in rheumatoid arthritis patients: an analysis of their occurrence and determinants, *Br J Rheumatology* (1998) **37**: 391–7.

Agrell B, Dehlin O, Comparison of six depression rating scales in geriatric stroke patients, *Stroke* (1989) **20**: 1190–4.

Alexander GE, Crutcher MD, Parallel organization of functionally segregated circuits linking basal ganglia and cortex, *Ann Rev Neurosci* (1986) **9**: 357–81.

Andersen G, Vestergaard K, Lauritzen L, Effective treatment of poststroke depression with the selective serotonin reuptake inhibitor citalopram, *Stroke* (1994) **25**: 1099–104.

Andersen G, Vestergaard K, Ingemann-Nielsen M, Lauritzen L, Risk factors for post-stroke depression, *Acta Psychiatr Scand* (1995) **92**: 193–8.

American Psychiatric Association, *Diagnostic and Statistical Manual of Mental Disorders.* 4th edn (DSM-IV). American Psychiatric Association, Washington, DC, 1994.

Åström M, Adolfsson R, Asplund K, Major depression in stroke patients. A 3-year longitudinal study, *Stroke* (1993) **24**: 976–82.

Bottomley A, Depression in cancer patients: a literature review, *Eur J Can Care* (1998) **7**: 181–91.

Burrus JW, Hurley RA, Taber KH et al, Functional neuroanatomy of the frontal lobe circuits, *Radiology* (2000) **214**: 227–30.

Bush BA, Major life events as risk factors for post-stroke depression, *Brain Inj* (1999) **13**: 131–7.

Callahan CM, Hui SL, Nienaber NA, Musick BS, Tierney WM, Longitudinal study of depression and health services use among elderly primary care patients, *J Am Ger Soc* (1994) **42**: 833–8.

Carson AJ, Ringbauer B, MacKenzie L, Warlow C, Sharpe M, Neurological disease, emotional disorder, and disability: they are related: a study of 300 consecutive new referrals to a neurology outpatient department, *J Neurol Neurosurg Psychiatry* (2000b) **68**: 202–6.

Carson AJ, MacHale S, Allen K et al, Depression after stroke and lesion location: a systematic review, *Lancet* (2000a) **356**: 122–6.

Cole MG, Elie LM, McCusker J, Bellavance F, Mansour A, Feasibility and effectiveness of treatments for post-stroke depression in elderly inpatients: systematic review, *J Geriatr Psychiatry Neurol* (2001) **14**: 37–41.

Cummings JL, Frontal-subcortical circuits and human behavior, *Arch Neurol* (1993) **50**: 873–80.

Cummings JL, Masterman DL, Depression in patients with Parkinson's disease, *Int J Ger Psychiatry* (1999) **14**: 711–9.

Currier MB, Murray GB, Welch CC, Electroconvulsive therapy for post-stroke depressed geriatric patients, *J Neuropsychiatry Clin Neurosci* (1992) **4**: 140–4.

Dahmen N, Marx J, Hopf HC, Tettenborn B, Roder R, Therapy of early poststroke depression with venlafaxine: safety, tolerability, and efficacy as determined in an open, uncontrolled clinical trial, *Stroke* (1999) **30**: 691–2.

Dam H, Pedersen HE, Ahlgren P, Depression among patients with stroke, *Acta Psychiatr Scand* (1989) **80**: 118–24.

Drevets WC, Neuroimaging studies of mood disorders, *Biol Psychiatry* (2000) **15**: 813–29.

Duman RS, Heninger GR, Nestler EJ, A molecular and cellular theory of depression, *Arch Gen Psychiatry* (1997) **54**: 597–606.

Evans S, Katona CLE, Epidemiology of depressive symptoms in elderly primary care attenders, *Dementia* (1993) **4**: 327–33.

Fazekas F, Chawluk JB, Alavi A, Hurtig HI, Zimmerman RA, MRI signal abnormalities at 1.5 T in Alzheimer's dementia and normal aging, *Am J Roentgenol* (1987) **149**: 351–6.

Folstein MF, Maiberger R, McHugh PR, Mood disorder as a specific complication of stroke, *J Neurol Neurosurg Psychiatry* (1977) **40**: 1018–20.

Fujikawa T, Yamawaki S, Touhouda Y, Incidence of silent cerebral infarction in patients with major depression, *Stroke* (1993) **24**: 1631–4.

Gainotti G, Azzoni A, Marra C, Frequency, phenomenology and anatomical-clinical correlates of major post-stroke depression, *Br J Psychiatry* (1999) **175**: 163–7.

Grade C, Redford B, Chrostowski J, Toussaint L, Blackwell B, Methylphenidate in early poststroke recovery: a double-blind, placebo-controlled study, *Arch Phys Med Rehabil* (1998) **79**: 1047–50.

Greenwald BS, Kramer-Ginsberg E, Krishnan KR et al, Neuroanatomic localization of magnetic resonance imaging signal hyperintensities in geriatric depression, *Stroke* (1999) **29**: 613–7.

Hachinski V, Post-stroke depression, not to be underestimated, *Lancet* (1999) **353**: 1728.

Herrmann M, Bartels C, Schumacher M, Wallesch C-W, Poststroke depression. Is there a pathoanatomic correlate for depression in the postacute stage of stroke? *Stroke* (1995) **26**: 850–6.

Herrmann N, Black SE, Lawrence J, Szekely C, Szalai JP, The Sunnybrook stroke study. A prospective study of depressive symptoms and functional outcome, *Stroke* (1998) **29**: 618–24.

House A, Dennis M, Warlow C, Hawton K, Molyneux A, Mood disorders after stroke and their relationship to lesion location, *Brain* (1990) **113**: 1113–29.

House A, Knapp P, Bamford J, Vail A, Mortality at 12 and 24 months after stroke may be associated with depressive symptoms at 1 month, *Stroke* (2001) **32**: 696–701.

Kauhanen M-L, Korpelainen JT, Hiltunen P, Brusin E, Mononen, H et al, Poststroke depression correlates with cognitive impairment and neurological deficits, *Stroke* (1999) **30**: 1875–80.

Kim JS, Choi-Kwon S, Poststroke depression and emotional incontinence: correlation with lesion location, *Neurology* (2000) **54**: 1805–10.

Kneebone II, Dunmore E, Psychological management of post-stroke depression, *Br J Clin Psychology* (2000) **39**: 53–61.

Kotila M, Numminen H, Waltimo O, Kaste M, Depression after stroke. Results of the Finnstroke study, *Stroke* (1998) **29**: 368–72.

Kreutzer JS, Seel RT, Gourley E, The prevalence of depression after traumatic brain injury: a comprehensive examination, *Brain Inj* (2001) **15**: 561–2.

Leeds L, Meara RJ, Woods R, Hobson JP, A comparison of the new executive functioning domains of the CAMCOG-R with existing tests of executive function in elderly stroke survivors, *Age and Ageing* (2001) **30**: 251–4.

Lincoln NB, Flannaghan T, Sutcliffe L, Rother L, Evaluation of cognitive behavioural treatment for depression after stroke: a pilot study, *Clin Rehabil* (1997) **11**: 114–22.

Lipsey JR, Robinson RG, Pearlson GD, Rao K, Price TR, Nortriptyline treatment of post-stroke depression: a double-blind study, *Lancet* (1984) **i**: 297–300.

Lipsey JR, Spencer WC, Rabins PV, Robinson RG, Phenomenological comparison of functional and post-stroke depression, *Am J Psychiatry* (1986) **143**: 527–9.

MacHale SM, O'Rourke SJ, Wardlaw JM, Dennis SM, Depression and its relation to lesion location after stroke, *J Neurol Neurosurg Psychiatry* (1998) **64**: 371–4.

Manji HK, Drevets WC, Charney DS, The cellular neurobiology of depression, *Nat Med* (2001) **7**: 541–7.

Miller AR, Isenberg KE, Reversible ischemic neurologic deficit after ECT, *J ECT* (1998) **14**: 42–8.

Morris PL, Robinson RG, Prevalence and course of depressive disorders in hospitalized stroke patients, *Int J Psychiatry Med* (1990) **20**: 349–64.

Morris PL, Robinson RG, Raphael B, Samuels J, Molloy P, The relationship between risk factors for affective disorder and post-stroke depression in hospitalized stroke patients, *Aust NZ J Psychiatry* (1992) **26**: 208–17.

Morris PL, Robinson RG, Andrzejewski P, Samuels J, Price TR, Association of depression with 10-year post-stroke mortality, *Am J Psychiatry* (1993) **150**: 124–9.

Morris PL, Robinson RG, Raphael B, Hopwood MJ, Lesion location and post-stroke depression, *J Neuropsychiatry Clin Neurosci* (1996) **8**: 399–403.

Musselman DL, Evans DL, Nemeroff CB, The relationship of depression to coronary heart disease: epidemiology, biology and treatment, *Arch Gen Psychiatry* (1998) **55**: 580–92.

Pohjasvaara T, Erkinjuntti T, Vataja R, Kaste M, Dementia three months after stroke, *Stroke* (1997) **28**: 785–92.

Pohjasvaara T, Leppävuori A, Siira I et al, Frequency and clinical determinants of post-stroke depression, *Stroke* (1998) **29**: 2311–7.

Pohjasvaara T, Vataja R, Leppävuori A, Kaste M, Erkinjuntti T, Depression is an independent predictor of poor long-term functional outcome poststroke, *Eur J Neurol* (2000) **8**: 315–9.

Ramasubbu R, Kennedy SH, Factors complicating the diagnosis of depression in cerebrovascular disease, Part II—Neurological deficits and various assessment methods, *Can J Psychiatry* (1994) **29**: 601–7.

Ramasubbu R, Flint A, Brown G, Awad G, Kennedy S, Diminished serotonin-mediated prolactin responses in nondepressed stroke patients compared with healthy normal subjects, *Stroke* (1998) **29**: 1293–8.

Reding MJ, Orto LA, Winter SW et al, Antidepressant therapy after stroke. A double-blind trial, *Arch Neurol* (1986) **43**: 763–5.

Robinson RG, Differential behaviour and biochemical effects of right and left hemisphere cerebral infarction in the rat, *Science* (1979) **205**: 707–10.

Robinson RG, *The Clinical Neuropsychiatry of Stroke* (Cambridge University Press: Cambridge, 1998a) 94–124.

Robinson RG, *The Clinical Neuropsychiatry of Stroke* (Cambridge University Press: Cambridge, 1998b) 254–81.

Robinson RG, Shoemaker WJ, Schlumpf M, Valk T, Bloom FE, Effect of experimental cerebral infarction in rat brain on cathecolamines and behaviour, *Nature* (1975) **255**: 332–4.

Robinson RG, Szetela B, Mood change following left hemisphere brain injury, *Ann Neurol* (1981) **9**: 447–53.

Robinson RG, Kubos KL, Starr LB, Rao K, Price TR, Mood changes in stroke patients: relationship to lesion location, *Compr Psychiatry* (1983) **24**: 555–66.

Robinson RG, Kubos KL, Starr LB, Rao K, Price TR, Mood disorders in stroke patients: importance of location of lesion, *Brain* (1984) **107**: 81–93.

Robinson RG, Sdhultz SK, Castillo C et al, Nortriptyline versus fluoxetine in the treatment of depression and in short-term recovery after stroke: a placebo-controlled, double-blind study, *Am J Psychiatry* (2000) **157**: 351–9.

Ron MA, Logsdail SJ, Psychiatric morbidity in multiple sclerosis: a clinical and MRI study, *Psychol Med* (1989) **19**: 887–95.

Schramke CJ, Stowe RM, Ratcliff G, Goldstein G, Condray R, Poststroke depression and anxiety: different assessment methods result in variations in incidence and severity estimates, *J Clin Exp Neuropsychol* (1998) **20**: 723–37.

Schwartz JA, Speed NM, Brunberg JA et al, Depression in stroke rehabilitation, *Biol Psychiatry* (1993) **33**: 694–9.

Sharpe M, Hawton A, House A et al, Mood disorders in long-term survivors of stroke: associations with brain lesion location and volume, *Psychol Med* (1990) **20**: 815–28.

Shimoda K, Robinson RG, The relationship between poststroke depression and lesion location in long-term follow-up, *Biol Psychiatry* (1999) **45**: 187–92.

Singh A, Herrmann N, Black SE, The importance of lesion location in poststroke depression: a critical review, *Can J Psychiatry* (1999) **43**: 921–7.

Sinyor D, Jacques P, Kaloupe DG et al, Poststroke depression and lesion location, *Brain* (1986) **109**: 537–46.

Soares JC, Mann JJ, The anatomy of mood disorders – review of structural neuroimaging studies, *Biol Psychiatry* (1997) **41**: 86–106.

Starkstein SE, Fedoroff JP, Price TR, Leiguarda R, Robinson RG, Apathy following cerebrovascular lesions, *Stroke* (1993) **24**: 1625–30.

Starkstein SE, Robinson RG, Price TR, Comparison of cortical and subcortical lesions in the production of poststroke mood disorders, *Brain* (1987) **110**: 1045–59.

Starkstein SE, Robinson RG, Berthier ML, Parikh MR, Price TR, Differential mood changes following basal ganglia vs thalamic lesions, *Arch Neurol* (1988) **45**: 725–30.

Steffens DC, Skoog I, Norton MC et al, Prevalence of depression and its treatment in an elderly population: the Cache County study, *Arch Gen Psychiatry* (2000) **57**: 601–7.

Stein PN, Sliwinski MJ, Gordon WA, Hibbard MR, Discriminative properties of somatic and nonsomatic symptoms for post stroke depression, *Clin Neuropsychologist* (1996) **10**: 82–7.

van der Werf SP, van der Broek HL, Anten HW, Bleijenberg G, Experience of severe fatigue long after stroke and its relation to depressive symptoms and disease characteristics, *Eur Neuro* (2001) **45**: 28–33.

Vataja R, Pohjasvaara T, Leppävuori A et al, Magnetic resonance imaging correlates of depression after ischemic stroke, *Arch Gen Psychiatry* (2001) **58**: 925–31.

Weintraub D, Lippmann SB, Electroconvulsive therapy in the acute poststroke period, *J ECT* (2000) **16**: 415–8.

Wiart L, Petit H, Joseph P, Mazaux JM, Barat M, Fluoxetine in early poststroke depression: A double-blind placebo-controlled study, *Stroke* (2000) **31**: 1829–32.

World Health Organization *The ICD-10 Classification of Mental and Behavioral Disorders: Clinical Descriptions and Diagnostic Guidelines* (WHO, Geneva, 1992).

14(ii)
Post-stroke depression

Sergio E Starkstein and Alejandro Serbanescu

Post-stroke depression and physical impairment

One of the first ideas coming to mind when trying to understand the mechanism of post-stroke depression is that depressed mood may be an understandable emotional reaction to the physical impairment. However, as is discussed in the following pages, the correlation between (more severe) physical impairment and (more severe) depression is rather low. It could also be hypothesized that depression after stroke may impair the recovery from physical impairments, and findings supporting this alternative explanation will be presented.

Robinson et al (1983) carried out a longitudinal study that included a consecutive series of 103 patients with an acute stroke lesion. When patients were divided into those with mild to moderate motor impairment vs those with severe motor impairment, no significant between-group differences were found in the severity of depression scores. Similar negative findings were obtained when patients were divided into those with right vs those with left hemiparesis.

Robinson et al (1983) developed the Johns Hopkins Functioning Inventory to measure deficits in activities of daily living (ADL) such as the ability to dress and feed oneself, to walk, to find one's way around, to express needs, to read and write, to keep living accommodation in order, and to maintain sphincter control. Using this instrument Robinson et al (1983) reported that patients with post-stroke depression had significantly more severe impairments in ADLs as compared to non-depressed stroke patients.

In a study that included a group of 87 stroke patients who were assessed with the Barthel Index between 2 and 3 months after stroke, Eastwood et al (1989) found those patients with major or minor depression to have significantly more impairments in ADLs as compared to non-depressed stroke patients.

Schwartz et al (1993) assessed a series of 91 stroke patients in a rehabilitation setting and found a significant correlation between depression and disability scores. Robinson et al (1987) reported a significant correlation between scores of depression and ADLs, but the amount of variance explained by the severity of deficits in ADLs was low (about 12%). During the first 6 months following stroke the correlation between depression scores and deficits in ADLs increased, but at 1 and 2 years follow-up the magnitude of the correlation decreased, suggesting that during the first 6 months after stroke the most severely impaired patients remain depressed, but by 1–2 years after stroke other factors besides ADLs may play a more prominent role in the mechanism of depression.

A few studies could not demonstrate a significant association between depression and deficits in ADLs. Morris et al (1992) assessed a consecutive series of 88 patients undergoing rehabilitation at 2–3 months following stroke. They found a weak and non-significant correlation between depression and impairments in ADLs as measured with the Barthel index. In a study of 80 stroke patients, Åstrom et al (1993) found no significant correlation between depression and disability scores during the acute stroke period and at 1, 2, and 3 years follow-up.

Several studies examined those factors associated with the long-term prognosis of ADLs in stroke. In their longitudinal study, Robinson et al (1987) examined in-hospital factors related to outcome at 3 and 6 months follow-up. They found a significant correlation between in-hospital measures of depression and deficits in ADLs both at 3 and 6 months follow-up, suggesting that the most depressed patients remained the most impaired in ADLs at follow-up. They also found a significant correlation between in-hospital deficits in ADLs and depression scores both at 3 and 6 months follow-up, suggesting that the most physically impaired patients remained the most depressed at follow-up.

Factors demonstrated to influence recovery from deficits in ADLs include baseline neurological deficits, early intervention, type of infarct, and use of physiotherapy (Robinson, 1998). Kotilla et al (1984) reported the presence of depression during the acute stroke period to be a significant predictor of poor outcome at 3 and 12 months after stroke. Sinyor et al (1986) reported that stroke patients with depression were significantly more impaired than non-depressed stroke patients both during the acute stroke period and 6 weeks after stroke. Parikh et al (1990) compared the longitudinal evolution of 25 depressed and 38 non-depressed stroke patients with comparable in-hospital impairment in ADLs. At 2 years follow-up, patients with in-hospital depression had significantly more severe impairments than patients without in-hospital depression, and this finding was true for patients with either major or minor depression. On the other hand, the correlation between in-hospital ADLs and depression scores 2 years later was not significant, demonstrating that the most severely impaired patients at the time of the acute stroke were not the most severely depressed patients at the 2 year follow-up.

Morris et al (1992) examined the association between depression and deficits in ADLs in a 15-month follow-up study that included 49 patients with an acute stroke lesion. Using the Karnofsky Scale and the Barthel Index as the main outcome measures, they found a significantly smaller recovery on overall functioning and physical disability, respectively, among stroke patients with in-hospital depression as compared to those without depression.

Herrmann et al (1998) assessed the effects of depressive symptoms on stroke recovery in a series of 136 patients. The main finding was that depressive symptoms correlated with functional outcome and handicap at both 3 months and 1 year after stroke. On the other hand, there were no significant correlations between severity of depression and age, lesion volume, and handicap.

Based on the finding that patients with either major or minor depression have a similar decrease in the magnitude of physical recovery as compared to non-depressed patients, Robinson (1998) suggested that the reduced physical recovery in depressed stroke patients may be mediated by psychological mechanisms. Thus, lack of energy and motivation to participate in rehabilitation activities, hopelessness about the future, and difficulties with concentration could result in less physical recovery. Another possibility is that the reduced physical recovery results from the persistence of depression, but Robinson et al (1987) found no association between the magnitude of recovery in ADLs and the severity of depression at follow-up.

To examine whether the persistence of depression over time may impair the recovery in ADLs among stroke patients, Chemerinski et al (2001) examined differences on recovery of ADLs between post-stroke depressed patients with remission of their depression ($N=21$), as compared to post-stroke depressed patients without mood recovery over the first 3–6 months after stroke. Whereas there were no significant between-group differences in demographic variables, lesion characteristics, and neurological symptoms, those patients who improved mood at follow-up had significantly greater recovery in ADLs at follow-up than patients without mood improvement. Interestingly, patients with either major or minor depression with mood improvement at follow-up had a similar amount of recovery in ADLs. Based on this finding the authors suggested that the poor recovery of ADLs in post-stroke depressed patients may be related to less motivation to engage in rehabilitation treatments, leading to slow recovery. On the other hand, Kimura et al (2000) reported that among patients who responded to treatment of post-stroke depression, recovery in cognitive functions was significantly greater among those with major as compared to those with minor depression, suggesting that cognitive recovery may be mediated by the mechanism of major, but not minor, depression.

The question now arising is whether the early treatment of post-stroke depression could decrease the influence of depression on recovery in ADLs. Reding et al (1986) demonstrated that stroke patients treated with the antidepressant trazodone showed greater improvement in ADLs as compared to patients treated with placebo. One limitation of this study was that depressed patients had a similar improvement while on trazodone as non-depressed patients. Gonzalez-Torrecillas et al (1995) compared 11 post-stroke depressed patients treated with nortriptyline, 26 depressed patients treated with fluoxetine, and 11 post-stroke depressed patients treated with placebo. After a 6-week treatment period, patients on either nortriptyline or fluoxetine had a significantly greater improvement on ADLs as compared to patients on placebo.

In a recent study, Gainotti et al (2001) examined the influence of post-stroke depression and antidepressant therapy on the improvement of motor scores and disability. A group of 49 patients with depression after stroke who received antidepressant treatment (N=24) or no treatment (N=25) were compared with 15 non-depressed stroke patients. Twenty-three of the 24 patients received fluoxetine monotherapy with dosages ranging from 20 to 40 mg/day. Main outcome measures were the Barthel Index, the Canadian Neurological Scale, and the Rivermead Mobility Index. There was a significant time x group interaction; the physical recovery of non-treated depressed patients was significantly lower than in non-depressed and depressed but treated stroke patients.

Palomäki et al (1999) examined whether post-stroke depression could be prevented with the use of the antidepressant mianserin. They carried out a study that included 100 consecutive patients admitted to hospital for an acute ischaemic stroke, who were randomized to receive 60 mg/day mianserin or placebo for 1 year. The main finding was that active treatment and placebo groups did not show significant differences in the frequency of depression at any time point during the 1 year follow-up period. There also were no significant between-group differences on both neurological status and functional outcomes, but the study may have been underpowered to detect true treatment differences given the low prevalence of post-stroke depression in this sample.

In conclusion, several studies demonstrated a significant albeit mild correlation between (more severe) depression, and more severe impairments in ADLs during the acute stage after stroke. On the other hand, post-stroke depression has been shown to be a significant predictor of worse recovery in ADLs. There is preliminary evidence that treatment of post-stroke depression with antidepressant medication may improve long-term recovery in ADLs.

Quality of life (QOL) and depression after stroke

QOL is one of the main outcome measures for medical disorders and their treatments, but few studies have examined the association between depression and QOL among stroke individuals. Kauhanen et al (2000) examined relevant QOL domains such as physical, social and role functioning, mental health, vitality, bodily pain, and general health. The authors identified depression as the most important correlate of impaired QOL.

Carod-Artal et al (2000) examined overall and domain-specific QOL in a cohort of 118 stroke patients 1 year after the cerebrovascular lesion. The main finding was that functional status and depression at the in-hospital evaluation were identified as significant predictors of QOL 1 year after stroke.

In a recent study, Bosworth et al (2000) examined long-term patient health status in a series of 1073 individuals with an acute stroke lesion. Twelve months after the acute event the authors found that living alone, being institutionalized, decreased physical function, and depression were independently associated with lower levels of patient health status. After adjusting for physical functioning, stroke patients with significant depressive symptoms reported lower health status, which persisted over time.

Depression and mortality after stroke

The presence of primary (i.e. no known brain injury) depression has been consistently associated with a higher mortality and this association was reported to be stronger among elderly patients with physical illness. Several studies examined this association in stroke patients.

Morris et al (1993a) carried out a 10-year follow-up study of a series of 103 patients with an acute stroke lesion. At 10 years follow-up those patients with in-hospital depression had a three-fold higher mortality as compared to non-depressed patients (odds ratio= 3.4; 95 CI= 1.4–4.8, $P<0.01$). A difference in the probability of survival between the depressed and non-depressed patients was evident as early as the first year after stroke, and continued during the first 5 years before the curves began to parallel each other. These findings remained significant after a multiple logistical regression which included measurements of social ties, general cognition, medical co-morbidity, marital status, age, gender, social class, impairment in ADLs and social functioning. Lesion volume was the CT variable most strongly associated with increased mortality: patients who died after the 10-year follow-up period had over twice the lesion volume as compared with patients who survived. However, the association between depression and a higher mortality remained significant after lesion volume was partialled out.

Morris et al (1993b) examined mortality rates among 99 patients with a stroke lesion that were admitted to a rehabilitation hospital. Fifteen months after the initial psychiatric evaluation, the mortality rate was 23% among patients with an initial diagnosis of major depression, 10% among those with minor depression, and 2% among non-depressed patients. Combining patients with major and minor depression, depressed patients had a seven-fold higher mortality rate than non-depressed patients.

A 12-month follow-up study Burvill et al (1995) reported a mortality of 7% among depressed stroke patients, 12% among stroke patients with an anxiety disorder, and 3% among those with no psychiatric disorder.

House et al (2001) examined whether mood symptoms at 1 month after stroke may be a risk factor for mortality at 12 and 24 months in a study that included a consecutive series of 448 acute stroke patients. Their main finding was that symptoms of depression during the first month after stroke were significantly associated with 12- and 24-months mortality after adjustment for age, cognitive impairment, urinary incontinence, and level of physical disability after stroke. They suggested that general psychological distress or negative thoughts may be the psychological factors most strongly associated with mortality after stroke.

The only negative study was reported by Ästrom et al (1993) in a 3-year follow-up study that included 21 patients. They reported that older age, disorientation, impairments in ADLs, and more severe cortical atrophy were significantly related to a higher mortality during the follow-up period. On the other hand, no significant association was found between post-stroke depression and a higher mortality.

In conclusion, several studies reported a strong association between depression and a relatively higher post-stroke mortality. Whereas the underlying mechanism of this association is unknown, the higher mortality among depressed patients may be related to a return to detrimental habits and non-compliance with treatment recommendations. Primary depression was reported to be related to autonomic changes, cardiac arrythmias, and enhanced plattelet aggregation may also be associated with the higher mortality reported in depressed stroke patients (Musselman et al, 1998).

Aphasia and depression after stroke

Benson (1979) suggested that depression after stroke could represent a psychological reaction to the loss of language function, and Gainotti (1972) suggested that aphasic patients may show a high frequency of the so-called 'depressive-catastrophic reaction'. The main limitation to the study of depression in aphasics is how to assess emotional changes among individuals with severe comprehension deficits, given that a psychiatric evaluation requires a verbal report with the patient. Ross et al (1986) suggested that specific behavioural signs (e.g. decreased sleep, decreased food intake) could be used to diagnose depression in aphasic patients, and Gainotti et al (1997) designed the Post-Stroke Depression Rating Scale which rates a variety of non-verbal behaviours, such as apathy, loss of interest, anhedonia, and diurnal mood variations. However, the validity of these criteria to diagnose depression in stroke patients has not been demonstrated. Other studies examined the usefulness of biological 'markers' of primary depression to diagnose depression in neurological disease, such as the dexamethasone suppression test and the growth hormone response to desipramine, but none of these screening tests showed adequate sensitivity or specificity (Robinson, 1998).

In their initial studies, Robinson et al (1983) required patients to score within 10 points following readministration of the Zung Depression Scale before attempting a structured psychiatric interview. In later studies they required their patients to perform part of the Token Test without error (this test examines the patient's ability to comprehend and follow verbal instructions of increasing complexity). This strategy excludes patients with moderate or severe comprehension deficits from a reliable psychiatric interview, and studies are needed to design alternative assessment strategies for patients in whom verbal interviews are not feasible.

In their initial study of 103 patients with acute stroke lesions, Robinson et al (1983) found a similar frequency of depression among aphasic as compared to non-aphasic individuals. When aphasic patients were divided into those with non-fluent (N=7), fluent (N=8), or mild global aphasia (N=9), those with non-fluent aphasia had a significantly greater severity of depression than fluent or global aphasic patients.

To examine the influence of lesion location upon the association between depression and aphasia, Starkstein and Robinson (1988) divided aphasic patients into types of aphasia based on findings on the Western Aphasia Battery. The main finding was a significant association between depression and left anterior hemisphere brain injury, regardless of the type of aphasia. Based on these findings, Starkstein and Robinson (1988) suggested that the strong association between Broca´s aphasia and post-stroke depression may result from lesions in similar locations.

Herrmann et al (1993) examined the frequency of depression in aphasic patients with either acute (N=21) or chronic (N=21) single stroke lesions of the left hemisphere. Among patients within the acute post-stroke period, those with a non-fluent aphasia had a significantly higher frequency of depression as compared to patients with fluent aphasia. On the other hand, this association between depression and type of aphasia was not found among patients within the chronic post-stroke stage. There also was a significant correlation between distance of the lesion to the frontal pole and depression scores (i.e. the closer the lesion to the frontal pole, the more severe the depression). These findings suggest that lesion location may be more relevant than type of aphasia to explain the association between post-stroke depression and aphasia. Similar findings were reported by Åstrom et al (1993) who found a significantly higher frequency of depression among aphasic patients within the first 3 months after the acute stroke lesion but not at 1, 2, or 3 year follow-ups. Damecour and Caplan's (1991) study was the only study not to find a significant association between type of aphasia and depression both at the acute and the chronic stages.

In conclusion, aphasic patients show a high frequency of depression. This association was reported to be significantly higher for patients with non-fluent aphasia as compared to those with fluent aphasia and may be related to both depression and non-fluent aphasia involving similar left frontal regions. Robinson (1998) reported that patients who were depressed immediately after stroke had significantly less recovery in language functions as compared to acute stroke patients without depression, suggesting that post-stroke depression may impact on the patient's recovery from aphasia.

Post-stroke depression and cognitive impairment

Robinson and co-workers reported a significant correlation between the severity of cognitive impairment [as measured with the Mini-Mental State Exam (MMSE)] and the severity of depression, as measured with specific depression scales (i.e. more severe depression was significantly correlated with more severe cognitive deficits) (Robinson, 1998). Moreover, patients with major depression had significantly lower MMSE scores as compared to patients with minor depression and those without depression (Robinson, 1998). Downhill and Robinson (1994) reported the frequency of cognitive impairment (as defined by a MMSE score < 23) to be 70% among patients with major depression, 43% among those with minor depression, and 43% among those without depression ($P < 0.01$). When stroke patients ($N = 276$) were divided into sub-groups based on the presence of depression and side of injury (i.e. right vs left hemisphere lesion), and MMSE scores were entered as the dependent variable, an ANOVA showed a significant effect for depression (i.e. depressed patients had significantly lower MMSE scores as compared to non-depressed patients), and a significant depression × hemisphere interaction, which resulted from patients with depression and left hemisphere lesions showing significantly lower MMSE scores as compared to the other sub-groups.

House et al (1990) reported that patients with major depression ($N = 10$) or any other DSM-III axis-I diagnosis ($N = 27$) had significantly lower MMSE scores than patients with no axis-I disorder. They also reported a significant inverse correlation between depression scores and cognitive deficits (i.e. higher depression scores were significantly related to lower MMSE scores), and this correlation was strongest among patients with left hemisphere lesions. In a study that included patients at 2-3 months following acute stroke, Morris et al (1990) reported a significant association between major depression and relatively lower MMSE scores.

Few studies examined the longitudinal course of cognitive deficits and depression among stroke patients. In a study that included a series of 140 stroke patients with at least one follow-up evaluation during the first 2 years post-stroke, Downhill and Robinson (1994) found significantly lower MMSE scores for major-depressed as compared to non-depressed individuals at the in-hospital evaluation and at both the 3 and 6 month follow-ups. Depressed patients with a left hemisphere lesion had significantly more severe cognitive impairments than non-depressed patients or depressed patients with right hemisphere lesions at the initial evaluation and at 3 and 6 months follow-up. The depressed and cognitively impaired patients were significantly more likely to remain depressed than the depressed patients without cognitive impairment, suggesting that major depression associated with cognitive dysfunction has a longer duration than that which is not associated with cognitive dysfunction. They also found that stroke patients with cognitive deficits were no more likely to develop depression during the follow-up period than stroke patients without cognitive impairment.

Murata et al (2000) assessed a consecutive series of patients with (N=41) or without major depression (N=135) who were evaluated for cognitive functioning during acute hospitalization and both 3 and 6 months later. The main finding was that patients with major depression whose mood improved at follow-up had significantly greater recovery in cognitive functioning than patients whose mood did not improve. Moreover, they also found that patients whose cognitive function improved at follow-up had significantly greater mood improvement than patients whose cognitive function did not improve, suggesting that post-stroke major depression may lead to cognitive impairment.

The association between depression and relatively lower MMSE scores could be related to lesion variables, such as larger lesion volumes or different lesion location. This issue was examined by Starkstein et al (1998) who matched depressed and non-depressed patients for lesion location and lesion volume. Of the 13 pairs of patients thus matched, 10 depressed patients had lower MMSE scores than their respective lesion-matched non-depressed control, two pairs had the same score, and only one depressed patient had a higher MMSE score as compared to the control individual These findings demonstrate that the presence of depression is related to cognitive impairment regardless of lesion characteristics.

Since the MMSE is heavily-dependent on language functions, which are primarily mediated by the left hemisphere, the above findings could be explained by an independent association between post-stroke depression and MMSE deficits with a relatively higher frequency of left hemisphere lesions. This issue was examined by Bolla-Wilson and co-workers (1989) in a study that used a comprehensive neuropsychological battery that included tests of orientation, language, remote memory, verbal memory, visual memory, recognition memory, visuoperception/visuoconstruction, executive motor functions, and 'frontal lobe' functions. Patients were divided into subgroups based on the presence of depression and side of lesion, and all four groups were comparable in terms of background variables, neurological deficits, and lesion volume. The summed Z scores for the neuropsychocological tasks showed a significantly greater cognitive impairment among those with left hemisphere lesions and depression as compared to those with left hemisphere lesions and no depression ($P<0.01$), or those with right hemisphere lesions with or without depression ($P<0.01$). On individual test analysis, patients with left hemisphere lesions and major depression were significantly more impaired on tasks assessing orientation, language, visuoperception and visuoconstruction, executive motor functions, and frontal lobe functions as compared to patients with left hemisphere lesions but no depression. On the other hand, no significant differences were found on any of the cognitive tasks between patients with right hemisphere lesions with or without depression. These findings suggest that left hemisphere lesions may produce both depression and deficits in cognitive functions related to both hemispheres. It is important to note that the profile of cognitive deficits associated with depression and left hemisphere lesions was similar to the profile of cognitive deficits reported among elderly individuals with 'primary' (i.e. no known brain injury) depression.

Kauhanen et al (1999) examined the neuropsychological correlates of post-stroke depression in a consecutive series of 106 patients with an acute first-ever ischaemic stroke. They found a significant association between more severe depression and more severe cognitive impairments. This association was strongest on tests of memory, non-verbal problem solving, and attention and psychomotor speed.

Most double-blind treatment trials of depression after stroke could not demonstrate a significant improvement in cognitive function among depressed stroke patients on active treatment. Based on those findings, Andersen et al (1996) suggested that the cognitive deficits could account for the presence of depression in stroke victims. However, Murata et al (2000) demonstrated that depressed patients whose mood spontaneously improved over the first 3 months after stroke showed a significantly greater improvement in cognitive function than depressed stroke patients whose mood did not improve. Moreover, depressed patients with spontaneous improvement in cognitive function showed an associated mood improvement. In a recent study, Kimura et al (2000) examined the response of cognitive function to treatment with nor- triptyline or placebo in a double-blind trial which included 33 patients with major and 14 patients with minor depression after an acute stroke lesion. The main finding was that patients whose post-stroke depression remitted (mostly after nortriptyline treatment) had significantly greater recovery on cognitive functions (as measured with the MMSE) as compared to stroke patients whose mood disorder did not remit (most of them on placebo treatment). Another interesting finding was that patients who responded to treatment who were on placebo showed the same cognitive impairment as patients taking nortriptyline; suggesting that the mechanism of depression, but not the mech- anism of notriptyline, was responsible for the cognitive improvement.

In conclusion, several studies reported a significant association between major depression and cognitive deficits among stroke patients. This associ- ation is mostly observed among patients with left but not right hemisphere lesions, and may persist for up to 6 months after the brain lesion. Cognitive deficits are primarily found on tests of orientation, language, remote memory, verbal memory, visual memory, recognition memory, visuoperception / visuo- construction, executive motor functions, and frontal-lobe related functions. Patients with remission of depression may show a significantly greater cog- nitive improvement as compared to patients without mood improvement.

Ischaemic risk factors and depression

Few studies examined the role of cerebrovascular pathology associated with carotid stenosis and peripheral vascular disease in the mechanism of depression in older people. Rao et al (2001) examined patients with either first anterior circulation stroke, carotid stenosis accompanied by transient ischaemic attack, peripheral vascular disease, and a non-vascular aged control group. One of the main findings of the study was that patients with either stroke or carotid stenosis had higher depression scores than the control group. Based on these findings the authors suggested a possible role for carotid stenosis in the pathogenesis of depressive disorder in older people.

Lyness et al (2000) examined whether cerebrovascular risk factors and depression were independently associated at 1-year follow-up in a consecutive series of 247 patients aged 60 years or older. They found that a cumulative severity of cerebrovascular risk factors was associated with the presence of depression at 1-year follow-up. Stewart et al (2001) examined the association between stroke, vascular risk factors and depression in a community-based Caribbean-born population of aged individuals. They found that a history of stroke was strongly associated with the presence of depression, and this association was independent of the severity of disablement. On the other hand, vascular risk factors were not associated with depression.

Ohira et al (2001) examined the relationship between depressive symptoms and the risk of stroke in a sample of 901 individuals during a 10-year follow-up period. The main finding was that age- and sex-adjusted prevalence of mild depression (as measured with the Zung Self-Rating Depression Scale) was 25% among subjects with incident stroke, and 12% among subjects without stroke. Similar findings were reported by Simons et al (1998) who found that elderly individuals with depressive symptoms in the high tertile as measured with the CES-D had 41% higher risk for ischaemic stroke than those in the low tertile. The mechanism for this association remains unknown, but recent studies reported a significant association between depressive symptoms and increased platelet activity due to sympathoadrenal hyperactivity, higher mean plasma levels of platelet factor 4 and beta-thromboglobulin, and increased platelet 5-hydroxytryptamine binding density (Musselman et al, 1998).

Fujikawa et al (1994) reported a high frequency of silent cerebral infarction among individuals with senile-onset major depression, and suggested that major depression with silent cerebral infarction may be a warning sign of cerebrovascular disease. Alexopoulos et al (1997) and Krishnan et al (1997) reported that a substantial proportion of individuals with late-onset depression had significant vascular disease, which may have predisposed or triggered the affective disorder. Depression was reported to increase after a myocardial infarction, and hypertension was reported to be associated with a three-fold increase in the frequency of major depression (Musselman et al, 1998). In a recent study, Thomas et al (2001) examined whether late-life depression was associated with atheromatous changes in brain vessels in post-mortem tissue from 20 individuals with a history of major depression, and 20 individuals without a history of psychiatric disorders. They found a significant increase in atheromatous disease in the depressed group, and suggested that altheromatous disease may predispose or perpetuate depression in elderly individuals.

In conclusion, cerebrovascular pathology is demonstrated to be significantly related to the presence of depressive symptoms in elderly individuals. Whether silent ischaemic brain lesions, ischaemic white matter degeneration, or other factors related to vascular pathology explain the association with depressed mood in the elderly remains to be determined.

General conclusion

Several studies demonstrate a significant association between post-stroke depression and impairments in ADLs. Depression is associated with a worse long-term recovery in ADLs, poorer QOL, and higher long-term mortality. Pharmacological treatment with antidepressants is demonstrated to improve recovery in ADLs among patients with a depressive syndrome, but may not influence recovery in non-depressed stroke patients, suggesting an aetiological role for depression in the mechanism of ADL recovery. Depression after stroke was also related to relatively worse cognitive impairments, and less recovery from cognitive deficits over time. Primary depression in elderly individuals is significantly associated with carotid pathology and 'silent' brain infarctions, suggesting an important role for cerebrovascular pathology in the mechanism of depression among the elderly.

References

Alexopoulos GS, Meyers BS, Young RC et al, Vascular depression hypothesis, *Arch Gen Psychiatry* (1997) **54**:915–22.

Andersen G, Vestergaard K, Riis JO, Ingeman-Nielsen M, Dementia of depression or depression of dementia in stroke?, *Acta Psychiatr Scand* (1996) **94**:272–8.

Åstrom M, Adolfsson R, Asplund K, Major depression in stroke patients: a 3-year longitudinal study, *Stroke* (1993) **24**:976–82.

Benson DF, *Aphasia, Alexia, and Agraphia* (New York: Churchill Livingstone, 1979).

Bolla-Wilson K, Robinson RG, Starkstein SE, Boston JD, Price TR, Lateralization of dementia of depression in stroke patients, *Am J Psychiatry* (1989) **146**:627–34.

Bosworth HB, Horner RD, Edwards LJ, Matchar DB, Depression and other determinants of values placed on current health state by stroke patients: evidence from the VA Acute Stroke (VASt) study, *Stroke* (2000) **31**:2603–9.

Burvill PW, Johnson GA, Jamrozik KD et al, Prevalence of depression after stroke: the Perth community stroke study, *Br J Psychiatry* (1995) **166**: 320–27.

Carod-Artal J, Egido JA, Gonzalez JL, Varela de Seijas E, Quality of life among stroke survivors evaluated one year after stroke: experience of a stroke unit, *Stroke* (2000) **31**: 2995–3000.

Chemerinski E, Robinson R, Kosier JT, Improved recovery in activities of daily living associated with remission of post-stroke depression, *Stroke* (2001) **32**:113–7.

Damecour CL, Caplan D, The relationship of depression to symptomatology and lesion site in aphasic patients, *Cortex* (1991) **27**:385–401.

Downhill JE, Robinson RG, Longitudinal assessment of depression and cognitive impairment following stroke, *J Nervous Ment Dis* (1994) **182**:425–31.

Eastwood MR, Rifat SL, Nobbs H, Ruderman J, Mood disorder following cerebrovascular accident, *Br J Psychiatry* (1989) **154**:195–200.

Fujikawa T, Yamawaki S, Touhouda Y, Background factors and clinical symptoms of major depression with silent cerebral infarction, *Stroke* (1994) **25**:798–801.

Gainotti G, Emotional behavior and hemispheric side of the brain, *Cortex* (1972) **8**:41–55.

Gainotti G, Azzoni A, Razzano C et al, The Post-Stroke Rating Depression Scale: a test devised to investigate affective disorders of stroke patients, *J Clin Exp Neuropsychol* (1997) **19**:340–56.

Gainotti G, Antonucci G, Marra C, Paolucci S, Relation between depression after stroke, antidepressant therapy, and functional recovery, *J Neurol Neurosurg Psychiatry* (2001) **71**:258–61.

Gonzalez-Torrecillas JL, Hidebrand J, Mdelwicz J, Lobo A, Effects of early treatment of post-stroke depression on neuropsychological rehabilitation, *Int Psychogeriatr* (1995) **78**:547–60.

Herrmann N, Black SE, Lawrence J, Szekely C, Szalai JP, The Sunnybrook Stroke Study: a prospective study of depressive symptoms and functional outcome, *Stroke* (1998) **29**:618–24.

House A, Dennis M, Warlow C, Hawton K, Molyneux A, The relationship between intellectual impairment and mood disorder in the first year after stroke, *Psychol Med* (1990) **20**:805–14.

House A, Knapp P, Bamford J, Vail A, Mortality at 12 and 24 months after stroke may be associated with depressive symptoms at one month, *Stroke* (2001) **32**:696–701.

Kauhanen ML, Korpelainen J, Hiltunen P et al, Poststroke depression correlates with cognitive impairment and neurological deficits, *Stroke* (1999) **30**:1875–80.

Kauhanen ML, Korpelainen JT, Hiltunen P et al, Domains and determinants of quality of life after stroke caused by brain infarction, *Arch Phys Med Rehab* (2000) **81**:1541–6.

Kimura M, Robinson RG, Kosier JT, Treatment of cognitive impairment after poststroke depression. A double-blind treatment trial, *Stroke* (2000) **31**:1482–6.

Kotila M, Waltimo O, Niemim L, Laaksonen R, Lempinen M, The profile of recovery from stroke in factors influencing outcome, *Stroke* (1984) **15**:1039–44.

Krishnan KR, Hays JC, Blazer DG, MRI-defined vascular depression, *Am J Psychiatry* (1997) **154**:497–501.

Lyness JM, King DA, Conwell Y, Cox C, Caine ED, Cerebrovascular risk factors and 1-year depression outcome in older primary care patients, *Am J Psychiatry* (2000) **157**:1499–501.

Morris PLP, Robinson RG, Raphael B, Prevalence and course of depressive disorders in hospitalized stroke patients, *Int J Psychiatry Med* (1990) **20**:349–64.

Morris PL, Robinson RG, Samuels J, Depression, introversion and mortality following stroke, *Aust NZ J Psychiatry* (1993a) **24**:443–9.

Morris PL, Robinson RG, Andrzejewski P, Samuels J, Price TR, Association of depression with 10-year poststroke mortality, *Am J Psychiatry* (1993b) **150**:124–9.

Morris PLP, Raphael B, Robinson RG, Clinical depression impairs recovery from stroke, *Med J Aust* (1992) **157**:239–42.

Murata Y, Kimura M, Robinson RG, Does cognitive impairment cause post-stroke depression? *Am J Psychiatry* (2000) **8**:310–7.

Musselman DL, Evans DL, Nemeroff CB, The relationship of depression to cardiovascular disease. Epidemiology, biology, and treatment, *Arch Gen Psychiatry* (1998) **55**:580–92.

Ohira T, Iso H, Satoh T et al, Prospective study of depressive symptoms and risk of stroke among Japanese, *Stroke* (2001) **32**:302–8.

Palomäki H, Kaste M, Berg A et al, Prevention of poststroke depression: 1 year randomized placebo controlled double blind trial of mianserin with 6 month follow up after therapy, *J Neurol, Neurosurg Psychiatry* (1999) **66**:490–4.

Parikh RM, Robinson RG, Lipsey JR et al, The impact of post-stroke depression on recovery in activities of daily over two year follow-up, *Arch Neurol* (1990) **47**:785–9.

Rao R, Jackson S, Howard R, Depression in older people with mild stroke, carotid stenosis and peripheral vascular disease: a comparison with healthy controls, *Int J Geriatr Psychiatry* (2001) **16**:175–83.

Reding MJ, Orto LA, Winter SW, et al, Antidepressant therapy after stroke: a double-blind trial, *Arch Neurol* (1986) **43**:763–5.

Robinson RG, *The Clinical Neuropsychiatry of Stroke* (Cambridge University Press, Cambridge, 1998).

Robinson RG, Starr LB, Kubos KL, Price TR, A two year longitudinal study of post-stroke mood disorders: findings during the initial evaluation, *Stroke* (1983) **14**:736–44.

Robinson RG, Bolduc PL, Price TR, Two-year longitudinal study of post-stroke mood disorders: diagnosis and outcome at one and two years, *Stroke* (1987) **18**:837–43.

Ross ED, Gordon WA, Hibbard M, Egelko S, The dexamethasone suppression test, poststroke depression, and the validity of DSM-III based diagnostic criteria, *Am J Psychiatry* (1986) **143**:1200–1.

Schwartz JA, Speed NM, Brunberg JA et al, Depression in stroke rehabilitation, *Biol Psychiatry* (1993) **33**:694–9.

Simons LA, McCallum J, Friedlander Y, Simons J, Risk factors for ischemic stroke: Dubbo study of elderly, *Stroke* (1998) **29**:1341–6.

Sinyor D, Amato P, Kaloupek P, Post-stroke depression: relationship to functional impairment, coping strategies, and rehabilitation outcome, *Stroke* (1986) **17**:112–7.

Starkstein SE, Robinson R, Aphasia and depression, *Aphasiology* (1988) **2**:1–20.

Starkstein SE, Robinson RG, Price TR. Comparison of patients with and without post-stroke major depression matched for size and location of lesion, *Arch Gen Psychiatry* (1998) **45**:247–52.

Stewart R, Prince M, Mann A, Richards M, Brayne C, Stroke, vascular risk factors and depression: Cross-sectional study in a UK Caribbean-born population, *Br J Psychiatry* (2001) **178**:23–8.

Thomas AJ, Ferrier IN, Kalaria RN et al, A neuropathological study of vascular factors in late-life depression, *J Neurol Neurosurg Psychiatry* (2001) **70**:83–7.

15
Mania and cerebrovascular disease

Kenneth I Shulman

Classification and nosology

Multiple terminologies and classifications have confounded the medical literature related to mania. The diagnostic classification 'bipolar disorder' as defined
in DSM-IV (American Psychiatric Association, 1994) is determined by the presence of a manic or hypomanic episode and is considered a primary mood
disorder whose spectrum is divided into bipolar I, II or III dependent on the
severity of manic symptomatology or the nature of the precipitation of mania
(Akiskal, 1986). Diagnosis of manic syndromes in the elderly is further confounded by the very high levels of comorbidity (Shulman and Singh, 1999). In
this context, it is often assumed that mania is a secondary phenomenon. For
example, DSM-IV has established a category of 'mood disorder due to a general medical condition' (293.83). The underlying assumption is that 'the
disturbance is a direct physiological consequence of a general medical condition'. However, when a condition is a 'direct consequence' rather than simply
a precipitant can be a vexed question. This is especially problematic in an
elderly population with a high prevalence of both medical and neurological
comorbidity (Shulman et al, 1992). A presumption of aetiology is also encom-
passed under the widely used term 'secondary mania' originally defined by
Krauthammer and Klerman (1978). Under this rubric, mania is due to cerebral
organic factors supported by a close temporal relationship between the med-
ical/neurological condition and a manic episode. Other associated conditions
include a trend towards a negative family history or negative personal history.
This is in contradistinction to primary bipolar disorder, which is strongly influenced by genetic (familial) factors (Goodwin and Jamison, 1990).

Finally, the concept of 'disinhibition syndromes', derived largely from the
neurology literature, implies that mania is a function of frontal disinhibition
resulting from a cerebral injury or insult. Disinhibition syndromes can also be
considered to be a precipitated mania associated with an underlying affective predisposition (genetic or acquired). Akiskal (1986) has suggested that
temperament may be one of the manifestations of a mood vulnerability along
the bipolar spectrum. Disinhibition syndromes may be associated with such
a spectrum that becomes manifest only after a specific cerebral injury
(Shulman, 1997), as described below.

The relationship of cerebrovascular disease to mania in old age must be considered in the light of these nosological debates. This chapter will review the literature relevant to this specific association, including the influence of age of onset of mania, neurological comorbidity, neuroimaging, outcome studies and treatment implications. The related concept of vascular mood disorder including mania and depression will also be reviewed. However, as a starting point, the question of classification is appropriate as it cuts to the fundamental understanding of mania. It is only then that one can make sense of the significance of cerebrovascular disease/pathology as found in association with manic syndromes. The greater the precision of our sub-types, the greater will be our capacity to understand the pathogenesis and ultimately the aetiology of these conditions. Moreover, the findings in elderly people, with a strong overlay of medical and neurological comorbidity, may help to shed light on the nature of bipolar disorder in younger people in whom the neuropathology is less obvious.

Age at onset

Age at onset of mania is a potentially important variable that may help to distinguish subtypes of mania and in turn lead to a better understanding of pathogenesis (Young and Klerman, 1992). Can age at onset help to elucidate the nature of cerebrovascular pathology? Elderly bipolar patients report a mean age of onset of mood disorder ranging from age 40 to 47 years and onset of mania from age 51 to 60 (Chen et al, 1998). In an epidemiological study examining the incidence of hospitalization for bipolar disorder in Finland, almost 20% of first admissions for mania occurred after the age of 60 (Rasanan et al, 1998). The late onset of mania in the elderly indirectly implicates cerebral-organic factors (Shulman et al, 1992). This is further highlighted by the long latency (mean 15 years) in the manifestation of mania in those elderly bipolar patients whose first episode was depression (Shulman and Post, 1980).

The cut-off for 'late onset' is generally accepted as approximately age 50 years. This is supported by Wylie et al (1999) who propose that the median age at onset of a mixed-age sample of patients with mania could be used to set the cut-off point between early and late onset. Depending on the definition of an elderly sample, the late onset cut-off may range from late 40s to mid-50s. Cerebrovascular risk factors were found to be present to a greater degree in a group of people with late-onset bipolar disorder (49 years cut-off) as compared with an early-onset group; 70% of these late-onset elderly bipolar patients had at least one risk factor for cerebrovascular disease compared to 37.5% of early-onset bipolar subjects matched for age and sex (Wylie et al, 1999). Similarly, Hays et al (1998), using a cut-off of 50 years for age at onset, found an increase in vascular comorbidity in a sample of elderly bipolar subjects whose mean age was 74 years. Despite the late age at onset, 83% of this subgroup reported a positive family history; only slightly less than the extremely high prevalence of 88% in early-onset elderly bipolar patients. While genetic factors have been considered less of an influence in late-onset cases, the bipolar group seems to have a strong genetic predisposition even in the face of late age at onset, cerebrovascular pathology and other neurological comorbidity (Shulman et al, 1992). Even in the very late onset group described by Tohen et al (1994), where almost universal neurological comorbidity applied, 30% of their sub-sample had a first degree relative with a mood disorder. This suggests that 'affective vulnerability' is an important predisposition in the multi-factorial nature of bipolarity even into old age when neurobiological forces play a larger role.

Neurological comorbidity

Studies of mania in late life have demonstrated a clear association with a heterogeneous group of neurological disorders (Shulman and Post, 1980; Shulman et al, 1992). However, comprehensive reviews of mixed-age populations with secondary mania also show a mixture of common and exotic systemic/neurological conditions (Strakowski et al, 1994; Verdoux and Bourgeois, 1995). In all age groups, cerebrovascular disease emerges as the most common condition to be associated with mania, with right-sided predominance affecting the orbito-frontal and temporal regions of the brain. Cerebrovascular pathology was especially pronounced in elderly people with very late-onset mania (Tohen et al, 1994).

Whether one focuses on the neurological literature associated with disinhibition syndromes or on the psychiatric literature describing mania, the majority of case reports and case series point to right-sided brain lesions involving a preponderance of cerebrovascular pathology (Jampala and Abrams, 1983; Starkstein et al, 1990; Fawcett, 1991; Cummings, 1993; Shulman and Herrmann, 1999). More specifically, it has been observed that the integrity of the frontal, limbic and basal ganglia circuits are necessary for 'normal mood' (Pearlson, 1999). This functional circuit, known as the orbital frontal circuit (OFC), integrates sensory information with motivational states (Zald and Kim, 1996). This in turn led Starkstein and Robinson (1997) to hypothesize that lesions of the baso-temporal and orbital frontal cortices lead to disinhibition syndromes and secondary mania. Volitional, motivational and psychomotor behaviours are modulated by connections to the frontal lobes; emotional drive and inhibition are modulated by limbic and paralimbic connections; and instinctive behaviours are influenced by the connections to the hypothalamus, amygdala and brain stem nuclei. It is hypothesized that manic syndromes are dependent on localization (right-sided OFC lesions) influenced by an affective predisposition (Robinson et al, 1988; Shulman et al, 1992).

While evidence for localization in mania is based exclusively on individual case reports and case series, Braun et al (1999) systematically pooled the available literature on focal unilateral cortical lesions. They confirmed the observed trend for right-sided lesions to produce mania and left-sided lesions to be associated with depression. Lesions were heterogeneous in nature with about half including cerebrovascular pathology, mainly cerebral infarcts.

Neuroimaging

The neuroimaging research in mania is focused on three main areas: (1) the relevance of subcortical hyperintensities; (2) the finding of silent cerebral infarctions; and (3) cerebral atrophy. Hyperintensities found on (magnetic resonance imaging) MRI are associated with hypertension, atherosclerotic heart disease and diabetes mellitus, thereby strengthening the relationship of mania to cerebrovascular pathology (McDonald et al, 1999). In order to control for age, Woods et al (1995) confirmed the association of hyperintensities with age in a bipolar population but not in a normal control group. The specificity of hyperintensities with bipolarity rather than age alone was recently addressed by McDonald et al (1999) who did not find a correlation of white matter hyperintensities with clinical evidence of cerebrovascular disease. Moreover, late-onset elderly bipolar patients had similar numbers of hyperintensities in deep white matter and subcortical grey nuclei to those found in age-matched early-onset bipolar subjects. Even young bipolar patients had equivalent numbers of hyperintensities, prompting the investigators to hypothesize that the neuroanatomical changes associated with mania as found on MRI are present early in the lifespan. Moore et al (2001) (see below) suggest that these early structural abnormalities in younger bipolar patients may reflect cerebrovascular pathology. Why some people with bipolar disorder do not manifest mania until later in life requires further exploration, especially for those whose first mania occurs after a prolonged latency from their first depression (Shulman et al, 1992).

Japanese investigators have reported evidence of a strong association between cerebrovascular disease, mania and age (Kobayashi et al, 1991; Fujikawa et al, 1995). An age-related increase in silent cerebral infarctions ranges from 6% in middle-aged individuals to over 20% in the elderly (Kobayashi et al, 1991). Clinically silent cerebral infarctions occurred with greatest frequency (65%) in late-onset mania compared to late-onset depression (55%) and early-onset mood disorder (25%) (Fujikawa et al, 1995). Relative to young bipolar subjects, these patients showed a relatively low incidence of family history in first degree relatives consistent with the concept of secondary mania. Not surprisingly, these patients were found to have higher prevalence of cerebrovascular risk factors.

Volumetric studies of bipolar patients show a trend towards global cerebral atrophy, especially in older patients (Steffens and Krishnan, 1998; Young et al, 1999). In a CT study comparing 30 elderly manic patients to age-matched controls, the manic patients showed greater cortical sulcal widening (CSW) and increased ventricle:brain ratios (VBR) (Young et al, 1999). CSW was associated with age at first mania, suggesting a relationship between brain structure and the manifestation of mania.

Outcome and cerebrovascular pathology

In the few long-term outcome studies of late-life bipolar patients, mortality has been high, ranging from 33 to 50% after a mean follow-up of 6 years (Dhingra and Rabins, 1991; Shulman et al, 1992). In a retrospective cohort study, elderly people with mania were found to have a significantly higher level of neurological comorbidity and associated mortality compared to age- and sex-matched individuals with depression (Shulman et al, 1992). In a 1-year follow-up, outcome was relatively poor among elderly manic patients, who suffered from higher prevalence of cognitive dysfunction and cerebrovascular disease (Berrios and Bakshi, 1991). Even in a younger sample of bipolar patients, poor outcome was associated with evidence of deep white matter lesions on MRI (Moore et al, 2001). Cerebrovascular pathology is implicated in these poor prognosis cases as white matter lesions are presumed to be due to perivascular abnormalities and possibly represent areas of microcystic infarcts in more severe cases. The robust finding of relatively poor prognosis of manic syndromes in old age may very well reflect the underlying cerebrovascular pathogenesis.

Defining vascular mood disorders

A subtype of late depression has been proposed based on the assumption that cerebrovascular disease may be associated with the predisposition, precipitation or perpetuation of some depressive syndromes (Krishnan and McDonald, 1995; Alexopoulos et al, 1997a). Cerebrovascular risk factors such as hypertension, coronary artery disease and diabetes are associated with a greater incidence of depression. Moreover, patients suffering from vascular dementia have more mood disturbances than Alzheimer patients (Sulzer et al, 1993). The 'vascular depression' hypothesis rests on a number of associations found in late-onset geriatric depression. Patients with late-onset depression compared to early depressed people show more cognitive dysfunction, and increased cerebral atrophy and deep white matter lesions on neuroimaging (Alexopoulos et al, 1997a). Furthermore, they demonstrate greater functional disability, medical morbidity and mortality, and there is a lower familial predisposition for mood disorders in first degree relatives among those with late-onset depression as compared with early-onset patients. The accumulation of findings points towards a neurobiological basis for these mood disorders, and cerebrovascular disease appears as the predominant condition constituting this neurobiological basis.

Depression has been associated with stroke (Robinson et al, 1998), silent cerebral infarcts (Fujikawa et al, 1995) and white matter hyperintensities (McDonald et al, 1999), all of which are considered to reflect vascular pathology. Lesion location in depression tends towards the left hemisphere involving the left head of caudate and left frontal pole (Alexopoulos et al, 1997a). The vascular depression hypothesis suggests that exceeding a threshold of vascular lesions disrupts prefrontal systems and their modulating pathways, which include the striatum and thalamus as well as cortical connections.

In comparing a group of elderly depressed people with clinically defined vascular disease (using the Cumulative Illness Rating Scale) to a group with depression but without vascular disease, a distinct symptom complex emerges (Alexopoulos et al, 1997b). Individuals with vascular depression have more cognitive impairment, including decreased word fluency and naming; more psychomotor retardation; and less guilt or insight. A marked similarity exists to the behavioural and mood abnormalities of vascular dementia.

This hypothesis and recent clinical findings led Steffens and Krishnan (1998) to propose criteria for a vascular subtype of mania similar to that proposed for vascular depression (Table 15.1). Longer-term follow-up studies are necessary, however, to ensure that this diagnostic category remains

Table 15.1   Proposed criteria for vascular mania subtype specifier.

Specify vascular subtype (can be applied to the current or most recent manic episode in bipolar disorder) if A and either B1 or B2 or B3:

A.   Mania occurring in the context of clinical and/or neuroimaging evidence of cerebrovascular disease or neuropsychological impairment.

B1.   Clinical manifestations may include history of stroke or transient ischaemic attacks, or focal neurological signs or symptoms (e.g. exaggeration of deep tendon reflexes, extensor plantar response, pseudobulbar palsy, gait disturbance, weakness of an extremity).

B2.   Neuroimaging findings may include white or grey matter hyperintensities (Fazekas et al, 1988 criteria >2; or lesion >5 mm in diameter and irregular in shape), confluent white matter lesions, or cortical or subcortical infarcts.

B3.   Cognitive impairment manifested by disturbance of executive function (e.g. planning, organizing, sequencing, abstracting), memory, or speed of processing of information.

The diagnosis is supported by the following features:

1)   Mania onset after 50 years of age or change in the course of mood disorder after the onset of vascular disease in patients with onset before 50 years of age.

2)   Lack of family history of mood disorders.

3)   Marked disability in instrumental or self-maintenance activities of daily living.

Reprinted with permission from Steffens and Krishnan (1998).

stable over time; that the homogeneity of prognosis is established; and that morbidity (cognition) and mortality levels are determined in comparison to other subtypes of mania.

Treatment implications of vascular mania

Mood stabilizers such as lithium, divalproex and the atypical neuroleptic olanzapine remain the mainstay of treatment for bipolar disorder (Shulman and Herrmann, 1999). However, the vascular subtype of mania may lend itself to specific therapies that target cerebrovascular disease. Taragano et al (2001) recently tested the hypothesis that calcium channel blockers which have been suggested as treatments for cerebrovascular disease might in turn be useful in treating the symptoms and the recurrence of depression in a subgroup of people with vascular depression. In a controlled double-blind randomized clinical trial in which the calcium channel blocker nimodipine was used as an augmenting agent to standard antidepressant therapy, there was a significant decrease in symptoms of depression and a lower rate of recurrence. If this is true for vascular depression, then a similar approach for the treatment of vascular mania may be a useful research line to pursue.

Case illustration

A 79-year-old married woman was brought into the emergency department by her husband who reported that she had a 1-month history of excessive energy, elevated mood and hypertalkativeness. The patient had packed all of her belongings in the previous week in order to dispose of them as she felt they were 'of no use'. She expressed ideas of poverty and worthlessness.

Her family history revealed that her father had died of suicide in old age and one brother suffered from alcoholism. As to her personal history, she reported a stable early family life and described a mutually gratifying marriage in which she was a homemaker raising two healthy sons. Tragically, her only daughter had died of muscular dystrophy at the age of 16.

Past psychiatric history included two prior suicide attempts in her 40s, yet she had never had any specific treatment for a mood disorder. Medical history revealed evidence of rapid atrial fibrillation and episodic congestive heart failure treated with frusemide, digoxin and coumadin.

Her clinical course included a brief hospitalization during which her mental state settled quickly within 4 days of neuroleptic therapy. A CT scan showed evidence of diffuse microangiopathic disease and a SPECT scan of her brain showed decreased perfusion in the bilateral parietal areas. Follow-up 1 year later revealed that she was euthymic, she had a Mini-Mental State examination score of 29/30 but showed subtle abnormalities of frontal functioning as detected on the clock-drawing test.

Discussion

This brief real-life vignette reflects a number of relevant practical issues related to bipolarity and cerebrovascular disease. The first clinical point is that this patient presented with a mixed affective state, a condition much more common than described in textbooks. Furthermore, typical of bipolar patients, she had an affective predisposition characterized by a positive family history in first degree relatives, including the suicide of her father and alcoholism in her brother. Consistent with the literature, her late-life manic episode was preceded many years earlier by what appeared to be two depressive episodes, which resolved and were followed by a long latency of over 30 years before her manic episode occurred.

Brief medical review and investigations reveal evidence of diffuse vascular disease treated with commonly used agents in the elderly: frusemide, digoxin and coumadin. The history of rapid atrial fibrillation certainly confers a significant risk of emboli and cerebrovascular pathology which was reflected on a CT scan by evidence of microangiopathic disease and on a SPECT scan by decreased perfusion. Cognitive assessment reveals subtle frontal impairment consistent with her neuroimaging pathology and literature suggesting that cognitive dysfunction is a significant aspect of manic episodes, particularly those occurring late in life. The initial diagnosis was considered to be bipolar disorder with secondary mania, but equal consideration could be given to a form of manic delirium given the relatively acute onset and resolution. This differential requires careful consideration given the high neurological comorbidity described in the literature (Weintraub and Lippmann, 2001).

A manic episode in late life warrants assiduous attempts to assess for underlying neurological disease, especially cerebrovascular pathology, and to optimize medical treatment. While attempting to treat the psychiatric symptoms with mood-stabilizing agents, additional vigorous efforts to address vascular disease are warranted. Further research should involve neuroimaging and neuropsychological assessment in prospective outcome studies. By defining subtypes more accurately we can address aetiology and hence treatment more effectively.

References

Akiskal H, The clinical significance of the 'soft' bipolar spectrum, *Psychiatr Ann* (1986) **16**: 667–71.

Alexopoulos GS, Meyers BS, Young RC et al, Vascular depression hypothesis, *Arch Gen Psychiatry* (1997a) **54**: 915–22.

Alexopoulos GS, Meyers BS, Young RC et al, Clinically defined vascular depression, *Am J Psychiatry* (1997b) **154**: 562–5.

American Psychiatric Association, *Diagnostic and Statistical Manual of Mental Disorders, 4th edn (DSM-IV)* (American Psychiatric Association: Washington, DC, 1994).

Berrios GE, Bakshi N, Manic and depressive symptoms in the elderly: their relationships to treatment outcome, cognition and motor symptoms, *Psychopathology* (1991) **24**: 31–8.

Braun CMJ, Larocque C, Daigneault S, Montour-Proulx I, Mania, pseudomania, depression, and pseudo-depression resulting from focal unilateral cortical lesions, *Neuropsych Neuropsychol Behav Neurol* (1999) **12**: 35–51.

Chen ST, Altshuler LL, Spar JE, Bipolar disorder in late life: a review, *J Geriatr Psychiatry Neurol* (1998) **11**: 29–35.

Cummings JL, Frontal-subcortical circuits and human behavior, *Arch Neurol* (1993) **50**: 873–80.

Dhingra U, Rabins PV, Mania in the elderly: a five-to-seven year follow-up, *J Am Geriatr Soc* (1991) **39**: 582–3.

Fawcett RG, Cerebral infarct presenting as mania. *J Clin Psychiatry* (1991) **52**: 352–3.

Fujikawa T, Yamawaki S, Touhouda Y, Silent cerebral infarctions in patients with late-onset mania, *Stroke* (1995) **26**: 946–69.

Goodwin FK, Jamison KR, *Manic-depressive Illness* (Oxford University Press: New York, 1990).

Hays JC, Krishnan KRR, George LK, Blazer DG, Age of first onset of bipolar disorder: demographic, family history, and psychosocial correlates, *Depres Anxiety* (1998) **7**: 76–82.

Jampala VS, Abrams R, Mania secondary to left and right hemisphere damage, *Am J Psychiatry* (1983) **140**: 1197–9.

Kobayashi S, Okada K, Yamashita K, Incidence of silent lacunar lesions in normal adults and its relation to cerebral blood flow and risk factors, *Stroke* (1991) **22**: 1379–83.

Krauthammer C, Klerman GL, Secondary mania: manic syndromes associated with antecedent physical illness or drugs, *Arch Gen Psychiatry* (1978) **35**: 1333–9.

Krishnan KRR, McDonald WM, Arteriosclerotic depression, *Med Hypotheses* (1995) **44**: 111–5.

McDonald WM, Tupler LA, Marsteller FA et al, Hyperintense lesions on magnetic resonance images in bipolar disorder, *Biol Psychiatry* (1999) **45**: 965–71.

Moore PB, Shephered DJ, Eccleston D et al, Cerebral white matter lesions in bipolar affective disorder: relationship to outcome, *Br J Psychiatry* (2001) **178**: 172–6.

Pearlson GD, Structural and functional brain changes in bipolar disorder: a selective review, *Schizophrenia Res* (1999) **39**: 133–40.

Rasanan P, Tiihonen J, Hakko H, The incidence and onset-age of hospitalised bipolar affective disorder in Finland, *J Affect Dis* (1998) **48**: 63–8.

Robinson RG, Boston JD, Starkstein SE, Price TR, Comparison of mania with depression following brain injury: causal factors, *Am J Psychiatry* (1988) **145**: 172–8.

Shulman KI, Disinhibition syndromes, secondary mania and bipolar disorder in old age, *J Affect Dis* (1997) **46**: 175–82.

Shulman KI, Herrmann N, The nature and management of mania in old age, *Psychiatr Clin North Am* (1999) **22(3)**: 649–65.

Shulman K, Post F, Bipolar affective disorder in old age, *Br J Psychiatry* (1980) **136**: 26–32.

Shulman KI, Singh A, Co-morbidity and mania in old age. In: Tohen M, ed, *Co-morbidity and Psychiatric Disorders* (Marcel Dekker, Inc.: New York, 1999) 249–261.

Shulman K, Tohen M, Satlin A, Mallya G, Kalunian D, Mania compared to unipolar depression in old age, *Am J Psychiatry* (1992) **149**: 341–5.

Starkstein SE, Robinson RG, Mechanism of disinhibition after brain lesions, *J Nerv Ment Dis* (1997) **185**: 108–14.

Starkstein SE, Mayberg HS, Berthier ML et al, Mania after brain injury: neuroradiological and metabolic findings, *Ann Neurol* (1990) **27**: 652–9.

Steffens DC, Krishnan KRR, Structural neuroimaging and mood disorders. Recent findings, implications for classification, and future directions, *Biol Psychiatry* (1998) **43**: 705–12.

Strakowski SM, McElroy S, Keck P, West S, The co-occurrence of mania with medical and other psychiatric disorders, *Int J Psychiatry Med* (1994) **24**: 305–28.

Sulzer DL, Levin HS, Mahler ME, High WM, Cummings JL, A comparison of psychiatric symptoms in vascular dementia and Alzheimer's disease, *Am J Psychiatry* (1993) **150**: 1806–12.

Taragano FE, Allegri R, Vicario A, Bagnatti P, Lyketsos CG, A double blind, randomized clinical trial assessing the efficacy and safety of augmenting standard antidepressant therapy with nimodipine in the treatment of 'vascular depression', *Int J Geriatr Psychiatry* (2001) **16**: 254–60.

Tohen M, Shulman KI, Satlin A, First-episode mania in late life, *Am J Psychiatry* (1994) **151**: 130–2.

Verdoux H, Bourgeois M, Manies secondaires a des pathologies organiques cerebrales, *Ann Med Psychology* (1995) **153**: 161–8.

Weintraub D, Lippmann S, Delirious mania in the elderly, *Int J Geriatr Psychiatry* (2001) **16**: 374–7.

Woods BT, Yurgelun-Todd D, Mikulis D, Pillay SS, Age-related MRI abnormalities in bipolar illness: a clinical study, *Biol Psychiatry* (1995) **38**: 846–7.

Wylie ME, Mulsant BH, Pollock BG et al, (1999) Age at onset in geriatric bipolar disorder, *Am J Geriatr Psychiatry* **7**: 77–83.

Young RC, Klerman GL, Mania in late life: focus on age at onset, *Am J Psychiatry* (1992) **149**: 867–76.

Young RC, Nambudiri DE, Jain H, de Asis JM, Alexopoulos GS, Brain computed tomography in geriatric manic disorder, *Biol Psychiatry* (1999) **45**: 1063–5.

Zald D, Kim SW, Anatomy and function of the orbital frontal cortex: I anatomy, neurocircuitry, and obsessive-compulsive disorder, *J Neuropsych Clin Neurosci* (1996) **8**: 125–38.

16
Management of affective disorder in cerebrovascular disease

Robert C Baldwin

Introduction

Co-morbidity, whether from cerebrovascular disease (CVD) or other pathology, does not in principle affect the management of affective disorder. In practice, CVD may influence the expression of depression, its detection and the outcome of treatment. The range of affective disorders includes mania, depression (major depression and dysthymia) and emotionalism ('pathological' laughing or crying). Management should address both assessment and treatment. It should be both collaborative, involving physicians and psychiatrists working together, and multidisciplinary. The aims of treatment are: resolution of depressive symptoms and signs; restoration of functioning; and prevention of relapse and recurrence.

There is evidence that depression may increase CVD morbidity in patients with vascular disease and delay recovery in stroke patients; and that CVD, when present, worsens the prognosis for major depression (Simpson et al, 1998; Ramasubbu, 2000). These findings suggest an interactive relationship. An accurate assessment of both physical and psychiatric domains is therefore essential.

Previous work, discussed elsewhere in this book has linked stroke risk to specific lesion sites within the brain. There are now doubts about this (Carson et al, 2000), so all stroke patients should be regarded as at risk. For pathological crying, the evidence suggests that stroke patients who are depressed are at most risk (Gustafson et al, 1995). Structurally, pathological crying may be associated with several mechanisms such as direct limbic damage or loss of cortical disinhibition to limbic structures (van Gijn, 1993). The important therapeutic question therefore is less the site of the lesion or lesions, but whether or not the patient has a mood disorder.

Unfortunately, there are many more studies of the relationship between depression and stroke than of treatment of depression in stroke (Gustafson et al, 1995). Such research as there is largely concerns antidepressant drug treatment. There is little published information regarding the role of psychological and social treatments despite the obvious devastating effects of diseases such as stroke on these domains.

The focus of this chapter is depression in stroke, but mention will be made of emotionalism and mania, as will reference, where relevant, to other forms of CVD.

Assessment

History

The main elements of assessment are summarized in Table 16.1. There is no substitute for taking a psychiatric history. The structure should cover current symptoms, their onset, duration, and severity, and special features such as diurnal variation; predisposing (vulnerability) factors, precipitants and perpetuating factors; cultural and social background; past personal and family psychiatric details and medical history; drugs taken (including alcohol and over-the-counter preparations); level of support and social circumstances. For example, an important risk factor for depression following stroke is whether the individual has ever had depressive episodes in the past. In cases where the diagnosis is difficult, a positive past history of depression may tip the balance in favour of prescribing antidepressants. A strongly positive family history of depression will also carry some weight. Irrespective of stroke location, adverse life events have been shown to predict depression at 6 months after stroke (Bush, 1999). An added unpleasant event in the life of a person recovering from a stroke may seem at first sight to be of lesser importance, but again it may tip the balance and precipitate a depressive disorder. Another example is alcohol. In the long term, excessive alcohol consumption facilitates atherosclerosis and may therefore be a risk factor for stroke. Depression following stroke may lead to an increase in alcohol consumption and to

Table 16.1   Assessment of affective disorder in cerebrovascular disease.

- Current symptoms – onset, duration, severity, diurnal variation
- Signs noted by others (e.g. tearfulness)
- Behavioural disturbances (positive such as aggression; negative such as withdrawal)
- Risk factors for affective disorder (e.g. family history)
- Cultural and religious factors
- Personal factors – employment, housing, leisure pursuits
- Adverse life events within preceding 6 months (besides stroke)
- Social support
- Medication (including over-the-counter)
- Alcohol history
- Illicit drug use
- Mental state examination
- Overall level of disability

therapeutic resistance to antidepressant treatment. Such obvious areas of enquiry are often overlooked.

Some prescribed drugs may precipitate depressive disorder. Among the many listed in the literature (Baldwin, 2000) are several antihypertensive agents, such as beta blockers, calcium channel blockers and methyldopa. Antihypertensive drugs are more commonly prescribed to patients with stroke because hypertension is a risk factor for stroke. Clearly the potential benefits of withdrawing a suspected drug must be balanced by the risks of destabilizing blood pressure.

Mental state

Cerebrovascular disease, particularly stroke, uniquely hampers the detection of depression because of its effect on language and communication. Performing a mental state examination may be particularly difficult. Yet patients with aphasia may be at increased risk of depression. In a study of over 100 patients with first-ever ischaemic stroke, a third had aphasia acutely, and of these 70% met DSM-III-R criteria for major depression at 3 months and almost 66% at 12 months (Kauhanen et al, 2000). In another study, the use of antidepressants in stroke patients ranged between 17 and 41% depending on whether the patient was aphasic, the latter being associated with the lower rate of treatment (Lim and Ebrahim, 1983).

Depression after stroke is also associated with cognitive impairment (Nieminen et al, 1999). Impaired cognition and other neurobehavioural sequelae of strokes can limit a patient's ability to describe or express emotion, can cause him or her to give 'yes' answers to the clinician who expects them, or may give rise to apathy or uncontrolled crying spells which are then mistaken for depressive disorder. Also, anosognosia for depressive signs can cause the patient to deny depressive signs that are objectively observable. These diagnostic confounders have not been adequately assessed in previous research on post-stroke depression (Black, 1995). For patients unable to answer questions related to cognition the interviewer will have to rely on the observations of others – does the patient show recognition of staff, family or friends? are basic instructions understood? Can the patient choose between two simple alternatives by gesturing yes or no?

Apathy is a frequent accompaniment of stroke and may co-exist with depression or arise separately (Starkstein et al, 1993). Apathy and depression are not the same. Apathy is associated more often with cognitive impairment and older age (Starkstein et al, 1993). There are rating instruments for apathy (e.g. Marin et al, 1991), but in routine clinical practice apathy can usually be distinguished from depression by the history and mental state examination. Thus depression is usually associated with anhedonia (reduced ability to experience pleasure) and apathy with reduced motivation; depression leads to depressive ideation (guilt, hopelessness, worthlessness, suicidal ideation) and apathy to poverty of thought and reduced insight. In severe cases depression is associated with delusions of guilt, hypochondriasis and nihilism, which are not features of apathy. Of course apathy and depressed mood can coexist.

Suicide is a risk in any patient with depressive disorder. Those most at risk are older males who are isolated (Baldwin, 2000). Although physical impairment may reduce the options that a severely depressed patient may have to end his or her own life, this should not lead to complacency – a determined patient will find a way. Embarrassment must not deter asking about self harm. A well-chosen phrase usually helps, e.g. 'Do you ever feel desperate?'; 'Does it ever feel so bad you do not feel like going on?' These 'lead-ins' allow rapport to develop so that the exact state of mind of the person can then be understood via more specific questions.

Given all these factors, an informant history is particularly important in eliciting and/or amplifying some of the factors in Table 16.1.

Other measures

In a study of over 600 patients (268 with stroke) admitted to hospital, measures of marked disability appeared to correlate most strongly with anxiety and depression (Bond et al, 1998). The authors also found that social contact appeared to protect against depression. Overall though, disability appeared a more robust measure of outcome than assessment of mental health alone, highlighting the need to assess the impact of illness in its entirety and not just mental health or physical health alone. There are a number of measures of disability in use. Given the relevance to prognosis, both of the stroke and of the mood disorder, at least one should be routinely performed on stroke patients and ideally repeated at intervals.

All illness causes behaviour and some illnesses lead to abnormal behavioural responses (so-called abnormal illness behaviour, AIB). In stroke it has been suggested that AIB and depression lead to differential effects, with depression leading to social withdrawal and AIB to poorer functional recovery (Clark and Smith, 1998). The nature and extent of all behaviours associated with stroke should therefore be clarified, with excessive or disproportionate behaviours being targeted for behavioural intervention. An example would be difficulty in engaging a stroke patient in self-care activities because of complaints of poor mobility out of keeping with the neurological deficit. Again, there are a number of behavioural techniques available, although some require training.

Screening may help with diagnosis, although most of the scales in use today have not been validated on older stroke patients. An exception is a study by Shinar et al (1986) who found satisfactory performance with the Center for Epidemiologic Studies for Depression (CES-D) scale in non-aphasic stroke patients. No scale is perfect in addressing the problems posed by communication difficulties. The Geriatric Depression Scale (Yesavage et al, 1983) was not validated in stroke patients, although there is no reason to suppose its properties alter in non-aphasic patients. An alternative to questionnaires reliant on the patients' answers is to use an informant rating scale. Given the association of depression, dysphasia and impaired cognition, the Cornell Scale for Depression in Dementia may be useful (Alexopoulos et al, 1988) as it utilizes information from an informant.

Harvey and Black (1996) reviewed the utility of the dexamethasone suppression test as an aid to the diagnosis of post-stroke depression. Reviewing several studies they found a median specificity of 87%, and a median sensitivity of 47%. This makes it unacceptable as a screening test.

Carers

Last, but by no means least, stroke exacts a high price on carers. In one study (Angeleri et al, 1993) partners of stroke patients experienced high levels of dissatisfaction, usually arising from the person with the stroke being irritable and unable to communicate properly. Sexual difficulties were almost universal. It is important therefore to ask the principal carer(s) questions about their own mood.

Vascular depression

The concept of 'vascular depression' (Table 16.2) has recently been proposed to account for depressed patients, usually with a late-onset depressive disorder. Vascular risk factors and ischaemic-like changes in cerebral white matter and subcortical grey matter nuclei may combine to produce depression with prominent psychomotor change, notably apathy, less depressive ideation such as guilt, and impaired executive function. Vascular depression may also be associated with relative resistance to antidepressant treatment (Simpson et al, 1998) but is responsive to electroconvulsive therapy (ECT), although ECT is more likely to provoke delirium in patients with extensive white matter and related change (Figiel et al, 1991). Furthermore, white matter and subcortical grey matter changes, especially when extensive, are associated with poorer recovery in the longer term, higher rates of relapse and the subsequent development of dementia (O'Brien et al, 1998; Baldwin et al, 2001).

Table 16.2   Main features of vascular depression.

- Late-onset depression
- Reduced depressive ideation (e.g. guilt)
- Reduced insight
- More overall morbidity
- Apathy and retardation
- More cognitive impairment (particularly executive dysfunction)
- Poorer recovery from depression

Treatment

Gustafson et al (1995) comment on the high rate of placebo response in the early phase (up to about 6 weeks) after a stroke. Starkstein et al (1988) also found a high prevalence of spontaneous recovery in those with either sub-cortical infarcts or mixed cortical/subcortical infarcts as opposed to pure cortical stroke.

Furthermore, functional independence is associated with reduced levels of depression and higher scores on quality of life measures (Robinson-Smith et al, 2000), while the process of rehabilitation itself may lead to an improve-ment of depression via increased independence, better social stimulation and other measures to counter boredom (Wade, 1992) . Hence it has often been taught that depression improves if the patient's physical condition improves. However, as Gustafson et al (1995) point out this is not a satis-factory line of reasoning because a substantial proportion of patients do not improve and do require intervention. As a rule, significant depressive symp-toms that persist 6 weeks beyond a stroke should be treated.

There is surprisingly little written about the efficacy of drug treatment for post-stroke depression and rates of antidepressant treatment seem to be very low (Rigler, 1999). In a small study of post-stroke depression using the antidepressants imipramine, amitriptyline, and amoxapine, the response rate was 13 out of 20 (Shima, 1997), a proportion not much different from the response rates to antidepressants among older depressed people (Wilson et al, 2001). However, in their review Gustafson et al (1995) do not recommend the use of the older tricyclic antidepressants because of the high rate of con-traindications and side effects.

Double-blind placebo-controlled studies

There have been very few double-blind placebo-controlled studies of antide-pressant drugs given to patients with stroke. Five of them are detailed in Table 16.3. In one of the few from which meaningful inferences can be made, Andersen et al (1994) examined 66 patients with mild to moderate depres-sion (Hamilton Depression Rating Score 19; range 18–29) from a pool of 285 stroke patients aged 25–80 years, 2–52 weeks after stroke. They were assigned to equal sized treatment and placebo groups. Up to 6 weeks after stroke the recovery rate was the same in both groups. This, the authors con-cluded, highlighted the high rate of spontaneous recovery in the placebo group, although another explanation is that depressive disorder may be very hard to distinguish from an acute reaction to the stress of having a stroke. Recovery in the placebo group was infrequent in patients who became depressed 7 weeks or more after stroke. In that group there was significant advantage to citalopram, but there were more drop-outs in the active group. The authors comment that citalopram was well tolerated with few serious adverse effects.

Table 16.3 Double-blind placebo-controlled studies of antidepressant drugs given to stroke patients.

Study	No. patients	Patient sample	Active treatment
Lipsey et al, 1984	39	Selected young in- & outpatients	Nortriptyline
Reding et al, 1986	27	Consecutive rehabilitation patients	Trazodone
Andersen et al, 1994	66	Consecutive hospital sample	Citalopram
Kimura et al, 2000	47	Stroke patients with major and minor depression	Nortriptyline
Wiart et al, 2000	31	Multi-centred recent stroke patients	Fluoxetine

Reding et al (1985) studied trazodone vs placebo in 27 patients, some depressed and some not, seen on average 44 days after their stroke. There was a trend for better scores on the Barthel measure of function and no difference in the drop-out rate. There was no separate evaluation of mood. Lipsey et al (1984) compared nortriptyline to placebo and found a significant beneficial effect by 3 weeks of treatment which persisted at 6 weeks. However, patients with aphasia and dementia were excluded, three of 17 patients treated with nortriptyline developed delirium and, in all, six of 17 withdrew because of side-effects. Only 11 patients completed the nortriptyline arm.

In a double-blind study comprising 31 patients, 16 were given fluoxetine and 15 placebo (Wiart et al, 2000). At 6 weeks twice as many patients in the active group responded, and the mean reduction in depression score (Montgomery Asberg Depression Rating Scale) was significantly greater in those treated with fluoxetine. However, the study group represented only a quarter of those screened. In a study of 47 patients given either placebo or nortriptyline, successful treatment of depression led to improvement of cognitive impairment associated with stroke (Kimura et al, 2000). This is an interesting finding which ought to be repeated in a larger cohort.

There is a limited body of evidence linking stroke damage to neuroamine systems known to be of importance in depressive disorder. A blunted prolactin response to buspirone in post-stroke depression and altered response to d-fenfluramine suggest a serotonergic deficit in some patients (Ramasubbu et al, 1998; Sevincok and Erol, 2000), as do lower levels of 5-hydroxy indoleacetic acid (5HIAA) in the cerebrospinal fluid of depressed stroke patients vs non-depressed patients (Bryer et al, 1992). Dam et al

(1996) reported a differential effect on recovery of fluoxetine (facilitatory) and marprotiline (possibly inhibitory) in stroke patients. Serotonergic drugs may produce different effects from noradrenergic ones.

Lauritzen et al (1994) gave either imipramine plus mianserin or desipramine plus mianserin to two groups of depressed stroke patients. No placebo group was included. There was a significant advantage in terms of reduction in depressive symptoms with the imipramine and mianserin combination. Unlike the study of Lipsey et al (1984), which used a tertiary tricyclic, this combination was well tolerated. Again, though, numbers were small. The authors speculate that imipramine is a 'broad spectrum' antidepressant, unlike desipramine which, along with mianserin, affects mainly noradrenergic neurones. The implication is that serotonergic antidepressants may be more effective than noradrenergic ones in post-stroke depression. Future studies might therefore exploit these differences.

With regard to other newer antidepressants, venlafaxine exerts both hypo- and hypertensive effects and can, in theory, exacerbate or cause ischaemia (Reznik et al, 1999), but it has been shown to be effective and well tolerated in an uncontrolled study (N=12) of depressed stroke patients (Dahmen et al, 1999). It also has a dual action, which is favoured by Gustafson et al (1995), but it requires further evaluation. Moclobemide has a reasonable safety record and is well tolerated. It has been recommended in stroke but there are no controlled trials (Tiller, 1992).

Stimulant drugs

Before the advent of selective serotonin reuptake inhibitors, psychostimu- lants were given to medically ill patients, including those with stroke, as they were deemed to cause fewer side-effects than the tricyclics, which were the only other available antidepressant drugs at the time. More recently, Grade et al (1998) showed that methylphenidate improved depression as well as a measure of functional independence in 21 patients randomly allocated either to the active drug or placebo. Methylphenidate has also been shown to be as effective as nortriptyline in improving depressive symptoms but with an earlier onset of action – between 2 and 4 days (Lazarus et al, 1994). There are concerns that stimulants may become addictive. Also, although the effect can be rapid, clinical experience suggests that it may not last. It is cer- tainly logical, and therefore quite possible, that the main therapeutic effect of psychostimulants is to improve stroke-related apathy. With the advent of a range of newer antidepressant drugs it is difficult to justify the use of psy- chostimulants to treat definite depressive disorder.

Augmentation therapy

This refers to the use of drugs adjunctively to antidepressants in cases of depression resistant to first-line treatment. The best studied of these is lithium (Baldwin, 1996). Although lithium is an effective agent in treatment-resistant depression, it has to be monitored by regular blood assay because of renal toxicity. Renal function is often impaired in stroke patients because of associated hypertensive or diabetic nephropathy. In patients with brain damage neurotoxicity, which is life-threatening, can develop at therapeutic lithium levels. It is therefore a treatment best left to specialists in psychiatry.

Electroconvulsive therapy (ECT)

This is usually indicated in patients with severe depression who are psychotic, actively suicidal, or who are refusing food or fluid. As a treatment it is the most potent in relieving the symptoms of depression and promoting recovery (Baldwin, 2000). There are, however, no controlled trials of ECT in depressed stroke patients. High recovery rates (over 80%) were reported in two retrospective studies of ECT in post-stroke depression. (Currier et al, 1992; Murray et al, 1992). There were, however, marked differences in the reported rates of serious adverse effects (one of 14 in the study of Murray et al, and 12 out of 20 in that of Currier et al). These included pulmonary oedema, ventricular arrhythmia, and delirium. Furthermore, seven out of 20 patients in the study of Currier et al relapsed on medical maintenance, a figure similar to rates found in psychiatric settings. In severe depression all the contraindications to ECT are relative, as untreated depression is itself life-threatening (Baldwin, 2000). Patients presenting the greatest risk are those with uncontrolled hypertension, raised intracranial pressure, cardiac irregularity (especially ventricular arrhythmia), aneurysm, or poorly controlled heart failure. The single most important pre-ECT investigation is the physical examination (Abramczuk and Rose, 1979).

Psychological therapies

There has been little evaluation of psychological therapies in post-stroke depression, although in one small UK study 10 of 19 patients offered cognitive-behaviour therapy (CBT) showed some benefit (Lincoln et al, 1997). It is also important to consider the effects of stroke on other family members who may themselves be candidates for problem-oriented therapy aimed at helping them to find adaptive modes of coping rather than 'self-defeating efforts' (Watzlawick and Coyne, 1980).

Response to treatment may be assessed by use of a rating scale. As proposed by Gustafson et al (1995), the Montgomery Asberg Depression Rating Scale is widely validated as a measure of change and keeps questions relating to somatic complaints to a minimum (Montgomery and Asberg, 1979). There are 10 questions with a maximum score of 60. It can be taught reliably to non-medical health personnel (Yohannes et al, 2000).

Prevention

Primary prevention

As post-stroke depressive disorder is so common, might the routine pre-scription of an antidepressant be justified? In the only study to have addressed this, prophylaxis with mianserin was not effective (Palomakió et al, 1999). Mianserin is a noradrenergic antidepressant and there may be some justification for conducting a preventative trial of a serotonergic agent or a dual-action drug such as venlafaxine.

Future treatments of 'vascular depression' may involve interventions to pre-vent the progression of vascular disease. Included among these are antihypertensives, but also antiplatelet treatment or even agents that reduce arterial spasm. In one recent trial in South America (Taragano et al, 2001) 84 patients with clinically defined vascular depression were allocated to either vitamin C or nimodipine, a drug with antihypertensive and calcium channel blocking actions, in combination with an antidepressant. More patients given the combination achieved full remission of depression and they also had fewer relapses over a year of follow-up compared to those on standard antidepressant treatment alone. This is exciting new research which clearly requires replication.

Secondary prevention

This refers to measures taken to prevent relapse, which is usually defined as reappearance of depression occurring in the period up to 6 months after recovery, and recurrence, the emergence of a new episode of depression. In the absence of specific data, the principles are the same as in any other group of patients with depression. They are outlined elsewhere (Baldwin, 2000). In brief: antidepressants should be continued at the same dosage as produced recovery for at least 6 months after recovery has been achieved. Thereafter the decision to discontinue (which should always involve a grad-ual tapering over 4 weeks and not an abrupt cessation) depends on the risk of further episodes and is an individual decision. This risk is increased in patients who have had three prior episodes of depression at any time over the preceding 5 years; who have had a severe depressive episode, for example, psychotic depression; whose symptoms were present for more than 2 years prior to depression diagnosis; or who have severe disability.

Mania

Mania is a rare primary disorder in the population most at risk of stroke, the elderly, but it may be provoked by a stroke, especially one involving the frontal lobe(s). The principles of management are the same as at any age and are described in Chapter 15 and elsewhere (Baldwin, 2000).

As with younger patients, the mainstays of acute treatment are neuroleptics and lithium, with anticonvulsants or ECT reserved for refractory cases. Some general points to consider are: 1) the greater inter-individual variability in drug metabolism, which makes predicting the therapeutic dose difficult. Rapid tranquillization with haloperidol 5–10 mg (often with 1–2 mg of lorazepam) can be used, but haloperidol has a long half-life and may lead to sudden immobility after a few days; 2) the increased risk of falls in the elderly when trying to balance treatment of overactivity with sedating tranquillizers; 3) the increased risk of confusion and delirium if anticholinergic drugs are given to counteract side-effects; 4) although lithium is seen as a 'kinder' treatment of milder mania, the risk of side-effects and toxicity is much increased in the elderly and those with brain injury; 5) thioridazine should not be used as it has been associated with ventricular arrhythmia; 6) sodium valproate is an acceptable first line treatment.

The advent of atypical antipsychotics (risperidone, olanzapine, quetiapine) is gradually having an impact on the treatment of mania. These drugs are not licensed for this use, but they do have some anti-manic properties and cause fewer extra-pyramidal side-effects.

Emotionalism

This disorder, which has already been described, should not be overlooked. First, it is very distressing to those who have it and frequently leads to social withdrawal. Second, it responds well to drugs that act principally on serotonergic neurones. There are data showing good response to amitriptyline, fluoxetine, and citalopram (summarized by Hanger, 1993; Gustafson et al, 1995) and, more recently, sertraline (Burns et al, 1999). The dosage is the same as for depressive disorder.

Conclusions

Depression is common in cerebrovascular disease. It is often hard to detect. There is a need for a reliable and valid screening instrument for post-stroke depression, especially in patients with aphasia. Currently there are no reliable alternatives to taking a structured psychiatric history, augmented by someone that knows the patient well. Treatment for depression should be considered in all cases where depressive symptoms have lasted for more than 6 weeks post-stroke.

The general principles of managing affective disorder apply to this patient group. However, post-stroke depression is increasingly being treated with newer antidepressants and there is some evidence that drugs acting on serotonergic neurones are the most effective. The older tricyclics are effective but side-effects markedly limit their use. ECT can be used but only in severe cases. Post-ictal delirium is not infrequent.

Mania is uncommon. It responds to antipsychotic drugs and the trend is for greater use of atypical agents to minimize extra-pyramidal effects. Lithium can be given but there is a risk of neurotoxicity even at therapeutic doses. Valproate is an alternative. Emotionalism is probably linked to altered serotonin mechanisms and responds well to selective serotonin re-uptake inhibitors.

Lastly, increased understanding of cerebrovascular disease will lead to novel approaches which not only limit brain pathology but also the increased risk of mood disorder that accompanies it.

References

Abramczuk JA, Rose NM, Pre-anaesthetic assessment and the prevention of post-ECT morbidity, *Br J Psychiatry* (1979) **134**:582–7.

Alexopoulous GS, Abrams RC, Young RC, Shamoian CA, Use of the Cornell scale in non-demented patients, *J Am Geriatr Soc* (1988) **36**:230–6.

Andersen G, Vestergaard K, Lauritzen L, Effective treatment of poststroke depression with the selective serotonin reuptake inhibitor citalopram, *Stroke* (1994) **25**:1099–104.

Angeleri F, Angeleri VA, Foschi N, Giaquinto S, Nolfe G, The influence of depression, social activity, and family stress on functional outcome after stroke, *Stroke* (1993) **24**:1478–83.

Baldwin RC, Treatment resistant depression in the elderly: a review of treatment options, *Rev Clin Gerontol* (1996) **6**:343–8.

Baldwin RC, Depression in the elderly. In: *Oxford Textbook of Geriatric Medicine*, ed J Grimley-Evans, 2nd edn (Oxford University Press, 2000) 987–99.

Baldwin RC, Walker S, Simpson S, Jackson A, Burns A, The prognostic significance of abnormalities seen on magnetic resonance imaging in late-life depression: clinical outcome, mortality and progression to dementia at three years, *Int J Geriatr Psychiatry* (2001) **15**:1097–104.

Black KJ, Diagnosing depression after stroke, *South Med J* (1995) **88**:699–708.

Bond J, Gregson B, Smith M et al, Outcomes following acute hospital care for stroke or hip fracture: how useful is an assessment of anxiety or depression for older people? *Int J Geriatr Psychiatry* (1998) **13**:601–10.

Bryer JP, Starkstein SE, Votypka V et al, Reduction of CSF monoamine metabolites in post-stroke depression: a preliminary report, *J Neuropsych Clin Neurosci* (1992) **4**:440–2.

Burns A, Russell E, Stratton-Powell H et al, Sertraline in stroke-associated lability of mood, *Int J Geriatr Psychiatry* (1999) **14**:681–5.

Bush BA, Major life events as risk factors for post-stroke depression, *Brain Injury* (1999) **13**:131–7.

Carson AJ, MacHale S, Allen K et al, Depression after stroke and lesion location: a systematic review, *Lancet* (2000) **356**:122–6.

Clark MS, Smith DS, The effects of depression and abnormal illness behaviour on outcome following rehabilitation from stroke, *Clin Rehab* (1998) **12**:73–80.

Currier MB, Murray GB, Welch CC, Electroconvulsive therapy for post-stroke depressed geriatric patients, *J. Neuropsych Clin Neurosci* (1992) **4**:140–4.

Dahmen N, Marx J, Hopf HC, Tettenborn B, Roder R, Therapy of early poststroke depression with venlafaxine: safety, tolerability, and efficacy as determined in an open, uncontrolled clinical trial, *Stroke* (1999) **30**:691–2.

Dam M, Tonin P, De Boni A, Effects of fluoxetine and marprotiline on functional recovery in post-stroke hemiplegic patients undergoing rehabilitative therapy, *Stroke* (1996) **27**:1211–4.

Figiel GS, Krishnan KRR, Doraiswamy PM et al, Subcortical hyperintensities on brain magnetic resonance imaging: a comparison between late age onset and early onset elderly depressed subjects, *Neurobiol Aging* (1991) **12**:245–7.

Grade C, Redford B, Chrostowski J, Toussaint L, Blackwell B, Methylphenidate in early post-stroke recovery: a double-blind placebo-controlled study, *Arch Phys Med Rehab* (1998) **79**:1047–50.

Gustafson Y, Nilsson I, Mattsson M, Astrom M, Bucht G, Epidemiology and treatment of post-stroke depression, *Drugs Aging* (1995) **7**:298–309.

Hanger HC, Emotionalism after stroke, *Lancet* (1993) **342**:1235–6.

Harvey SA, Black KJ, The dexamethasone suppression test for diagnosing depression in stroke patients. [Review] *Ann Clin Psychiatry* (1996) **8**:35–9.

Kauhanen ML, Korpelainen JT, Hiltunen P et al, Aphasia, depression, and nonverbal cognitive impairment in ischaemic stroke, *Cerebrovasc Dis* (2000) **10**:455–61.

Kimura M, Robinson RG, Kosier JT, Treatment of cognitive impairment after poststroke depression: a double-blind treatment trial, *Stroke* (2000) **31**:1482–6.

Lauritzen I, Brendsen BB, Vilmar T, Poststroke depression: combined treatment with imipramine or desipramine or Mianserin, *Psychopharmacology* (1994) **114**:119–22.

Lazarus LW, Moberg PJ, Langsley PR, Lingham VR, Methylphenidate and nortriptyline in the treatment of post-stroke depression: a retrospective comparison, *Arch Phys Med Rehab* (1994) **75**:403–6.

Lim ML, Ebrahim SB, Depression after stroke: a hospital treatment survey, *Postgrad Med J* (1983) **59**:489–91.

Lincoln NB, Flannaghan T, Sutcliffe L, Rother L, Evaluation of cognitive behavioural treatment for depression after stroke: a pilot study, *Clin Rehab* (1997) **11**:114–22.

Lipsey JR, Robinson RG, Pearlson GD, Rao K, Price TR, Nortriptyline treatment of post-stroke depression: a double-blind study, *Lancet* (1984) **333**:297–300.

Marin RS, Biedrzycki RC, Firinciogullari S, Reliability and validity of the Apathy Evaluation Scale, *Psychiatry Res* (1991) **38**:143–62.

Montgomery S, Asberg M, A new scale designed to be sensitive to change, *Br J Psychiatry* (1979) **134**:382-9.

Murray GB, Shea VM, Conn DK, Electroconvulsive therapy for post stroke depression, *J Clin Psychiatry* (1992) **47**:258-60.

Nieminen P, Sotaniemi KA, Myllyla VV, Poststroke depression correlates with cognitive impairment and neurological deficits, *Stroke* (1999) **30**:1875–80.

O'Brien JT, Ames D, Chiu E et al, Severe deep white matter lesions and outcome in elderly patients with major depressive disorder: a follow-up study, *BMJ* (1998) **317**:982–4.

Palomäkió H, Kaste M, Berg A et al, Prevention of poststroke depression: 1 year randomised placebo controlled double blind trial of mianserin with 6 month follow up after therapy, *J Neurol, Neurosurg Psychiatry* (1999) **66**:490–4.

Ramasubbu R, Flint A, Brown G, Awad G, Kennedy S, Diminished serotonin-mediated prolactin responses in nondepressed stroke patients compared with healthy normal subjects, *Stroke* (1998) **29**:1293–8.

Ramasubbu R, Relationship between depression and cerebrovascular disease: conceptual issues, *J Affect Disord* (2000) **57**:1–11.

Reding M, Haycox J, Blass J, Depression in patients referred to a dementia clinic, *Arch Neurol* (1985) **42**:894–6.

Reznik I, Rosen Y, Rosen B, An acute ischaemic event associated with the use of venlafaxine: a case report and proposed pathophysiological mechanisms, *J Psychopharmacol* (1999) **13**:193–5.

Rigler SK, Management of poststroke depression in older people, *Clin Geriatr Med* (1999) **15**:765–83.

Robinson-Smith G, Johnston MV, Allen J, Self-care efficacy, quality of life and depression, *Arch Phys Med Rehab* (2000) **81**:460–4.

Sevincok L, Erol A, The prolactin response to buspirone in poststroke depression: a preliminary report, *J Affect Disord* (2000) **59**:169–73.

Shima S, The efficacy of antidepressants in post-stroke depression, *Keio J Med* (1997) **46**:25–6.

Shinar D, Gross CR, Price TR et al, Screening for depression in stroke patients: the reliability and validity of the Center for Epidemiologic Studies Depression Scale, *Stroke* (1986) **17**:241–5.

Simpson S, Baldwin RC, Jackson A, Burns AS, Is subcortical disease associated with a poor response to antidepressant treatment? Neurological, neuropsychological and neuroimaging findings, *Psychological Med* (1998) **28**:1015–26.

Starkstein SE, Robinson RG, Price TR, Comparison of spontaneously recovered versus nonrecovered patients with poststroke depression, *Stroke* (1988) **19**:1491–6.

Starkstein SE, Fedoroff JP, Price TR, Leiguarda R, Robinson RG, Apathy following cerebrovascular lesions, *Stroke* (1993) **24**:1625–30.

Taragano FE, Allegn R, Vicario A et al, A double blind randomized clinical trial assessing the efficacy and safety of augmenting antidrepressant therapy with nimodipine in the treatment of 'vascular depression', *Int J Geriatr Psychiatry* (2001) **16**:254–60.

Tiller JW Post-stroke depression, *Psychopharmacology* (1992) **106** (Suppl):S130–3.

Van Gijn J, Treating uncontrolled crying after stroke, *Lancet* (1993) **342**:816–7.

Wade D, Stroke rehabilitation and long-term care, *Lancet* (1992) **339**:791–3.

Watzlawick P, Coyne JC, Depression following stroke: brief, problem-focused family treatment, *Fam Pro* (1980) **19**:13–8.

Wiart L, Petit H, Joseph PA, Mazaux JM, Barat M, Fluoxetine in early post-stroke depression: a double-blind placebo-controlled study, *Stroke* (2000) **31**:1829–32.

Wilson K, Mottram P, Sivanranthran A, Nightingale A, Antidepressant versus placebo for depressed elderly (Cochrane Review). In: *The Cochrane Library* Issue 2 (Oxford: Update Software, 2001).

Yesavage JA, Brink TL, Rose TL, Lum O, Development and validation of a geriatric depression screening scale: a preliminary report, *J Psychiatr Res* (1983) **17**:37–49.

Yohannes AM, Baldwin RC, Connolly MJ, Depression and anxiety in elderly outpatients with chronic obstructive pulmonary disease: prevalence, and validation of the BASDEC screening questionnaire, *Int J Geriatr Psychiatry* (2000) **15**:1090–6.

Concluding Chapter

17

Thinking through the relationship between vascular pathology and affective disorders – direction for further research and practice

Edmond Chiu, David Ames and Cornelius Katona

Over the last decade a new sub-type of depressive disorders has gradually emerged in the literature. There is a rapidly growing body of evidence to support the inclusion of 'vascular depression' into psychiatric nosology. This concept and the ability to use neuro-imaging data to support its diagnosis in individual cases can be of tangible utility in clinical management. It also provides a better understanding of the neuropathological and neuro-biochemical substrate of this depressive disorder. The challenge is to demonstrate whether the management and assertive treatment of vascular risk factors can reduce the incidence of vascular depression and make it less treatment resistant. The ability to locate the site(s) of the vascular pathology may also lead to more specific pharmacological targets in treatment.

The basal ganglia have been for many physicians a rather poorly understood part of the brain. The proposed circuits of Alexander which has been made more understandable by Cummings recently has provided us with a better understanding of the neuro-mechanism of late life depression and of depression in subcortical disease. The motor disorders that often present in depressive states can now be better understood. Further research in the area of the neuro-circuitry and its neuro-biochemical function will yield an abundance of new knowledge in fundamental understanding and clinically relevant information to assist clinicians in the treatment of depressive disorders.

One of the difficulties clinicians face in using the evidence base in this area is that many published studies have not fully addressed the methodological problems inherent in carrying out successful research in the context of very complex comorbidity. Two of the chapters in this book provide guidance around the many elephant traps. Schramke identifies the many areas in the stroke literature where research conclusions remain conflicting. She highlights the difficulties of distinguishing between vascular dementia and Alzheimer's disease and provides useful advice on identifying appropriate cohorts for study. Perhaps most important of all, she stresses the need to make full allowance for the language impairments so common in vascular brain disease. Stewart focuses on the gap between demonstrating the (well-known) association between vascular disease and depression and being clear on either the direction of or the possible mechanisms for such an association. Optimistically but (surely) correctly, he urges tomorrow's researchers to see these obstacles as challenges that can and should be overcome.

Post-stroke depression (PSD) is more important than physicians have thought. The editors' view is that the subject merits contribution from two groups to present a very comprehensive analysis to educate clinicians in the diagnosis and management of this disorder, which increases morbidity and mortality. However, although it is quite clear that PSD has led to excess disability in activities of daily living (ADLs) and impaired recovery, definite evidence for treatment-related recovery in function awaits further research. Whether treatment will improve quality of life is not certain at this time. What physical and psychosocial treatment will reduce morbidity, improved quality of life, restore ADL skills and reduce morbidity will be a challenge for us all. Another very cogent question is the relationship between PSD and cognitive decline. Longitudinal studies elucidating this question have very important implications. If, in some patients, PSD does *predict* cognitive decline then the location of the stroke lesion, type of stroke, premorbid risk factors, genetic contributions are all issues which demand attention in the early management of such patients in order to prevent vascular cognitive impairment or full-blown vascular dementia.

The relationships between cardiovascular disease (CaVD), depression and quality of life are crucial. Treatment of CaVD and depression must lead to improved quality of life (QOL) in our patients. What are the roles of psychosocial factors and social support in giving better QOL? Or is CaVD itself more influential? The interface between CaVD and the immune system requires further clarification. Is depression *per se* the culprit in this scenario or is depression a 'proxy' for other factors? Now that we have relevant neuro-imaging data we can hypothesize mechanisms linking cerebro-vascular disease (CVD) and depression. In contrast, we still know all too little about the mechanisms linking CaVD and depression. The increased risk of depression after myocardial infarction (MI) in those with previous mental disorder may suggest a genetic contribution, but what then is the mechanism, which leads to persistence and recurrence of post-infarction depression to be associated with younger age history of depression, high BDI and lower social class?

Depression in older people is all too often undetected and undertreated – this is even more the case where the depression occurs in the context of CVD. As Baldwin points out, we badly need a good screening instrument for use in patients whose communication is impaired. Equally important we need to remain optimistic about the prospects of treatment. Systematic assessment is crucial and the principles of treatment are the same as in 'simple' depression (not that depression is ever really simple, especially in older people). Treatment is also effective although safety considerations are particularly important. In this context the emerging evidence that serotonergic antidepressants are both effective and relatively safe in the context of cerebrovascular disease is particularly important.

Almost all treatment studies in this group are short-term. We still need to know what are the long-term effects of the novel antidepressants in this context? Even if we can anticipate improved outcome in depression, does antidepressant treatment reduce the risk of CaVD? Outcome of CaVD and CVD after treatment of depression is an area requiring more answers. Does it really matter, as far as the outcome of CaVD and CVD are concerned, if we aggressively treat the depression? Can we assume from early data in the outcome of antidepressant treatment that it can alter the course of CaVD and CVD by delaying myocardial infarction, and other vascular disease-related morbidity?

Lavretsky and Kumar, in their review of the literature on cerebrovascular disease and depression, point out the four-fold potential relationship between depression and CVD. These four explanations are not mutually exclusive and probably operate to different degrees in different individuals. They comprise: depression as an 'understandable' response to neurological deficit; depression as a direct consequence of neurological lesions; depression as a potentially causative risk factor for stroke disease; and the coincidental coexistence of both cerebrovascular disease and an affective illness. That each of these explicative models should have some evidence in its favour is hardly surprising, but what is most useful is the fronto-subcortical nature of impairments seen both in depression and in some patients with cerebrovascular disease. There is a clear link between these ideas and Gordon Parker's (2000) view of melancholic depression as a psychomotor disturbance driven by physiological changes in circuits connecting the prefrontal cortex with the basal ganglia and again, this research field is generating testable hypotheses, the investigation of which should drive the acquisition of useful knowledge which may permit us to target our current effective but crude biological treatments for severe depressive disorders better.

In Chapter 11, Lyness and Caine offer a multifactorial model to illustrate how a range of cardiovascular risk factors may, in an individual case, affect mood via small vessel disease, cytokine release, and other influences while simultaneously interacting with other biological, psychological and social factors to produce a particular outcome (from normal mood to depressive psychosis) in a specific individual. Although some might argue that such complex models are of limited value in yielding testable hypotheses and effective interventions, the brain is the body's most complicated organ system and it seems unlikely that a profound understanding of any of its functions, including the maintenance of mood, can be attained unless we comprehend in detail a whole concatenation of determinants such as those proposed by Lyness and Caine.

Evidence to indicate that the presence of a depressive disorder immediately after MI predisposes to an increased risk of subsequent death continues to accumulate. Encouragingly, informal reports on the as yet unpublished SADHART study investigating the safety and efficacy of sertraline in the treatment of depression associated with myocardial infarction indicate that this SSRI seems to be both safe and well tolerated in individuals with post-MI depression and that those who have had previous episodes of depression or have pronounced biological features of depression are most likely to experience a significant improvement in mood with treatment. What is needed next is a study large enough to have the statistical power to determine whether or not drug treatment of post-MI depression has an impact on mortality in the medium to long term.

Much of the literature on vascular disease and affective disorders focuses exclusively upon depression, but for most of us who know a little medicine, the first emotional response to a central crushing chest pain is likely to be one of anxiety rather than misery, reinforced by the sense of urgency and loss of autonomy inherent in the necessary medical response to a possible acute ischaemic event. Thus, we view the chapter on anxiety by Lautenschlager and the contribution by Rushton et al as two elements of our text which are likely to be of considerable value to those who work with people who get cardiac disease. Differential diagnosis and appropriate management of *both* panic/anxiety symptoms *and* cardiac disease must go hand in hand. There is little point in cardiac revascularization if the patient remains crippled by fear and unable to resume activity. Excellent evidence exists for the efficacy of both cognitive–behavioural and pharmacological treatments for panic. What is needed is a workforce, which can detect and assess panic symptoms, a subset of whom can then tackle the treatment and psychological rehabilitation of the affected individual. At present too few people who could be helped by existing treatments for panic disorder receive them, a stark contrast with the generally good availability of high-tech interventions for cardiac disease in most relatively affluent societies. Similar considerations apply to the depression and anxiety commonly experienced following cardiac surgery. Stratford and Ames stress the very emotive nature of surgery on the heart (which renders much post-operative psychological morbidity 'understandable') and the need for strategies that identify people at high risk of post-operative depression or anxiety in order to prevent affective symptoms or illness rather than having to treat them.

An exclusive focus upon the more common depressive syndromes can obscure the clinical importance of the rarer but extremely disruptive manic disorders that may also occur in the context of vascular disease. Yet if one asks the relatives of a bipolar patient whether they would prefer for their relative to be manic or depressed it is our experience that the vast majority prefer to deal with them in a miserable rather than insightlessly elated state. The relative rarity of mania and the distractible lack of judgement shown by many in the grip of a manic illness also make it harder to suffer. (As the late, great David Marsden was once heard to say in a tutorial 'If we cannot get the treatment of breast cancer right despite the number of cases we see and learn from, how are we ever to know how best to manage a rare malignancy like ependymoma?') Nevertheless a few diligent souls including Ken

Shulman, John Snowdon and Robin Jacoby have displayed an ongoing dedication to studying this appalling and destructive affective disorder and at least it seems that standard effective treatments for 'purely functional' mania may also benefit those unfortunate individuals who develop the disorder in the context of a cerebrovascular injury.

Perhaps the most exciting of all our chapters to edit was Horrobin's provocative account of the possible relationships between impaired fatty acid and phospholipid metabolism and affective disorders. If Horrobin is right (and he adduces a strong body of evidence in favour of his arguments) then potentially correctable deficits in omega-3 fatty acids may explain many of the observed links between affective disorders and vascular disease. In Popperian terms this elegant hypothesis has the virtue of being eminently testable and, even if only partly correct, offers the possibility of tremendous public health benefits which could flow from cheap and simple community interventions. We fervently hope that a future edition of this book might carry a chapter on 'How to stop yourself from getting cardiac disease or depression by eating more mackerel' or something similar!

Reference

Parker G, Classifying depression: should lost paradigms be regained? *Am J Psychiatry* (2000) **157**:1195–203.

Index